Advance Praise for *Good Reasons for Bad Feelings*

"To quote a renowned geneticist, 'Nothing in biology makes sense except in the light of evolution.' A quarter century ago, Randolph Nesse bravely helped apply this dictum to medicine. Now, in *Good Reasons for Bad Feelings*, he tackles the deeper evolutionary question of why we, our minds, and our brains are so vulnerable to mental illness. He navigates the dangers of either too much or too little adaptationism, deftly handles the false dichotomy between psychological and biological perspectives, and bridges abstract intellectualizing with pressing clinical need. This is a wise, accessible, highly readable exploration of an issue that goes to the heart of human existence."
—Robert M. Sapolsky, author of *Behave*

"Those powerful feelings that fill our day, that give us the oomph to act one way or another are the guardrails to living and this wonderful book explains all of them. Randolph Nesse has done it again."
—Michael S. Gazzaniga, director, Sage Center, UC Santa Barbara; author of *Tales from Both Sides of the Brain*

"A masterful, groundbreaking book that persuasively challenges standard clinical wisdom and provides a road map for the transformation of our conceptually confused psychiatric nosology. With crystal clarity, Nesse reviews what we know of our biologically designed emotions and argues for unflinching acceptance of our evolved nature as a baseline for understanding both normal and disordered suffering. . . . Anyone interested in mental health—laypeople, students, clinicians, and scholars—will be grateful for the novel insights to be gained from this important book."
—Jerome C. Wakefield, professor of psychiatry, New York University; coauthor of *The Loss of Sadness*

"What is the nature of suffering, its origin and its adaptive significance? *Good Reasons for Bad Feelings* may well become a legend, as it is a book about psychology, psychiatry, biology and philosophy that is also a good read, and it opens the door to deep questions in a manner that is tender, quizzical and industrious."
—Judith Eve Lipton, MD, coauthor of *Strength Through Peace*

"Randolph Nesse's new book vividly demonstrates how careful thinking using principles of natural selection leads to new and profound insights into why humans sometimes suffer mental disorders; the key question is why our minds are fragile. His writing style is clear and engaging, and the narrative reflects a masterful blend of history, novel ideas, and clinical experience in an insightful and coherent manner. I hope it is widely read and discussed."
—Eric Charnov, Distinguished Professor Emeritus of Evolutionary Ecology, University of Utah; MacArthur Fellow

"Prompted by the distress of his patients and confusion within his own field, psychiatrist Randolph Nesse set out to combine years of clinical experience with new insights gleaned from evolutionary biology, allowing him to view the entire landscape of human obsessions, anxieties, and compulsions through the lens of deep time, placing traits that contribute to depression and mental illness into evolutionary perspective. The result is a book as wise and illuminating as it is relevant to our daily lives."

—Sarah Blaffer Hrdy, professor emerita of anthropology,
UC Davis; author of *The Woman that Never Evolved*
and *Mother Nature*

"Nesse's book is hugely important for the future of mental health care, and Nesse is the preeminent person to write it. It provides a personalized and lively but well-documented treatise on how we humans function as we do and on needed changes in the way psychiatry thinks about troublesome mental experiences and behavior. It draws on an impressive range of knowledge, from not only psychiatry, including extensive case descriptions, but also psychology, biology, philosophy, and humanistic literature. Many readers will find it hard to put the book down."

—Eric Klinger, professor emeritus of psychology,
University of Minnesota

"Two sets of ideas inform this fine book: one, the coldhearted logic of natural selection; the other, the practical wisdom of a compassionate psychiatrist. The tension is palpable. The result is riveting."

—Nicholas Humphrey, professor emeritus of psychology,
London School of Economics; author of *Soul Dust*

"*Good Reasons for Bad Feelings* by Randy Nesse is a delightful book. It is insightful about the human condition, sanguine and not overstated. And it is written in a straightforward and delightful manner, personal and professional, and with humor. Neese is one of the originators of the field of evolutionary medicine. This is a welcome book in evolutionary psychiatry and on the biological basis of the emotions and our cultural evolution."

—Jay Schulkin, research professor of neuroscience,
Georgetown University

"In *Good Reasons for Bad Feelings*, leading evolutionary theorist, psychiatrist Randolph Nesse, begs us to ask the right question: Why did natural selection make us so prone to mental disorders of so many kinds and intensities? It is no exaggeration to say that he opens the door to a new paradigm in thinking about human beings and their conflicted lives. A path-breaking book by a man who is truly humane and caring. A privilege to share time with him."

—Michael Ruse, Lucyle T. Werkmeister Professor of Philosophy,
Florida State University; author of *On Purpose*

"In this highly accessible, scholarly and deeply illuminating book the internationally acclaimed evolutionary psychiatrist Randolph Nesse guides us through the implications of being gene-built and contextually epigenetically fine-tuned for our states of mind. From depression to anxiety to issues of moral behavior, we are guided to new understandings of the algorithms of the human mind and the contexts in which they can play out, for better or worse. This paradigm offers fundamental, new ways of thinking about mental states and moral behaviours, illuminating new means and opportunities to gain insight to and work with some of the dark sides of our nature. This will become a treasured classic not just for clinicians but for all those interested in how to facilitate well-being and create more moral communities and societies."
—Professor Paul Gilbert OBE, author of
The Compassionate Mind and *Living like Crazy*

"How did we end up recognizing that every system in the body has a function shaped by evolutionary selection and yet thinking that systems in the mind do not? How did physical and mental health drift so far apart? Randolph Nesse explains, in this highly readable book, how 'symptoms' in psychiatry should be seen in their evolutionary context, and that anxiety and depression for example have functions, just as do inflammation, blood clotting, or a cough. Nesse is a pioneer of evolutionary psychiatry, which has the potential to revolutionize mental health care."
—Simon Baron-Cohen, professor of developmental psychopathology,
Cambridge University

"This book sets out to show how evolution underpins (or should underpin) psychiatry. In doing so, it will surely change the face of medicine—and deservedly so."
—Robin Dunbar, emeritus professor of evolutionary psychology,
University of Oxford

"Randy Nesse has brought a new and important synthesis to the study of illnesses that psychiatrists deal in. This engagingly accessible, pioneering book provides a wide range of answers for how something as maladaptive as bipolar disorders could have evolved. It provides a wide range of answers for why natural selection has left us vulnerable to so many mental disorders, and the 'mystery of missing heredity' is identified as a key problem. Nesse shows that by taking into account complex pleiotropic effects, natural selection may push some useful trait close to a fitness peak near a 'cliff edge' despite the disabling consequences for a few individuals who go over the edge. Thus a gene may be useful to many, but with bad luck contributes to victimizing the few. This complex problem surely will yield to further research."
—Christopher Boehm, professor of biological sciences, USC Dornsife

ALSO BY RANDOLPH NESSE

Why We Get Sick: The New Science of Darwinian Medicine
(with George C. Williams)

GOOD REASONS
for BAD FEELINGS

Insights from the Frontier of
Evolutionary Psychiatry

RANDOLPH M. NESSE, MD

DUTTON

DUTTON

An imprint of Penguin Random House LLC
penguinrandomhouse.com

LIBRARY OF CONGRESS CATALOGING-IN-PUBLICATION DATA
Names: Nesse, Randolph M., author.
Title: Good reasons for bad feelings : insights from the frontier of evolutionary psychiatry / Randolph M. Nesse, MD.
Description: New York, New York : Dutton, [2019]
Identifiers: LCCN 2018045094| ISBN 9781101985663 (hardcover) |
ISBN 9781101985687 (ebook)
Subjects: LCSH: Mental illness—Etiology. | Mental illness—Genetic aspects. |
Psychiatry—History.
Classification: LCC RC454.4 .N47 2019 | DDC 616.89—dc23
LC record available at https://lccn.loc.gov/2018045094

Printed in the United States of America
1   3   5   7   9   10   8   6   4   2

BOOK DESIGN BY Elke Sigal

To my patients, who have taught me so much

CONTENTS

PREFACE

When I first realized that evolutionary biology could provide a new kind of explanation for mental disorders, I immediately wanted to write this book. It was soon clear, however, that understanding why bodies are vulnerable to diseases in general had to come first. That project was the focus of my collaboration with the great evolutionary biologist George C. Williams. We wrote a series of technical papers and *Why We Get Sick: The New Science of Darwinian Medicine*, a popular book that helped inspire much new work in what is now the thriving field of evolutionary medicine. Ever since then, my career has been committed equally to bringing evolutionary biology to medicine and to helping my patients with mental disorders. The two missions are connected deeply.

Practicing psychiatry is enormously satisfying. Patients are grateful for effective treatment. Providing it is intellectually interesting as well as emotionally fulfilling. Each patient poses a puzzle. Why did this individual get these symptoms now? What treatment will work best? However, sometimes looking out the window from my cozy office, I have visions of a tsunami sweeping millions of people with mental disorders to oblivion, with no help or high ground in sight. Such dark apparitions inspire asking different larger questions: Why do mental disorders exist at all? Why are there so many? Why are they so common? Natural selection could have eliminated anxiety, depression, addiction, anorexia, and the genes that cause autism, schizophrenia, and manic-depressive illness. But it didn't. Why not? These are good questions. The aim of this book is to show that asking why natural selection has left us vulnerable can help make sense of mental illness and make treatment more effective.

The possible answers suggested here are examples, not conclusions; some will turn out to be wrong. That should not be discouraging at an early stage in a new field so long as ideas are tested. As Darwin put it, "False views, if supported by some evidence, do little harm, for every one takes a salutary pleasure in proving their falseness: and, when this is done, one path towards error is closed and the road to truth is often at the same time opened."[1]

Continuing controversies and slow progress in psychiatry have inspired many calls for new approaches to mental disorders. Evolutionary biology is not new; it is the well-established scientific foundation for understanding normal behavior, but its relevance for abnormal behavior is finally being recognized. Evolutionary medicine is providing new explanations for why our bodies are vulnerable to diseases and is now being applied systematically to mental disorders. The time is ripe to explore the frontier of evolutionary psychiatry.

I wish the field could have some other name. Evolutionary psychiatry is not a special method of treatment, and professionals in other mental health fields will also appreciate an evolutionary perspective. A more accurate descriptor would be "Using the principles of evolutionary biology to improve understanding and treatment of mental disorders in psychiatry, clinical psychology, social work, nursing, and other professions." But that is unwieldy, so this book is a report from the frontier of evolutionary psychiatry, viewed broadly.

Mental disorders are such a plague on our species that we all want solutions right now. Evolutionary psychiatry offers some practical benefits now, but the big payoffs will come as researchers, clinicians, and patients ask and answer new questions inspired by a fundamentally new perspective. In the meanwhile, evolutionary psychiatry offers philosophical insights. Nearly everyone has wondered why human life is so full of suffering. Part of an answer is that natural selection shaped emotions such as anxiety, low mood, and grief because they are useful. More of an answer comes from recognizing that our suffering often benefits our genes. Sometimes painful emotions are normal but unnecessary because the costs of not having the emotion could be huge. There are also good evolutionary reasons why we have desires we cannot fulfill, impulses we cannot control, and relationships full of conflict. Perhaps most profound of all, however, evolution explains the origins of our amazing capacities for love and goodness and why they carry the price of grief, guilt, and, thank goodness, caring inordinately about what others think about us.

July 2018

GOOD REASONS
for BAD FEELINGS

PART ONE

Why Are Mental Disorders So Confusing?

CHAPTER 1

A NEW QUESTION

If I had an hour to solve a problem and my life depended on the solution, I would spend the first fifty-five minutes determining the proper question to ask, for once I know the proper question, I could solve the problem in less than five minutes.

—Albert Einstein

I knew something was up when the psychiatry resident knocked on my office door five minutes before I was scheduled to meet with him and his new patient.

"I just wanted to warn you," he said. "This one wants answers."

"What are her questions?" I asked.

"She wants to know why everyone she sees gives her different explanations and different advice. She's skeptical about the whole shrink thing. She got up at five a.m. to drive here from upstate to get answers from the big shots at the Big U." He was referring, sardonically but with a smile, to me and our prestigious university hospital.

I asked him to summarize the case. He gave a quick case presentation:

"She's a thirty-five-year-old married mother of three grade-school-age children whose chief complaint is increasing worry about nearly everything for the past year. Her health, her kids, the economy, driving, everything. She often has a bad feeling in the pit of her stomach, and once or twice a month she has bouts of nausea, but she hasn't lost any weight.

She says she's irritable and fatigued and has trouble getting to sleep. She is less interested in things, but she's not suicidal, and she doesn't have other symptoms of depression. Anxiety runs in her family, but nothing dramatic. Her family doctor couldn't find any medical causes. I think it's generalized anxiety disorder, but it could be dysthymia or somatization disorder. I'll be curious to see what you think. And how you answer her questions."

When we joined Ms. A in the exam room, she greeted us warmly. When I asked how we could help, however, her voice took on an edge. "I take it that the young doctor already told you about my problems. I drove five hours from up north to get some answers."

Trying to be empathic, I said, "I understand you have had trouble getting help." It was as if I had pushed the play button.

"Not only have I gotten no help, but every expert I talk to gives me a different explanation. I started with our minister. He is a nice man, and he was sympathetic, but mainly he just suggested praying and accepting God's plan for me. I tried, but I guess my faith just isn't strong enough. Then I talked to my family doctor. He didn't even do any tests; he just said it was nerves. He said pills for worry are addicting, so he prescribed pills for my stomach, but they didn't help.

"He sent me to this therapist doctor who wanted me to come twice a week, which I couldn't afford. He didn't talk much, and when he did, he kept asking about my childhood and hinting like I had some sexual thing for my father, which I definitely do not! When I told him I was getting worse, he said I was avoiding getting in touch with my memories. I quit going, but he still sends bills for the session I skipped.

"I still felt awful, so I found a psychiatrist in the phone book who was far enough away that people wouldn't find out. He said my problem was an inherited brain abnormality and that I would have to take medications to correct a chemical imbalance. But he didn't do any blood tests, either, and when I looked up the pills, it said they might cause suicide. So I decided to get myself down here to the university to get some answers. All I do is worry, and I can hardly sleep or eat, and my husband has had it with my calling him about the kids all the time, so I hope you have some answers."

"No wonder you are frustrated," I said. "Four different explanations and recommendations from four different professionals! And we may well have yet other ideas. Could we ask a few more questions to figure out the best plan?"

She was glad to provide more details. She said she had always been a worrier and that her mother had often been nervous. She had never been abused, but her father had often been critical. When she was young her family had moved every few years, so she had always felt out of it at school. Her marriage was stable, but she and her husband fought a lot, especially about his frequent business trips and what to do about their oldest son's ADHD. She often drank "a few glasses" of wine to help her get to sleep. She said the anxiety had worsened two years previously, about the time her youngest son had started kindergarten and she had started trying to lose weight. Without a pause she went on to say, "But all that has nothing to do with my problem. What I came here to find out is whether it is neurosis or brain disease or stress or what."

I started to explain that her symptoms resulted from a combination of inherited tendencies, early life experiences, her current life situation, and drinking. She frowned. As I went on to explain that anxiety can be useful but that most people have more than they need because too little can result in disaster, she brightened and said, "That makes sense." When I told her that several kinds of treatment could be safe and effective and that an excellent cognitive behavior therapist near her home would likely be able to help, she relaxed and said, "Maybe this trip will be worth it." However, later, as she stepped out of the office, she stared at me and shared a parting comment that still rings in my ears: "Your whole field is confused. You know that, right?"

I had never quite admitted it to myself that clearly. Psychiatrists are supposed to help their patients get in touch with things they are trying to avoid, but Ms. A turned the tables on me. For all case reports, I have modified details so that patients cannot be recognized by friends, relatives, or even themselves, but if Ms. A reads this and recognizes her visit thirty years ago, she will likely be pleased to learn that her pointed observation shattered my denial and set me on a quest to transcend the confusion.

Embedded Shrink

During my early years as an assistant professor of psychiatry, I was embedded, like a journalist in a war zone, in a medical clinic staffed by internal medicine professors, medical residents, and nurse clinicians. Many patients in medical clinics have mental problems, so my help was appreciated. There was also a hope that my presence would encourage resident doctors to have greater sensitivity to patients' emotional lives. We accomplished that to some degree, but the bigger impact was on me. As I saw and experienced the emotional strains of treating a steady stream of sick patients, I came to appreciate how growing a thick skin can protect the psyche.

The internists often asked me to talk with troubled patients who had tried seeing a psychiatrist and vowed "never again." Some complained about spending fruitless months with a therapist who said little. Others complained about seeing a doctor for only a few minutes before being sent away with a prescription for a drug that caused side effects. A few told me that their lives had been transformed by a patient, caring therapist, and some described working closely with a doctor for months until finally finding a medication that worked. However, most patients who got good results never told anyone about their treatment, and I was rarely invited to see patients who were doing fine, so I saw many skeptics. I listened to them for hours each week for years, but I was so intent on convincing them to accept help that I never really heard their collective wail of frustration until Ms. A put it in a nutshell: the field of psychiatry is deeply confused.

That does not mean that psychiatric treatment is ineffective. When I told fellow medical students about my career choice, several put on sympathetic faces and said something like "Someone has to care for patients who can't be helped." That misconception is as unfounded as it is common. Almost all psychiatric problems can be helped, and treatment remarkably often provides an enduring cure. Patients with panic disorder and phobias get better so reliably that treating them would be boring if it were not for the satisfaction of watching them return to living full lives.

The woman whose agoraphobia had kept her from leaving her trailer for a year was, a few months later, driving to see her sister an hour away. The carpenter who came in with social anxiety so intense he could not eat lunch with coworkers came back a year later to tell us how much he enjoyed his new job giving public presentations all around the state. Even some patients with severe disorders get dramatic benefits. Last week I got an email out of the blue from a patient I saw twenty-five years ago, with a heartfelt spontaneous thank-you, saying that treatment of her severe obsessive-compulsive disorder had transformed and very likely saved her life.

Many books attack the field of psychiatry. This is not one of them. Yes, big money from big pharma results in more corruption in psychiatry than in some other medical specialties. And industry-funded advertising and professional "education" promote the profit-maximizing simplistic view that all emotional disorders are brain diseases needing drug treatment. However, the vast majority of psychiatrists I have known are caring, thoughtful doctors who work hard to help their patients by whatever means works. I recall one psychiatry resident who came in at 6 a.m. every day so his patients, who were mostly struggling with alcoholism, could get to work on time; he was still there at 7 p.m. Another psychiatrist friend took on the toughest borderline patients, despite knowing he would get midnight calls threatening suicide. Then there are the many psychiatrists who treat desperately depressed or psychotic patients, knowing that some will commit suicide and they will be blamed. Most of us lie awake some nights worrying about a patient in a crisis and wondering how to help. However, most patients get better, and the challenge of helping them makes the practice of psychiatry profoundly satisfying.

The challenge of understanding mental disorders is, by contrast, deeply unsatisfying. Several years into my work teaching psychiatry, I was frustrated as well as confused. The field seemed to be narrowing to the slogan "Mental disorders are brain diseases." The phrase is great for marketing drugs, decreasing stigma, and soliciting donations, but it short-circuits clear thinking. Sometimes it is accurate, but it excludes valuable insights from behaviorism, psychoanalysis, cognitive therapy, family dynamics, public health, and social psychology. Practicing psychiatry based on only one perspective is like living within the walls of a medieval town. Trying to understand different perspectives is like visiting a series of walled towns. To see the whole landscape of mental illness requires a view from a mile high using special glasses that show changes across evolutionary as well as historical time.

What Causes Mental Disorders?

Like the six blind men each touching a different part of an elephant, each different approach to mental disorders emphasizes one kind of cause and a corresponding kind of treatment. Doctors who look for hereditary factors and brain disorders recommend drugs. Therapists who blame early experience and mental conflicts recommend psychotherapy. Clinicians who focus on learning suggest behavior therapy. Those who focus on distorted thinking recommend cognitive therapy. Therapists with a religious orientation suggest meditation and prayer. And therapists who believe most problems arise from family dynamics usually recommend, predictably, family therapy.

The psychiatrist George Engel recognized the problem in 1977 and proposed an integrated "bio-psycho-social model."[1] Every year since has brought renewed calls for such integration, for the unfortunate reason that psychiatry's fragmentation has, if anything, increased. The messy realities of mental disorders are ignored to fit them into the procrustean bed of one or another schema. Learned panels plead for integration, but committees that decide on grant funding and tenure only support projects that fit into narrow disciplines.

Plans for a recent revision of the diagnostic system aroused hope for greater coherence, but the result was increased conflict and confusion. The distinguished psychiatrist Allen Frances chaired the committee that wrote the previous edition of the book that defines each mental disorder, *Diagnostic and Statistical Manual of Mental Disorders* (*DSM*).[2] The title of his recent book captures his dissatisfaction with the revised edition of the *DSM*: *Saving Normal: An Insider's Revolt Against Out-of-Control Psychiatric Diagnosis*, DSM-5, *Big Pharma, and the Medicalization of Ordinary Life*.[3] Debates about diagnosis are so rancorous that they spill onto newspaper editorial pages. The crowning blow was the US National Institute of Mental Health (NIMH) abandoning the official *DSM* diagnoses for mental disorders.[4,5] So much for a common diagnostic system creating consensus!

The search for brain abnormalities that cause mental disorders has offered another hope for reducing confusion. In a medical school admission interview in 1969, I revealed, perhaps unwisely, that I planned to become a psychiatrist. "Why would you want to do that?" the interviewer asked. "They're going to find the brain causes for mental disorders soon, and it will all become neurology." If only that prediction had come true! However, four decades of research by thousands of smart scientists, supported by billions of dollars, has still not found a specific brain cause for any of the major mental disorders, except for those such as Alzheimer's disease and Huntington's chorea in which brain abnormalities have long been obvious. For other mental disorders, we still have no lab test or scan that can make a definitive diagnosis.

This is as astounding as it is disappointing. The brains of people with bipolar illness and autism must somehow be different from those of other people. But brain scans and autopsy studies have identified only small differences. They are real, but small and inconsistent. It is hard to say which are causes and which are results of the disorders. None comes close to providing a definitive diagnosis of the sort radiologists provide for pneumonia or pathologists provide for cancer.

Hope for diagnosis based on genetics has also collapsed. Having schizophrenia, bipolar disorder, or autism depends almost entirely on what genes a person has, so most of us engaged in psychiatric research at the turn of the millennium thought the specific genetic culprits would soon be found. However, subsequent studies have shown that there are no common genetic variations with large effects on these disorders.[6] Almost all specific variations increase the risk by 1 percent or less.[7] This is the most important—and most discouraging—discovery in the history of psychiatry. What it means, and what we should do next, are big questions.

Leading psychiatric researchers deserve credit for acknowledging the failure and the need for new approaches. In a recent article in the journal *Science*, several of them wrote, "There have been no major breakthroughs in the treatment of schizophrenia in the last 50 years and no major breakthroughs in the treatment of depression in the last 20 years. . . . This frustrating lack of progress requires us to confront the complexity of the brain. . . . This calls for a new perspective."[8] A recent meeting of the Society of Biological Psychiatry solicited presentations on the topic "Paradigm Shifts in the Treatment of Psychiatric Disorders." And in 2011 the director of the National Institute of Mental Health, Thomas Insel, said, "Whatever we've been doing for five decades, it ain't working. . . . When I look at the numbers—the number of suicides, the number of disabilities, the mortality data—it's abysmal, and it's not getting any better. Maybe we just need to rethink this whole approach."[9]

Psychiatrists recognize patients' life crises as opportunities for them to make major changes. Could the same be true for psychiatry?[10]

Finding the Future in the Evolutionary Past

The Museum of Natural History was a block south of our medical center. Opening the heavy iron door between two big lion sculptures brings you into the exhibit museum, a place I knew well from taking my kids to see dinosaur fossils. But this time I had an invitation to go through the doors marked STAFF ONLY to join a group of scientists who met weekly to discuss animal behavior. In the first hour, it became clear that their approach was completely different from anything I had learned before.

Instead of asking only about brain mechanisms, they also asked how natural selection shapes the brain and how behavior influences Darwinian fitness. Fitness is the technical term biologists use to refer to how many offspring an individual has that grow up to reproduce themselves. Some individuals have more offspring than others do, so their genetic variations become more common in future generations. Other individuals have fewer than the average number of offspring, so their genetic variations become less common. This process of natural selection shapes bodies and brains that work very well indeed to maximize Darwinian fitness in the natural environment.

Usually traits at some middle value are best. Rabbits vary in boldness. Exceptionally bold rabbits become fox dinners. Timid rabbits flee so fast they don't get much to eat. Rabbits with intermediate levels of anxiety have more baby bunnies, so their genes become more common. Some people get so-called Darwin Awards for doing stupid things that eliminate them and their genes. The adventurous young man who strapped a rocket booster to his car was going 300 mph when he and his car flattened into a thin layer on a cliff side. Other people fear leaving the house. They don't die young, but neither do they have many children. People with more moderate degrees of anxiety have more children, so most of us have intermediate levels of caution.

My new colleagues at the museum relied on a simple principle to explain why animals do what they do: selection shapes organisms to behave in ways that maximize their reproductive success. This is not a hypothetical theory; it is a principle that must be true. It provides what I was looking for—a new kind of biological explanation, not just for behavior but also for why organisms are the way they are.

After mostly listening for a few weeks, I finally got up my nerve and shared a theory I had come up with as an undergraduate. Aging is useful, I suggested, to ensure that some individuals die each year so the species can evolve faster when the environment changes. The group got suddenly quiet, but one biologist, Bobbi Low, laughed so hard she was sputtering as she said, "You really don't know anything about evolution, do you?" It was a friendly laugh, the kind elicited by watching a puppy try to climb stairs. Bobbi and others explained that genes that benefit a species will nonetheless be eliminated if individuals with those genes have fewer than the average number of offspring.

Bobbi suggested that I read a 1957 paper by the evolutionary biologist George Williams. I stopped by the library on the way home and made a copy. As for so many before me, reading it transformed my view of life. Williams pointed out that a gene causing aging could become universal if it gives benefits early in life, when selection is stronger because more individuals are alive then.[11] For instance, a genetic variation that causes coronary artery calcification that kills many people by age ninety could nonetheless become universal if it also makes broken bones heal faster in childhood. His paper was so influential that a retrospective was published on its recent sixtieth anniversary.[12] Williams offered a completely different kind of explanation, not just for aging but also for diseases in general. If aging has an evolutionary explanation, what about schizophrenia, depression, and eating disorders?

Over the ensuing weeks, my new evolutionary biology colleagues helped me to recognize that everything in the natural world needs two kinds of explanations. The usual approach describes the body's mechanisms and how they work; biologists call these proximate explanations. The other kind of explanation describes how those mechanisms came to be the way they are; biologists call these evolutionary or ultimate explanations.[13,14,15,16] My medical education had been entirely about the proximate half of biology, which describes mechanisms, none about the half that explains how bodies got to be the way they are.

Failure to recognize that evolutionary explanations are essential complements to proximate explanations causes enormous confusion. If you ask for an explanation of eyebrows, one person is likely to say they are explained by genes that induce synthesis of certain proteins in certain locations. Another might point out that you also need to describe the process by which eyebrows develop. Another will likely say you need to know about eyebrows in other primates. Someone will likely note that eyebrows keep sweat out of the eyes. And someone will likely raise an eyebrow to demonstrate its utility as a signaling device. The first two explanations describe proximate mechanisms; the others are about evolution.

The Nobel Prize–winning ethologist Niko Tinbergen expanded the distinction in a 1963 article that described what have come to be known as "Tinbergen's Four Questions": What is the mechanism? How does the mechanism develop in an individual? What is its adaptive significance? And what is its evolutionary history?[17] After relying on them for years, I finally saw that two are proximate and two are evolutionary and that two are about a slice in time, while two are about change across time. They fit nicely into a neat two-by-two table. When I added a slide showing the table in my lectures, the audience was more interested in the table than in my talk. When I put a PDF of the table on my website, it spread fast.

TINBERGEN'S FOUR QUESTIONS, ORGANIZED[18]

	PROXIMATE	EVOLUTIONARY
SLICE IN TIME	What is the mechanism?	What is its adaptive significance?
SEQUENCE ACROSS TIME	How does it develop in an individual?	What is its evolutionary history?

Tinbergen's questions made me recognize that some late-night debates with medical school classmates arose from mistakenly thinking the questions are alternatives. They aren't. Answers to all four are necessary for a full explanation. The questions also made me realize that many things I had thought of as abnormal were actually useful. My medical education taught the details of the mechanisms in stomach cells that secrete acid and their role in causing ulcers but nothing about how stomach acid kills bacteria and digests food and why too little acid is as big a problem as too much. We learned all about the causes of diarrhea but little about its role in clearing toxins and infections from the GI tract. Coughing clears foreign matter from the respiratory tract. Fever is a carefully controlled response that fights infection. Even pain needs to be understood in terms of its function as well as its mechanisms; people born without the ability to experience pain usually die in early adulthood.[19] I started to think about the utility of anxiety and low mood.

While many things that seem useless turn out to have a function, others are abysmal designs. The eye would be better without a blind spot. The birth canal is too narrow. Cancer protection mechanisms are insufficient, as are those that protect against infection. Ability to regulate eating is weak. Anxiety and pain are often excessive. I started wondering full-time about why selection left the body riddled with such imperfections.

When George Williams visited for a conference, he was easy to recognize; he looked remarkably like Abraham Lincoln. I knew his 1957 paper was admired, but no one had told me that he was one of the leading biologists of the twentieth century, certainly not Williams himself. He didn't talk much, but when he did, everyone paid attention. Over beer, he explained how he had come up with his idea that selection can preserve the genes that cause aging. I saw a way to test his theory. It predicts that mortality rates should increase with age for some animals in the wild. The alternative theory, that genes for aging are outside the reach of selection, predicts that mortality rates should stay the same across the adult life span.

A few months of library work would be needed to find data on mortality rates for animals in the wild. I told my psychiatry department chair, John Greden, about my idea. He was new in the job and eager to encourage creativity, so he said I could devote half time to the project for the summer. By fall, I had found the data and a way to calculate how strongly selection was acting on aging in wild animals: *very* strongly indeed.[20] George's theory was right: genes that speed aging are not all unfortunate mutations whose effects come too late in life to be eliminated by natural selection; some give advantages that increase reproduction earlier in life. The idea has been confirmed in many studies that bred beetles and fruit flies for longer or shorter life spans.[21,22] Selecting for earlier reproduction results in a shorter life span. Selecting for longer life span results in fewer offspring, especially in the wild. Aging has an evolutionary explanation.[23]

By the next time George visited, I knew enough about evolutionary biology to have a coherent conversation, and my research on aging had been published. I told George I thought that evolution could offer a new kind of explanation not just for aging but for diseases. He had been thinking the same thing. We decided to write a paper about how evolution could be useful for medicine.

During the first several months of our work, we made a fundamental mistake: we tried to find evolutionary explanations for diseases. Why, we asked, did natural selection shape coronary artery disease? Why did it shape breast cancer? Why did it shape schizophrenia? Finally we recognized our mistake. We were Viewing Diseases As Adaptations (VDAA). VDAA is a serious error that remains common in evolutionary medicine. But diseases are not adaptations. They do not have evolutionary explanations. They were not shaped by natural selection. However, aspects of the body that make us *vulnerable* to diseases do have evolutionary explanations. Shifting the focus from diseases to traits that make bodies vulnerable to diseases was the crucial insight that became a cornerstone for evolutionary medicine.

We spent days discussing the appendix, wisdom teeth, inflammation in the coronary arteries, cancer, and, of course, the human back. George saw the implications more clearly than I did and insisted on giving our article the grand title "The Dawn of Darwinian Medicine." Our book, *Why We Get Sick: The New Science of Darwinian Medicine*, reached a wider audience and encouraged the growth of what is now called evolutionary medicine. There are now a dozen books on the topic, a scientific society, a journal, international conferences, and classes in most major universities.

Evolutionary medicine is not a method of practice or in any way an alternative to standard medicine. It just uses the principles of evolutionary biology to solve health problems the same way we use genetics and physiology. Evolutionary psychiatry is the part of evolutionary medicine that asks why natural selection left us vulnerable to mental disorders.

The New Question

The usual questions in medicine are those of a mechanic: How does the body work? What is broken? Why did it break? How can we fix it? These are proximate questions about how bodily mechanisms work and how they differ in people with a disease: What immune system mechanisms cause multiple sclerosis? What brain abnormalities explain why some people have schizophrenia? Answers to these questions advance the most important goal: finding causes and ways to fix problems. Asking such questions and finding their answers has vastly improved human health. If medicine is to use only one-half of biology, this is the half with the big practical payoffs.

The other, evolutionary half of biology poses questions that take an engineer's point of view: How did the body get to be the way it is? What selection forces shaped this trait? How do variations influence reproductive success? What trade-offs limit its reliability? In its general form, the new question asks, *Why did natural selection leave our bodies with traits that make us vulnerable to disease?*

The question is new, but it is close to one of the oldest questions. Why is life so full of suffering? Debated in religious and philosophical contexts for millennia as "the problem of evil," answers have proved elusive.[24,25,26] The Greek philosopher Epicurus recognized the conundrum 2,400 years ago; a slight adaptation of David Hume's terse summary is widely quoted: "Is God willing to prevent evil, but not able? Then He is not omnipotent. Is He able, but not willing? Then He is malevolent. Is He both able and willing? Then whence cometh evil? Is He neither able nor willing? Then why call Him God?"[27]

Ever since, philosophers and theologians, especially those in the Abrahamic tradition, have struggled to explain evil and suffering. Possible explanations have a special name, "theodicies." There are many of them, because none is fully satisfying.[28] The problem is also central to Buddhism, whose first noble truth is "Life is suffering."[29,30] Its second noble truth is that suffering is caused by desire, more specifically the inability of ever fully satisfying desire. The third is that relief from suffering requires recognizing that desire is an illusion. An evolutionary view explains why we have desires, why we can't satisfy them, and why it is so hard to set them aside: our brains were shaped to benefit our genes, not us.[31,32,33]

Reconciling the ways of God to man is far beyond the scope of this book. Explaining the prevalence of evil and suffering in general is also out of reach. However, most suffering is emotional suffering. Anxiety and low mood exist for the same reason as pain and nausea: because they are useful in certain situations. They are often excessive for good evolutionary reasons. There are also good reasons why we are vulnerable to addiction, schizophrenia, and all the other mental maladies. Reasons plural, because several are relevant in different combinations depending on the disorder.

Trying to explain why mental life is so often painful, and why thinking and behavior so often go awry, reveals another equally profound question. How can mindless selection that maximizes only reproductive success have shaped brains that make committed loving relationships and meaningful happy lives possible? Most people's lives are nothing like the selfish competition for money and sex imagined by naive Darwinians. People meditate, pray, cooperate, love, and care for others, even strangers. Our species is remarkably endowed, not only intellectually but also socially, morally, and emotionally. Understanding the origins of love and morality is a crucial foundation for understanding social anxiety and grief and the deep relationships they make possible.

Jonas Salk, the inventor of the polio vaccine, said, "What people think of as the moment of discovery is really the discovery of the question." We have a new question.

CHAPTER 2

ARE MENTAL DISORDERS DISEASES?*

There is little reason to believe that these diagnostic categories are valid.[1]
—A comment about the *DSM* diagnostic
categories on the first page of
the leading psychiatry textbook

There is no point in trying to explain mental disorders without first describing and defining them. That seems simple enough. The current edition of *Diagnostic and Statistical Manual of Mental Disorders* describes more than three hundred different ones. Problem solved? Hardly. The diagnostic system generates interminable debate—and intense controversy.

Definitions of diagnostic categories make mental disorders seem like diseases. Many are, but they are a bit different from most other diseases. They don't have specific causes we have been able to identify, such as the bacteria that cause pneumonia. They can't be diagnosed with blood tests the ways diabetes can. They don't have definitive tissue abnormalities, such as the dying neurons in multiple sclerosis. Instead, mental disorders are defined by clusters of symptoms. People who say that food tastes like cardboard are often depressed and suicidal. Paranoid people often hear voices. Dangerously thin people who think they are fat are often high-achieving

---

* This chapter is adapted from Nesse RM, Stein DJ. Towards a genuinely medical model for psychiatric nosology. BMC Medicine. 2012;10(1):5.

young women. Each disorder is defined by a list of symptoms. If a person has enough symptoms on the list for long enough, the diagnosis applies.

This checklist approach has vastly increased agreement about who has what, but at a high price. It encourages the assumption that the diagnosis contains all information needed and a corresponding neglect of the life situations that set off many disorders. Combined with an age of computer-accessible records, it discourages recording relevant but potentially embarrassing details. So clinical records now tend to provide a few sterile paragraphs that describe the symptoms and justify the diagnosis. For instance, here is a summary of Ms. B's psychiatric evaluation.

Ms. B is a 37-year-old white, married mother of three, who is referred by her general physician for depression. She was well until four months ago, when she experienced the sudden onset of early-morning awakening, decreased appetite, low motivation, and feelings of guilt and hopelessness. She lost ten pounds in the past two months. Sometimes she wishes she were dead, but she has no plans to commit suicide. Symptoms are present every day, but they are much worse on some days than others, and they vary diurnally, worse in the morning. She reports chronic anxiety for several months, characterized by worry, sweating, and gastrointestinal symptoms. She also has periods of more intense anxiety lasting for hours, with trembling, shortness of breath, and a bad feeling in the pit of her stomach, but no panic attacks and no agoraphobia. She says that she has developed an intense discomfort in social situations, which she now avoids. She drinks one or two glasses of wine nightly, but she has no history of substance abuse. She attributes the onset of symptoms to marital conflicts. There is no previous history of psychiatric disorder. She is physically healthy, takes no medications, and has no allergies. There is a history of alcoholism in the father and anxiety in the mother. Her sister takes antidepressants. She grew up in a stable home. She denies abuse and traumatic events in childhood. She has three children ages 3, 5, and 9, who are doing well. Her husband is a manager at a local manufacturing plant. They live in a suburban neighborhood. She previously taught elementary school full-time, but she now works part-time as a teacher's aide. Diagnosis: Major depression. Treatment Plan: Initiate antidepressant treatment and cognitive behavioral therapy, return in two weeks for follow-up.

The case report summarizes the facts that justify the diagnosis, but it gives no inkling of what brought on her symptoms. That came flooding out when she described seeing her former lover in a grocery store.

I was trying to buy groceries, but it was like I was walking in a swamp. I could hardly put one foot in front of the other. I had a list, but it didn't help. Nothing seemed to matter. But the boys needed food, so I went. Halfway through, I saw Jack wheeling his cart around the far end of the aisle. For months, I thought I saw him all the time, like a ghost. But this time I was almost sure it was him. My heart started pounding and I froze and had a flashback to six months ago sitting in Starbucks.

We were going to meet at seven the way we always did, then move our stuff into the apartment where we had been meeting. We promised each other that at midnight on November second I would tell Sam and he would tell Sally. We wanted to do it November first, but we postponed it because of the kids and Halloween. I will always remember the sparkling flakes of snow as I opened the door to our Starbucks; they seemed like symbols of our new life together.

I told Sam I was leaving at midnight. He blew up, but I knew he would. He yelled so loud a car slowed down outside. That made it easier to go through with it. We were done a long time ago. Enough of living a lie. All I wanted was to be with Jack. I brought him a bouquet of freesias. But he didn't come. I texted him at 7:30, thinking that maybe Sally had tried to jump out a window or something. Nothing. I called him. No answer. I couldn't believe it. I just went numb and sat there staring at the table so long the flowers got all wrinkled and limp, like fossils in the marble tabletop. That was pretty much the end of my life, right then.

I finally snapped out of my flashback and got up my nerve to follow where Jack had gone. Nothing. I went to check out. He wasn't in line. So I tried to track him. There was a cart by the pork ribs with all his usual things in it, organic Mr. Coffee Filters, those little sugar cubes, Sominex, unwaxed dental floss. I am sure it was his. He must have seen me and snuck out. I don't know what I would have said to him anyhow.

Ms. B's story provided more insight into her problem than the entire case report and vastly more than her diagnosis. Nonetheless, diagnosis is essential. It provides a shorthand description of symptom patterns. Recognizing common patterns can make even ordinary clinicians seem like mind readers. Asking a patient who reports lacking hope, energy, and interest, "Does your food taste like cardboard, and do you awaken at four a.m.?" is likely to elicit "Yes, both! How did you know?" Patients who report excessive hand washing are astounded when you guess correctly, "Do you ever drive around the block to see if you might have hit someone?" If a student has weight loss and a fear of obesity, she will likely be astonished when asked, "You get all A's, right?" Clinicians recognize these clusters of symptoms as syndromes: major depression, obsessive-compulsive disorder, and anorexia nervosa. After seeing thousands of patients, expert clinicians recognize different syndromes as readily as botanists recognize different species of plants. If only different illnesses were as distinct as different kinds of plants!

When I started in psychiatry, diagnoses were defined by the opinions of expert clinicians. The good part was that professors insisted on case presentations that included every symptom and historical detail, even heart-wrenching grocery store visits. The embarrassing part was their endless disagreements. They disagreed not only about the diagnosis for specific patients but even about how to define diagnoses. At a staff meeting to discuss a newly admitted hospital patient, one senior psychiatrist proclaimed that the diagnosis was recurrent endogenous depression, another that it was anxiety neurosis, and a third that the problem was obviously pathological guilt following the death of an ambivalently loved father. Brilliant professors wielded extraordinary clinical and rhetorical skills in defense of diagnoses that were little more than opinions.

Such diagnostic inconsistency was an embarrassment for the field. A 1971 study asked psychiatrists in the United States and United Kingdom to watch the same videos of diagnostic interviews.[2] For one of the cases, schizophrenia was diagnosed by 69 percent of American psychiatrists but only 2 percent of British psychiatrists. Such wild unreliability made research hopeless. The problem hit the fan in 1973, with publication of an article by the Stanford University psychologist David Rosenhan in the prestigious journal *Science*. He sent twelve mentally normal "pseudopatients" to emergency rooms, where they reported hearing hallucinated voices saying "empty," "hollow," and "thud." All were admitted to mental wards. They acted normal after admission, but all nonetheless received a diagnosis of schizophrenia.[3] Although fake patients could also have duped neurologists or cardiologists, the article made psychiatry a laughingstock. The last straw was in 1974, when the controversial status of homosexuality as a mental disorder was settled—by a vote of APA members. Psychiatry awoke from its long dream to find itself drifting on a psychoanalyst's couch half afloat in the backwaters of medicine.

A New Diagnostic Manual to the Rescue

Desperate to join the medical mainstream, psychiatry recognized that its diagnostic system was grossly inadequate. For instance, in the 1968 second edition of *Diagnostic and Statistical Manual of Mental Disorders* (*DSM-II*), depressive neurosis was defined as "An excessive reaction of depression due to an internal conflict or to an identifiable event such as the loss of a love object or cherished possession."[4] Is moderate depression a week after the loss of a favorite cat "excessive"? One diagnostician would say, "No, not at all, people love their cats"; another, "After a week, it is obviously excessive!" Such disagreements made psychiatry's scientific aspirations laughable.

The solution was a radical revision, *DSM-III*, published in 1980.[5] Written by a task force of the American Psychiatric Association under the leadership of psychiatry researcher Robert Spitzer, it purged psychoanalytic theory from *DSM-II* and replaced its 134 pages of clinical impressions describing 182 disorders with 494 pages of symptom checklists that defined 265 disorders. "Depressive neurosis" was eliminated. The definition of a new diagnosis, "major depressive disorder," said nothing about internal conflict; it only required the presence of at least five of nine possible symptoms for at least two weeks. Every diagnosis was now defined by a checklist of necessary and sufficient symptoms.

DSM-III transformed psychiatry.[6] It made possible standardized interviews that epidemiologists could use to measure the prevalence of specific disorders.[7] Neurobiologists could now search for brain abnormalities for specific disorders. Clinical researchers at different sites could compare outcomes of alternative treatments, providing the data needed to create treatment guidelines. Regulatory agencies, insurance companies, and funding agencies soon demanded *DSM* diagnoses. Psychiatrists could finally diagnose specific disorders, just like other physicians. As a solution to the diagnostic unreliability crisis of the 1970s, *DSM-III* succeeded beyond all expectations.

Controversies Erupt

Despite providing the objectivity so essential for research and scientific respectability, *DSM-III* aroused vociferous criticism. Instead of fading with time, dissatisfaction has grown. Clinicians say that *DSM* categories ignore important aspects of many patients' problems. Teachers of clinicians report that excess reliance on the criteria leads students to neglect careful observation of their patients' problems.[8] Researchers protest that *DSM* categories do not map well to their hypotheses.[9] Physicians in other areas of medicine wonder why psychiatric diagnosis is such a problem. And people outside of medicine who read about these controversies all too often conclude that the whole field of psychiatry is just a bunch of hooey.

DSM-III increased objectivity dramatically, at the cost of discouraging careful clinical evaluations. If Ms. B has five or more symptoms for two weeks or more, she has major depression, too bad about Jack abandoning her the day they were to run away together. Even leading biological researchers are appalled. Nancy Andreasen, the author of *The Broken Brain: The Biological Revolution in Psychiatry* and the former editor of a leading psychiatry journal, described the "unintended consequences" of *DSM-III*. "Since the publication of *DSM-III* in 1980, there has been a steady decline in the teaching of careful clinical evaluation based on a deep general knowledge of psychopathology, and attending to the individual person's problems and social context. Students are taught to memorize *DSM* rather than to learn complexities from the great psychopathologists of the past."[10]

The problem is not merely theoretical. A psychiatrist in training concluded a grand rounds case presentation by saying, "This patient has sleep problems, low interest, low energy, poor concentration, low appetite, and a seven-pound weight loss, so she qualifies for a diagnosis of major depression. We will begin antidepressant treatment." When asked, "What set this all off?" the young doctor replied, "Family problems." "What kind of family problems?" "Her husband left her." Did she see warning signs about his leaving? Don't know. Was this her first marriage? Don't know. Does she have a relationship with another man? Don't know. Was she abused in childhood? "I didn't ask about those things because they aren't relevant. The diagnosis is major depression, and the treatment plan follows established evidence-based guidelines for this brain disorder." The excessive confidence in and commitment to a narrow ideology were as breathtaking as the willful ignorance about the patient.

DSM-III's objectivity also exposed other problems. Many patients with one *DSM* disorder also qualify for several other diagnoses. This problem is so pervasive that the leading psychiatric epidemiologist Ronald Kessler, my former colleague at the University of Michigan, called his biggest project the "National Comorbidity Survey."[11] Not only do many patients meet the criteria for multiple disorders, patients in the same diagnostic category often have very different symptoms. Adding this "heterogeneity" on top of huge comorbidity makes many people wonder if the *DSM* categories correspond to real natural entities.

The blurry boundaries between different disorders raise still more concerns. For instance, most patients with depression also have anxiety, and vice versa.[12,13,14,15] Furthermore, the boundaries that separate disorders from normality are arbitrary. No laboratory tests like those that diagnose cancer or diabetes are available. The authors of *DSM-III* assumed, in 1980, that better categories would soon be based on new discoveries of brain abnormalities. Almost four decades of intensive research later, no laboratory test is yet available to diagnose any of the major psychiatric disorders.

To their great credit, the leaders of American psychiatry forthrightly acknowledge the problem. Allen Frances, the chair of the task force that wrote *DSM-IV*, said, "We are at the epicycle stage of psychiatry where astronomy was before Copernicus and biology before Darwin. Our inelegant and complex current descriptive system will undoubtedly be replaced by explanatory knowledge that ties together the loose ends. Disparate observations will crystallise into simpler, more elegant models that will enable us not only to understand psychiatric illness more fully but also to alleviate the suffering of our patients more effectively."[16]

Thomas Insel, a recent director of the NIMH, says, "It is time to rethink mental disorders, recognizing that these are disorders of brain circuits"[17] and "Our resources are more likely to be invested in a program to transform diagnosis by 2020, rather than modifying the current paradigm."[18]

Frances is less hopeful, saying, "The *DSM-V* goal to effect a 'paradigm shift' in psychiatric diagnosis is absurdly premature. . . . There can be no dramatic improvements in psychiatric diagnosis until we make a fundamental leap in our understanding of what causes mental disorders. The incredible recent advances in neuroscience, molecular biology, and brain imaging that have taught us so much about normal brain functioning are still not relevant to the clinical practicalities of everyday psychiatric diagnosis. The clearest evidence supporting this disappointing fact is that not even 1 biological test is ready for inclusion in the criteria sets for *DSM-V*."[19]

The courage and integrity of these scientists are as remarkable as their vision. All agree that new approaches are essential. The major proposals so far, however, have been to further revise the diagnostic categories and to look yet harder for biomarkers to validate them.

DSM-III was the focus of most complaints, so it was revised to *DSM-III-R* in 1987, *DSM-IV* in 1994, and *DSM IV-TR* in 2000. The task of writing the big revision, *DSM-5*, was pursued over the course of a decade by a twenty-nine-member APA task force that coordinated the work of six study groups and thirteen work groups.[20,21,22,23] After years of sometimes bitter controversies, *DSM-5* was finally published in 2013.[24] It made a few small structural changes, such as moving personality disorders into the same category as other disorders. It also combined some categories (for example, substance dependence and substance abuse were merged into substance use disorder) and split others (for example, agoraphobia is now separate from panic disorder). These and others sensible changes make *DSM-5* more coherent and useful.

Calls for sweeping changes were rejected, however. A proposal to replace categories with scales ranging from mild to severe was rejected as impractical. "The diagnosis is major depression" is simple and definitive compared to "The score on the depression scale is 15." Categories make for efficient communication and statistical recordkeeping. They also satisfy the human lust for making things seem simpler than they are. We have been trying to map the landscape of mental disorders by drawing lines around clusters of symptoms as if they were islands, but mental disorders are more like ecosystems: areas of arctic tundra, boreal forest, and swamp blend into one another, defying crisp boundaries.

The second strategy has been to push yet harder to find genes, blood tests, or scans that can define diagnoses. No one imagined that we would still have no tests for schizophrenia, autism, and bipolar disorder thirty-seven years after the publication of *DSM-III.* Continuing the search is essential; it offers our best hope for finding cures. However, after decades of consistently negative results, it is time to step back to ask why specific physical causes for mental disorders are so elusive compared to those for other medical disorders.

The consensus answer is that we have not looked hard enough in the right places. Many neuroscientists suggest that we should shift the focus from molecules and brain locations to "brain circuits."[25] This reflects the growing recognition that diverse brain areas and neurotransmitters are involved even in functions as specific as recognizing faces. Considering circuits highlights adaptive functions, but it perpetuates the misleading analogy of evolved brain systems with human-designed electronic circuits. Circuits designed by engineers have discrete modules with specific functions and defined connections that are all necessary for normal operation. Evolved information-processing systems have components with indistinct boundaries, distributed overlapping functions, intrinsic robustness, and innumerable connections that make them different from anything that an engineer could even imagine. Shifting the focus from molecules and neurons to circuits is a good idea, but neuroscience will succeed faster when it acknowledges that those circuits are organically complex in ways that make them very different from anything an engineer could design.

Revising the diagnostic criteria will not solve the problem. Looking harder for biomarkers will eventually provide a definitive diagnosis for only some disorders. The dilemma has provoked deep thinking about what mental disorders are.

Accepting the Reality of Organic Complexity

The question "What is a mental disorder?" has been addressed by Jerome Wakefield, a social worker, clinician, researcher, and philosopher at New York University.[26,27,28] His pithy conclusion is that mental disorders are characterized by "harmful dysfunction." "Dysfunction" means a malfunction in a useful system shaped by natural selection. "Harmful" means that the dysfunction causes suffering or other harm to the individual. Wakefield's analysis grounds psychiatric diagnosis in an evolutionary understanding of the normal functions of brain/mind, the same way the rest of medicine understands pathology in the context of normal physiology.[29] His cogent analysis has, however, had little influence on how psychiatrists make diagnoses.

The South African psychiatric researcher Dan Stein and I decided to see if a systematic evolutionary analysis could suggest ways to improve the *DSM*.[30] After wrestling with the problem for several months, we came to a conclusion that surprised us: *DSM* describes most mental disorders pretty well. We identified some big problems, especially the failure to distinguish symptoms from diseases. But most of the dissatisfaction with *DSM* diagnoses arises not because they fail to describe clinical realities but because they describe the messy reality of mental disorders all too well. Problems overlap. One disorder can have many causes. One cause can result in many different symptoms. No specific gene or brain abnormality has yet been found to define a mental disorder. Now what?

Toward a Genuinely Medical Model

The so-called medical model in psychiatry usually refers to the view that specific disorders are caused by specific brain abnormalities that are best treated with drugs and other physical therapies. The actual model of disease used in the rest of medicine is subtler. It does not just dive in looking for specific causes for presumably specific diseases. Instead, it tries to understand pathology in the context of normal functioning. Three examples illustrate how a more genuinely medical model could advance psychiatric diagnosis.

First, the rest of medicine recognizes symptoms, such as pain and cough, as protective defenses and carefully distinguishes them from the disorders that arouse them. In psychiatry, by contrast, extremes of emotions, such as anxiety and low mood, are categorized as disorders, irrespective of any situation that might be arousing them. This error is so basic and pervasive that it deserves a name: Viewing Symptoms As Diseases (VSAD). Reforming psychiatric diagnosis will require recognizing negative emotions as responses that can be useful in certain situations—at least for our genes.

Second, the rest of medicine recognizes many syndromes, such as congestive heart failure, which are defined not by specific causes but by failures of functional systems. Physicians know that heart failure can have a dozen different causes. If schizophrenia and autism result from similar system failures, searching for *the* specific cause is senseless.

Finally, the rest of medicine does not hesitate to diagnose some conditions, such as tinnitus and essential tremor, which have no identifiable specific cause or tissue pathology. Most result from dysregulated control systems. The same may be true for eating disorders and mood disorders.

The core problem for psychiatric diagnosis is the lack of a perspective on normal useful functions that physiology provides for the rest of medicine. Internal medicine doctors know the functions of the kidneys. They don't confuse protective defenses such as cough and pain with diseases such as pneumonia and cancer. Psychiatrists lack a similar framework for the utility of stress, sleep, anxiety, and mood, so psychiatric diagnostic categories remain confusing and crude.

Carefully distinguishing symptoms from both syndromes and diseases is crucial for making psychiatric diagnosis like diagnosis in the rest of medicine. Like fever and pain, anxiety and low mood are useful normal responses to some situations. It is time to give up the fantasy that each mental disorder has a specific cause. Instead, many mental disorders are, as in the rest of medicine, extremes of symptoms. Others are system failures that can have many different causes. This does not mean we should give up looking for specific brain abnormalities; they will be found, eventually, for some disorders, and the sooner the better. But the search will be sped by adopting a genuinely medical model.

CHAPTER 3

WHY ARE MINDS SO VULNERABLE?

If the immediate and direct purpose of our life is not suffering, then our existence is the most ill-adapted to its purpose in the world.

—Arthur Schopenhauer, 1851[1]

If the mind were a machine, we would praise its designer to the heavens for creating the most extraordinary device in the universe. It can recognize a thousand faces and instantly come up with names—except for that of the client you want to introduce to your boss at a party. It can learn Chinese, Finnish, or English by age three with no special effort, even tenses, genders, and verb conjugations. The cello virtuoso Yo-Yo Ma plays the thousands of notes in Edward Elgar's Cello Concerto in E minor in order, fast, from memory. The science rap artist Baba Brinkman makes up hilarious songs on the fly on any topic. A high school student learns calculus. An elderly man recalls the exact rusty pail he and his mother used one sunny morning seventy years ago when they picked blueberries on a sandy hill. A young man rehearses a dozen strategies for getting the beautiful one to go with him to the prom. A young woman, anticipating his invitation and hoping for a better offer, tries to figure out how to postpone giving an answer. What incredible information processing!

The mind's emotional abilities are equally astounding. They connect us to our partners, flooding us with love when with them, longing when they are away, sympathy when they suffer, and grief when they die. When they betray us, the mind fires us with rage. When we betray them, it racks us with guilt and motivates reparations. The mind works day and night, planning, ruminating, fantasizing, dreaming. Was Joe's apparently friendly josh really a subtle insult? Could I really have great sex with . . . Who was that in my dream? The mind is the most extraordinary device that we know of in the universe.

The mind's vulnerabilities are as extraordinary as its abilities. It goes awry so often in so many ways that any hosannas for the designer would soon be transformed into fury and lawsuits. Some failures occur early. Just when love is cementing emotional bonds with parents, some children pull back into an autistic shell, never to reemerge. Some three-year-olds learn the word "No" and never look back, defying every parental instruction. Most parents make extraordinary sacrifices for their children's welfare, but a few lock their children in closets, hold their hands over gas burners, or force them to perform sexual acts. Such experiences are awful beyond measure, but why, thirty years later, do they often still have more influence than all subsequent events?

The elementary school years offer a respite. Energies go mainly into growth and learning; conflicts and new onset mental disorders are rare. Then puberty jolts the mind/brain with the force of a fist coming down hard on a laptop keyboard. Social sensitivity blossoms in sync with acne that amplifies it. For some children, social fears make dating difficult, and assignments to speak in class cause nightmares and school dropout.

Other minds ruminate on an infinite sequence of dire "What if?" scenarios. What if I come home from school and my parents have moved? What if I catch HIV from a toilet seat? Some have the opposite problem, anxiety deficits that cause risky behavior, including adventures with alcohol and drugs that result in addiction. Some addicts can stop completely. The lives of others circle around drugs or alcohol like moths around a flame, in ever narrower spirals down to death. Some young people, mostly women, go on diets that spin out of control; they see rolls of fat where others see protruding ribs. Others, mostly men, cannot understand how others get sexually aroused by people; they are turned on only by shiny black rubber.

Six Reasons Why Natural Selection Left Us Vulnerable to Disease

If the mind had been designed, we could ask if its flaws resulted from incompetence, carelessness, or malevolence. But the mind is not a machine. There was no designer. There was never a plan. There are no blueprints for the brain. There is not even one exactly normal version. Like every other part of the body, the brain was shaped by natural selection. Genetic variations among our ancestors caused differences in brains that caused variations in behavior that influenced how many children they had. The result is brains that have extraordinary capabilities—and many vulnerabilities.

The annual Italian science festival Festa di Scienza e Filosofia in Spoleto is a cultural gem that glitters each July in a small town in Umbria. The theme of the 1998 festival was evolutionary medicine. As the applause died down after my talk on evolution and mental disorders, I stepped off the podium to see another speaker approaching, the famous biologist Stephen Jay Gould. He was notoriously critical of evolutionary applications to human behavior, so I was apprehensive. When he said, "Nice talk, Randy," I was elated, but he quickly went on, "Of course, they had no idea what you were talking about." I protested, and he explained, "Most people have no idea about how natural selection works, and most of the ideas they do have are wrong. There is no point in talking about how evolution applies to something like mental disorders without first explaining evolution." Then, in the most engaging talk at the festival, he did just that. Lesson learned. Following Gould's advice, here are a few fundamentals that are crucial to our enterprise.

Do you put random coins from your pocket into a jar? If you do, the jar is soon a mélange of copper and silver. As you take out mostly silver coins, the glint of silver coins fades until it is hardly worth fishing for them in the sea of copper. The principle of selection explains the change in the jar. Natural selection is the same process occurring in living organisms over the generations. If genetic variations influence the number of offspring who survive to reproduce, then a species will change over the generations, and the average individual will become more and more like those who had the most offspring. This is not a theory; it is a deduction that must be true if the assumptions are satisfied.

Natural selection shapes traits that work well. The beaks and tongues of individual woodpeckers vary slightly. Those that extract insects more efficiently from trees get more food and fledge more chicks. This process shaped sharp-edged beaks that slice swiftly through wood and long barbed tongues that extract wriggling insects. Dogs provide a more familiar example. Choices people made about which individuals to feed and, more recently, to breed have, in just a few thousand years, shaped dogs that are remarkably adept at herding sheep, retrieving birds, digging out rodents, attacking intruders, and cuddling on laps while looking adorable.

Some behaviors that seem stupid turn out to be smart. In a lunch conversation, a neurosurgeon said he didn't think animals behaved adaptively at all based on his recent observation of seagulls feasting on scores of turtles that had all hatched at once on a Florida beach. However, hatching en masse gives at least some turtles a chance of making it to the ocean safely, the same way that a military charge is more likely to get some soldiers to an enemy line than if soldiers marched forward one by one.

Selection shapes brains that maximize the number of offspring who survive to reproduce themselves. This is very different from maximizing health or longevity. It is also different from maximizing matings. That is why organisms do things other than having sex. Especially humans. Having the most offspring requires allocating plenty of thought and action to getting resources other than mates and matings, especially social resources, such as friends and status. Everyone else is doing the same thing, creating constant conflict, cooperation, and vast social complexity whose comprehension requires a huge brain.[2]

While the principle of natural selection is simple, its process and products are unimaginably complex. Genes interact with one another and environments to create bodies and minds that maximize Darwinian fitness, but this is not as simple as it sounds. Individuals sometimes make drastic sacrifices that benefit others. When honeybee drones sting, they die, giving their lives to protect the hive. The mystery preoccupied the genius British biologist William Hamilton. He finally recognized, in 1964, that genetic variations that decrease an individual's survival and reproduction can nonetheless become more common if they benefit relatives who have some of the same genes.[3] His discovery was presaged in the biologist J. B. S. Haldane's succinct reply to the question "Would you sacrifice your life for your brother?" "No," he said, "but I would for two brothers—or eight cousins." Genes that induce individual animals to help relatives can nonetheless become more common over the generations if they give sufficient benefits to the relative compared to the costs to the actor.

Hamilton proposed a simple formula that transformed the study of behavior: $C < B \times r$.[4,5,6,7] A trait (or a gene associated with a trait) will become more frequent if the cost to the actor, C, is less than the benefit to the relative, B, times the proportion of genes in common by direct descent, r. Cousins have one-eighth of their genes identical, so a hypothetical allele that gives cousins a benefit ten times the cost will become more common over the generations, but one that induces helping when the benefit is five times the cost will be eliminated. The principle of kin selection revolutionized the study of behavior. When I am asked for an example of something evolution can explain about human behavior, I reply, "People love their children and make major sacrifices for them."

Within a year of Hamilton's discovery of kin selection, and not knowing about it, George Williams wrote a slim book entitled *Adaptation and Natural Selection*.[8] Before its publication, biologists routinely assumed that selection acted for the good of groups and species. Williams explained why this is a mistake. Biology has not been the same since.

The idea that selection works to benefit groups was illustrated in the 1958 Walt Disney film *White Wilderness*. It showed scores of lemmings jumping into a fjord, as a mellifluous narrator explains that the self-sacrifice by some is necessary to ensure that there is enough food that the species can survive. A 1962 book by the zoologist V. C. Wynne-Edwards described examples of animals that stopped breeding when food supplies were short, to support his thesis that such tendencies evolve to prevent the demise of the entire group.[9]

Williams pointed out that this makes no sense. Genetic variations that induced an individual to stop breeding would be selected out, even if they benefited the group, even if they could save the species from extinction. Individuals that stop breeding for the good of the group will have fewer offspring than those that carry on, so such sacrifices must have other explanations. As for the lemmings, the Disney film crew could not find any lemmings jumping into fjords. So they bought brooms, paid locals to trap lemmings, then secretly but literally swept them into the sea.[10]

Evolutionary theory was transformed by the recognition that group selection is weak and that kin selection offers a powerful explanation for altruistic behavior. These are only two of many evolutionary reasons why natural selection didn't do a better job of making organisms resistant to disease. Traits that make us vulnerable are legion. Why do we have an appendix? Why do we have wisdom teeth? Why is the birth canal narrow? Why are the coronary arteries prone to blockage? Why are so many people nearsighted? Why haven't we evolved immunity to influenza? Why is there menopause? Why does breast cancer occur in one woman out of eleven? Why are so many of us obese? Why are mood and anxiety disorders so common? Why do genes for schizophrenia persist? Every trait or gene that makes an organism vulnerable to disease poses an evolutionary mystery.

The old answer was that there are limits to what natural selection can do—for instance, eliminating all mutations. That is one important kind of explanation, but the central insight of evolutionary medicine is that there are also at least five other evolutionary reasons why we are vulnerable to diseases.[11,12,13,14,15] Evolution explains not only why the body works so well but also why some parts are prone to failure. Brief examples provide illustrations for disease in general, as well as mental disorders.

SIX EVOLUTIONARY REASONS WHY BODIES/MINDS ARE VULNERABLE TO DISEASE

1. Mismatch: our bodies are unprepared to cope with modern environments.

2. Infection: bacteria and viruses evolve faster than we do.

3. Constraints: there are some things that natural selection just can't do.

4. Trade-offs: everything in the body has advantages and disadvantages.

5. Reproduction: natural selection maximizes reproduction, not health.

6. Defensive responses: responses such as pain and anxiety are useful in the face of threats.

1. Mismatch

Most of the chronic diseases that plague us now result from living in modern environments.[16,17,18,19] This does not mean we would be better off in the environments of our ancestors. Life back then was worse than just nasty, brutal, and short. Imagine having an infected impacted wisdom tooth in a time without dentists. Even minor infected wounds caused death or the slow loss of a limb. The standard treatment, pouring boiling oil on the wound, was only sometimes effective. When steel tools made amputations possible they were swift, because there was no anesthesia. Pregnancy with a large baby meant an agonizing death. Then there was simple starvation. We are far healthier than our ancestors were.

Many of our current health problems result, nonetheless, from the environments we have created to satisfy our desires.[20,21,22,23,24] Most people in developed societies live better now physically than the kings and queens of just a century ago. We have a surfeit of delicious food, protection from the elements, time for leisure, and relief from pain. These accomplishments are spectacular, but they also cause most chronic disease.

If you get a chance to join a doctor making hospital rounds, ask which patients would be there if they had been living in an ancestral environment. Those with cancer and heart and lung diseases caused by smoking would not be there; neither would those whose diseases are caused by alcohol or drugs. Most patients with diabetes, high blood pressure, coronary artery disease, and obesity-related diseases would not be there.[25] The majority of breast cancer patients would never have gotten cancer.[26,27] There would be few if any patients with multiple sclerosis, asthma, Crohn's disease, ulcerative colitis, and other autoimmune diseases that have become epidemic only in recent years.[28,29]

The greatest boon of modern life is also the greatest villain: the availability of plentiful food.[30,31,32,33,34,35] Or, rather, foodlike substances manufacturers concoct with the exact combinations of sugar, salt, and fat that we most desire. Those desires were helpful on the African savanna, where sugar, salt, and fat were scarce; now our preferences make us obese and ill. Addiction to tobacco was not much of a problem until the breeding of milder strains and the invention of cigarette papers; now smoking causes a third of all cancers and much heart disease. Fermented beverages were sometimes available, but now readily available beer, wine, and spirits cause alcoholism worldwide. Advances in chemistry and transport make concentrated drugs such as heroin and amphetamine available everywhere; in combination with novel means of administration such as needles, they cause massive modern epidemics.[36,37,38,39,40]

Better nutrition makes children mature faster; many women now start menstruating at ages eleven or twelve, half a decade before their bodies and minds are fully prepared for pregnancy, to say nothing of being prepared to care for infants.[41] More subtle aspects of our environment also increase the burden of disease. Exposure to light at night blocks the normal release of melatonin and increases cancer rates.[42] Birth control results in modern women having four times as many menstrual cycles, and proportionally higher hormonal exposure and cancer rates, than women living in ancestral environments.[43]

Living in modern environments explains the prevalence of some mental disorders. Substance abuse, eating disorders, and attention disorders are problems mostly in modernized societies. Depression and anxiety disorders are often blamed on modern life, but their prevalence in earlier times remains unclear. Schizophrenia and obsessive-compulsive disorder do not seem to be much more common now. Mismatch is the first of six reasons why we are vulnerable to disease. It is an important explanation for some mental disorders.

2. Infection

When most people think about disease, they think about infection. It is a wonderfully simple schema. When germs get into the body and grow, they cause disease. Doctors prescribe antibiotics to kill them. The reality is far more complex, interesting, and discouraging.

A human generation is about twenty-five years. A generation for bacteria is just a few hours—about 30,000 times faster. From this perspective, it is amazing that large, slow-evolving organisms such as humans have survived. Life on a tiny scale existed on earth for 3 billion years before anything bigger evolved. We may well discover other planets where larger organisms never evolved because they were soon consumed by smaller organisms that evolved much faster.

The threat of antibiotic resistance is now familiar. Those few bacteria that survive exposure to an antibiotic soon take over. This is an ordinary evolutionary process, but interestingly, medical journals rarely use the "e-word." Instead they use euphemisms such as "emerge" or "arise" or "spread."[44] This circumlocution matters. Well-meaning would-be evolutionary doctors have sometimes tried to prevent antibiotic resistance in their hospitals by all agreeing to use the same antibiotic as their first choice, shifting to a new one every few months. While intuitively attractive, sequential exposure to different agents may speed the evolution of multiple drug resistance.[45] Many doctors also tell their patients that they should take every pill in the bottle of antibiotics to prevent resistance; however, recent studies show that if pneumonia is already under control, taking an antibiotic longer increases selection for resistant strains without shortening a person's illness.[46,47] The lack of evolutionary knowledge in the medical profession harms health.

Bacteria and hosts coevolve; every time the host evolves new defenses, the pathogen evolves ways to get around them. Streptococci, the bacteria that cause strep throat, disguise themselves as human cells.[48] So the antibodies our immune system creates to attack them are likely to damage our own cells. Damage to the kidney causes glomerular nephritis. Damage to joints and heart valves causes rheumatic fever. Damage to neurons in a part of the brain called the basal ganglia causes abnormal movements called Sydenham's chorea and some cases of obsessive-compulsive disorder.[49]

Sometimes hosts and bacteria help each other. The old idea that bacteria are usually bad is being replaced by an evolutionary view of a complex microbiome that is essential to health. Disruptions of the microbiome are strongly implicated in our modern epidemic of obesity as well as autoimmune diseases such as multiple sclerosis, type 1 diabetes, and Crohn's disease.[50,51,52] Something about modern environments is causing excesses of inflammation that cause these diseases and atherosclerosis. Is antibiotic disruption of our microbiomes responsible?[53] If so, our ability to avoid and kill bacteria comes at a high price.

3. Constraints

There are many things that natural selection just can't do. No system can replicate genetic information with perfect accuracy, so mutations happen. Natural selection cannot upend the laws of physics, so there will never be flying elephants. Selection cannot make bodies that generate their own energy. These constraints apply to any system, natural or mechanical.

Path dependence also limits the perfection of machines as well as bodies. Once things have gone down a certain path, there may be no starting over. Your computer keyboard is an example. You could shift to a more efficient key arrangement, but only at a great cost of relearning and incompatibility with existing keyboards.

Changing substandard aspects of the body is even less likely. The vertebrate eye is often held up as a model of perfection, but it has gross design flaws. Vessels and nerves come through a hole in the back of the eyeball, creating a blind spot; then they run between the light and the retina. They could just come through the back of the eye wherever they are needed, as they do in the octopus eye. But they don't. Natural selection cannot fix the design defect in the eyes of vertebrates because any such transition would create thousands of generations of blind individuals.

Our brains are also jury-rigged. They are prone to all kinds of thinking errors.[54,55] Some persist for the same reason that the eye has a blind spot; it is impossible to start over and do it right. Even aside from path dependence, much of our vulnerability to mental disorders results from the limits of what selection can do. Mutations happen.

4. Trade-offs

Nothing in the body can be perfect, because making one trait better will make something else worse. You can buy a car that accelerates to 60 mph in four seconds, but it won't get fifty miles per gallon and it will not carry eight people. You can get a sunroof on your car, but only at the risk of rain leaking in. You can get tires made with sticky rubber that are fabulous on ice—I highly recommend them for Michigan winters—but they are expensive and short-lived and they make handling squishy.

The body is a bundle of trade-offs.[56,57,58,59,60] Everything could be better, but only at a cost. Your immune system could react more strongly, but at the cost of increased tissue damage. The bones in your wrist could be thick enough that you could safely skateboard without wrist guards, but then your wrist would not rotate and you could throw a rock only half as far. You could have an eagle's ability to spot a mouse from a mile away, but only at the cost of eliminating color vision and peripheral vision. Your brain could have been bigger, but at the risk of death during birth. Your blood pressure could be lower, at the cost of weaker, slower movement. You could be less sensitive to pain, at the cost of being injured more often. Your stress system could be less responsive, at the cost of coping less well with danger.

In every case, both extremes pose disadvantages. The best cost-benefit ratio comes at some middle level. Too much sensitivity to pain or anxiety is bad, but so is too little. Natural selection is not usually changing things; it is usually keeping things the same, at some middle level. Life without pain or anxiety seems attractive, but it would often be short.

5. Reproduction

The body is not shaped for maximum health or longevity; it is shaped for maximum transmission of its genes. Alleles (different versions of a gene) that increase the number of offspring become more common over the generations, even if that shortens life and increases suffering. This is not merely theoretical. Half of the human population has been shaped by selection to live fast and die young.[61] I mean, of course, the fragile sex. On the average, men die seven years sooner than women do. From ages zero to ten in developed countries, for every 100 girls who die, 150 boys die. At puberty and shortly thereafter, the ratio is 300 men for every 100 women.[62,63] Why? The proximate explanation involves testosterone and its effect on tissues, immunity, and risk taking. The evolutionary explanation is that allocating effort and resources to competition instead of tissue repair increases reproduction more for males than females; males who win competitions get more mates and have more offspring.

The costs are not, however, only for men. Females also sacrifice health for reproduction, just not as much as men do. All organisms are shaped to behave in ways that increase fitness even if that decreases health and happiness. Did you ever desperately want to have sex with someone even though you knew that could lead to disaster? Most people have, with sometimes dire consequences. Then there are the rest of our desires and the inevitable suffering because they cannot all be fulfilled. We want so badly to be important, rich, loved, admired, attractive, and powerful. For what? The good feelings from succeeding are just about balanced by the bad feelings from failure. Our emotions benefit our genes far more than they do us.

6. Defensive Responses

People seek help mainly for symptoms, not diseases. Pain, fever, malaise, cough, nausea, vomiting, and diarrhea are protective responses. So are anxiety, jealousy, anger, and low mood. They are set off when something bad is happening. They are unpleasant but useful. If you have pneumonia, you had better hope that your cough reflex works well; otherwise you are likely to die. You had also better hope that your doctor knows that cough is useful and does not prescribe too much medication that blocks your cough excessively.

Nonetheless, doctors routinely prescribe drugs to block normal defense responses. Thank goodness! Blocking unnecessary pain, nausea, cough, and fever makes life much better. However, there is a mystery here. If defenses are useful responses shaped by natural selection, you would expect that blocking them would usually make people sicker. Why don't people die like flies after taking medications that block normal defenses?

I thought about this for several years before finally finding a solution— the Smoke Detector Principle.[64,65] Most of the responses that cause human suffering are unnecessary in the individual instance but still perfectly normal because they have low costs but protect against huge possible losses. They are like false alarms from smoke detectors. The occasional wail when you burn the toast is worth it to ensure that you are warned early about every real fire. An occasional experience of unnecessary vomiting or pain is worth it to ensure protection against poisoning or tissue damage. This is why it is usually safe to use drugs to block vomiting and pain.

If you are a lumper, you may have already noticed that these six reasons for vulnerability can be collapsed to three. Mismatch and coevolution cause problems because bodies evolve too slowly to keep up with changing environments. The next two reasons are things selection just can't do; selection is constrained, and everything is subject to trade-offs. The last two are not exactly reasons why we are vulnerable to disease; they are misunderstandings about what natural selection shapes. Selection maximizes reproduction, not health, and the unpleasantness of defenses such as pain, cough, and anxiety is just part of their utility.

Disease and Evolution, *Not*

Trying to find evolutionary explanations for vulnerability to disease is a challenging enterprise prone to mistakes. As mentioned in chapter 1, Viewing Diseases As Adaptations (VDAA) is the most common and most serious mistake in evolutionary medicine. So several cautions bear repeating. Diseases themselves do not have evolutionary explanations. They are not adaptations shaped by natural selection. Genes or traits associated with some diseases provide advantages and disadvantages that influence natural selection. However, proposals about the utility of diseases themselves, such as schizophrenia, addiction, autism, and bipolar disorders, are wrong before they start. The correct question is *Why did natural selection shape traits that make us vulnerable to disease?*

Such vulnerabilities need an evolutionary explanation using some combination of these six factors. There is a tendency to seek a single explanation, for instance, blaming all problems on modern environments or on trade-offs or constraints. Usually, however, multiple factors contribute. For instance, an evolutionary explanation for atherosclerosis includes modern diets, the role of infection in causing inflammation, and the benefits and costs of immune activation in arteries. Finally, evolutionary explanations are not alternatives to explanations that describe mechanisms; both are necessary. Evolutionary explanations for vulnerability to disease are crucial to helping us understand why mental disorders exist at all and how to find their causes and better cures.

PART TWO

Reasons for Feelings

CHAPTER 4

GOOD REASONS FOR BAD FEELINGS

There is . . . a time to weep and a time to laugh, a time to mourn and a time to dance . . . a time to love and a time to hate.
—Ecclesiastes 3:4 (New American Standard Bible)

One of the pleasures of antique shopping is trying to fathom the functions of mysterious machines. The one I am looking at is mottled cast iron. A crank on one side rotates a vertical slotted disk through a little cup. Even after examining all the parts and cranking the handle, I can't figure out what it is for, so I ask the seller. "It's a cherry pitter," he explains. Of course! Knowing its function makes instant sense of its form. Cherries fall into the slots, and a plunging rod pokes out the pits. Knowing that purpose reveals that this one is broken—the crank does not turn smoothly. Even in working condition, it would not help much nowadays; the slots in the wheel are far too small for modern megacherries.

Emotions provoke perplexity for the same reason as the cherry pitter. They have been described in extraordinary detail, but what they are for remains uncertain. Basic questions remain controversial. What *are* emotions? Ten experts will give you ten different answers. How many basic emotions are there? Pick any answer, and you can find an expert who will agree. How can we decide when an emotion is abnormal? Agreement on an answer is impossible without knowing the benefits and costs of each emotion in different situations. What causes emotional disorders? Some blame the brain, others blame diet, infection, conditioning, thinking habits, psychodynamics, or social structures. Debates about emotions generate emotions: fury and frustration. Stepping back to observe the fray arouses others: alienation and hopelessness.

Several obstacles make understanding emotions difficult. Failing to recognize that negative emotions are useful is a big one. Another is failing to realize that emotions were shaped to benefit our genes, not us. A fundamental obstacle is not recognizing that describing mechanisms provides only one-half of a full explanation. However, perhaps the biggest obstacle is thinking about emotions as if they were part of a designed system. That makes it seem as if each emotion should have a different function. However, each emotion has many functions, and many functions are served by multiple emotions. Different emotions correspond not to different functions but to the different situations each was shaped to cope with.

Pain and Suffering Are Useful

People usually seek treatment not because they know they have a disease but because they are suffering. They go to general physicians seeking relief from pain, cough, nausea, vomiting, and fatigue. They go to mental health professionals seeking relief from anxiety, depression, anger, jealousy, and guilt. The clinical approach to such symptoms differs dramatically.

Imagine that you are a doctor working in a medical clinic, evaluating a young woman who complains of abdominal pain that has become gradually worse over the past couple of months. She says the pain is cramping or aching in the mid to lower part of her abdomen. It tends to be worse at night but doesn't seem to be related to when or what she eats or her menstrual cycles. She is generally healthy and takes no medications. You ask more questions and schedule tests to try to discover the cause. Is it cancer, constipation, irritable bowel syndrome, or an ectopic pregnancy? You assume that the pain is a symptom and that finding the cause will provide the key to a cure.

Now you are working in a mental health clinic, evaluating a young woman who complains of constant worry, poor sleep, lack of energy, and loss of interest in most activities, even caring for her previously spectacular garden. The symptoms began a couple of months ago but worsened enough in the past few weeks that she finally came for help. She is generally healthy and takes no medications. She denies drug use, drinking, and recent major life stressors. You are likely to assume that the negative emotions themselves are the problem and to prescribe treatment to relieve the symptoms.

It is deeply ironic that so-called biological psychiatry, with its commitment to what is called "the medical model," uses only half of biology and a model very different from that in the rest of medicine. In general medicine, symptoms such as pain or cough are recognized as useful responses that indicate the presence of a problem. They spur a search for the cause. In psychiatry, symptoms such as anxiety and low mood are often presumed to be the problems themselves. So instead of searching for what might be arousing anxiety or low mood, many clinicians instead assume that they are pathological products of a broken brain or distorted thinking.

The general human tendency to ignore the effects of situations and to attribute problems to characteristics of individuals is so pervasive that social psychologists have a name for it: "The fundamental attribution error."[1] It is exemplified by the *DSM*, in which symptoms of anxiety or depression that are intense enough for long enough are sufficient to diagnose an emotional disorder, no matter what life situation a person is in.

Social scientists Allan Horwitz and Jerome Wakefield suggested a way to reduce this error. They pointed out that the *DSM-IV* excluded the diagnosis of depression after the recent loss of a loved one, so they suggested including similar exclusions for other severe life events.[2] The *DSM-5* authors acknowledged the inconsistency, but their solution was to eliminate *all* exclusions, even the one for recent loss of a loved one.[3] They said this was necessary for consistency and because intense bereavement symptoms sometimes indicate depression that needs treatment. They also wanted to avoid the unreliability that would result if diagnosis required judging the severity of life events.

The tendency to assume that symptoms are disorders is also a problem in the rest of medicine, where it has been called "the clinician's illusion."[4] Symptoms seem as though they are the problem because they are so distressing and disabling. Pain can make life agony. Diarrhea can cause fatal dehydration. Such symptoms seem unnecessary because it is usually safe to use medications to block them. However, pain, diarrhea, fever, and cough are all useful in certain situations. Each is expressed normally when the relevant situation is present and, as the Smoke Detector Principle points out, when it might be present. Excessive expression is abnormal. Deficient expression is less obvious but equally abnormal. Whether a response is normal depends on the situation.[5,6,7]

Many responses adapt bodies to changing situations.[8,9,10] Physiologists study the mechanisms that adjust breathing, heart rate, and body temperature to changing situations.[11,12,13] Behavioral ecologists study how cognition, behavior, and motivation changes adapt organisms to shifting situations.[14,15,16] Like sweating, shivering, fever, and pain, capacities for fear, anger, joy, and jealousy are useful in certain situations.[17]

The very idea that negative emotions can be useful can seem preposterous to those who are experiencing them. To get beyond such understandable skepticism, here are four good reasons for thinking that symptoms have evolutionary origins and utility. First, symptoms such as anxiety and sadness are, like sweating and coughing, not rare changes that occur in a few people at unpredictable times; they are consistent responses that occur in nearly everyone in certain situations. Second, the expression of emotions is regulated by mechanisms that turn them on in specific situations; such control systems can evolve only for traits that influence fitness. Third, absence of a response can be harmful; inadequate coughing can make pneumonia fatal, inadequate fear of heights makes falls more likely. Finally, some symptoms benefit an individual's genes, despite substantial costs to the individual.

Emotions Are for Our Genes, Not Us

It was a warm summer evening in 1975, and I was settling in for a night in the hospital as the doctor on call. There were no problems on the ward and the ER was calm, so I started reading Edward O. Wilson's new book, *Sociobiology*. It was nearly midnight when I encountered a sentence that left me gobsmacked:

> Love joins hate; aggression, fear; expansiveness, withdrawal; and so on; in blends designed not to promote the happiness of the

individual, but to favor the maximum transmission of the controlling genes.[18]

In a flash, I realized that my view of behavior and emotions was wrong.
I had thought that selection shaped us to be healthy, happy, nice, cooperative members of a community. Alas, no. Natural selection does not give
a fig about our happiness. In the calculus of evolution, only reproductive
success matters. I had been treating emotional disorders full-time for a
decade without knowing much about normal emotions. After a night of
unsettled sleep, I decided to educate myself. The next day I looked up
emotions in my psychiatry textbooks. I found only vague smatterings that
aroused confusion and boredom. Those emotions did their job, and I
turned my interests elsewhere.

Soon after, a student came for help in controlling his jealousy. It was
urgent, he said, because "My girlfriend is gorgeous, and I will never get
another chance to have a woman like her. We have been living together
for a few months, but she says she will leave if I don't stop acting so jealous.
I have got to stop it." He vividly imagined her kissing another man but
said he had no reason to suspect that she was unfaithful. He sometimes
followed her to see if she was really going to work, and he made up excuses
to call and check on her whereabouts. He was not psychotic or depressed.

I asked about his parents' relationship, his early life and previous relationships, and symptoms of other disorders but found nothing relevant.
So we started cognitive behavioral therapy to try to correct his irrational
thoughts. He made little progress. He insisted that his girlfriend was
getting ready to leave, so we reassessed his problem.

I now knew him well enough to ask him again about a common cause
of pathological jealousy; "No," he said, "I'm not having an affair, why would
you think that?" However, when I asked again if he had any reason to suspect
that his girlfriend might be having an affair, he said, "No, not at all. When
she stays out, it is only with her best friend." "How late does she stay out?"
I asked. "Well," he said, "she is with me at least five or six nights a week,
but sometimes she stays out all night." "And she swears it is just with her
girlfriend?" I asked. "Oh, it's not a girlfriend," he said. "It is her best friend,
a guy she has known for practically her whole life. They are just friends." I
paused to take this in and then said quietly, "We need to talk."

Sexual jealousy is an especially nasty emotion. In the 1960s, many people living in communes tried to eradicate it, advocating free love on the assumption that jealousy was a social convention that could be set aside. None of those communes survived. Despite all attempts to suppress it, jealousy grows back like a weed. It has dire effects on relationships. The expert on evolution and jealousy, David Buss, reports that 13 percent of all homicides are committed by a spouse.[19] Of homicide victims in the United States from 1976 to 2005, 34 percent of women, but only 2.5 percent of men, were killed by an intimate partner. Murder is dramatic, but the everyday scourge of accusations, violence, and relationships ruined by jealousy is pervasive. Why hasn't natural selection eliminated this awful emotion?

Imagine two men, one with a tendency for jealousy when he senses his partner straying, another who is mellow with whatever goes down. Which one would have more children? The mellow one might well have a happier life, but his partner would be at a higher-than-average risk of becoming pregnant by someone else. That would make her infertile during the pregnancy and for several years more if she breastfeeds the baby. So men who lack jealousy tend to have fewer children than men whose jealousy—obnoxious, dangerous, and aversive as it is to all parties and society—makes such pregnancies less likely. If only emotions always benefited us! Alas, they were shaped to benefit our genes.

Remedial Education

As the utility of emotions became more obvious, I began to worry that my efforts to eliminate anxiety and depression might be like prescribing cough medicine to treat pneumonia. Renewed recognition of my ignorance about emotions aroused new emotions: embarrassment, confusion, low self-esteem, and, thankfully, curiosity. They were effective motivators. I examined my psychiatry textbooks more carefully. Of the 4,500 pages in the most widely used psychiatry textbook, normal emotions get only half a page.[20] But hundreds of other books and articles describe emotions in detail. I embarked on a project to study them.

After a month, I felt like a mountain climber pulling up over a ledge, expecting to be at the peak, only to discover higher peaks looming in the distance. After six months and ledge after ledge, I had had it. Instead of a clear view from a commanding peak, I saw a foggy landscape of jumbled facts and clashing factions. I found nothing remotely like a periodic table of the emotions. Instead, most writings about emotions rehashed debates that had persisted for decades or centuries. How many basic emotions are there? Four? Seven? Thirteen? Or are emotions better described as positions on continuous dimensions, such as positive ←→ negative, and aroused ←→ calm? Which aspect of emotions is primary: Physiology, thinking, feeling, facial expression, or behavior? What is the function of anger? Of sadness? And, most fundamental of all, what *are* emotions? Scores of books and articles offered conflicting answers.[21,22,23,24,25,26,27,28,29,30,31]

In frustration, I turned to William James and his classic 1890 book, *The Principles of Psychology.*

> As far as "scientific psychology" of the emotions goes, I may have been surfeited by too much reading of classic works on the subject, but I should as lief read verbal descriptions of the shapes of the rocks on a New Hampshire farm as toil through them again. They give one nowhere a central point of view, or a deductive or general principle. They distinguish and refine and specify *in infinitum*, without ever getting on to another logical level.[32]

It was satisfying to find such good company but discouraging to realize how little progress had been made in a hundred years. It is not for any lack of effort by smart people. If a periodic table of the emotions existed, the legions of emotions researchers would have found it. Unanswerable questions often turn out to be wrong questions. Does the object of the search even exist? What if emotions are organically complex in ways that make any simple description a gross misrepresentation? What if emotions are not at all like the components of a designed machine? Who had taken an evolutionary approach to emotions?

I turned first to Charles Darwin's book *The Expression of Emotions in Man and Animals.*[33] It emphasizes the similarities of emotional expression in humans and other animals. Many emotion experts see it as a touchstone,[34] but it seemed to me to be mostly about evolutionary history of the emotions, with little to say about their functions. Finally, I found a book chapter by the psychologist Alan Fridlund, whose title captured my misgivings: "Darwin's Anti-Darwinism in *The Expression of the Emotions in Man and Animals.*"[35]

Fridlund explained that Darwin wrote his book as a rebuttal to the neurologist and artist Charles Bell (of Bell's palsy renown in medical circles), who claimed that the thirty-two muscles in the human face had been arranged there by the deity for the purpose of communication.[36,37] Darwin countered this thesis by showing remarkable continuities in emotional postures and facial expressions across many species. Darwin so emphasized the continuities that he neglected how emotions have been customized to the needs of a species in a specific situation. He emphasized communication but neglected physiological, cognitive, and motivational functions. In short, Darwin's book about emotions really is anti-Darwinian. The legacy lives on in continued emphasis on communication via facial expression and relative neglect of questions about exactly how emotions give a selective advantage.

A second evolutionary approach was proposed in the 1960s by the neuroscientist Paul MacLean. He described what he called the "triune brain," with three components he viewed as having been added sequentially in the course of evolution.[38] The oldest and lowest, the reptilian brain, was said to be the source of instinctual behavior. The middle part, the limbic system, he viewed as the source of emotions. The newest module, the cortex, was said to serve abstraction and to be present only in primates. However, neither the allocation of separate functions to different parts of the brain nor the evolutionary sequence has held up.[39] More significant, the theory does not address explicitly how the emotions give selective advantages.

Modern neuroscientists, such as Joseph LeDoux, use new methods to show how specific sites in the brain, such as the amygdala, contribute to specific emotions, such as fear. His research has found two routes for fear, a fast-reacting "low road" and a slower "high road" that involves more cognitive processing.[40] These approaches are much more explicit about the functions of emotions, even if not about how they increase fitness.

Another evolutionary approach addresses functions explicitly by trying to specify a function for each emotion. One website on mental health says, "The sole function of anger is to stop stress. It does this by discharging or blocking awareness of painful levels of emotional or physical arousal."[41] Another says, "we have recycled the primary function of anger from the protection of life, loved ones, and fellow tribesmen to protection of the ego."[42]

Even some careful scientists say, "each emotion has an inherently adaptive function."[43] The function of sadness is said to be "strengthening social bonds," "slowing mental and motor activity" and "communication to the self that there is trouble."[44] Anger "decreases aggression in others, mobilizes energy, and increases blood flow to muscles."[45] "Shame or the anticipation of shame motivates the individual to accept his or her share of responsibility for the welfare of the community."[46]

This approach gets closer to explaining how emotions are useful, and newer work focused on functions is increasingly sophisticated and explicitly evolutionary.[47] However, it seems to me that most such approaches misrepresent emotions as if they were components of a designed machine. It is sensible to seek the function of each part in a machine. The crank, the wheel, and the moving rod on the cherry pitter all have specific functions. But emotions were not designed; they evolved. Instead of one function, each emotion has many.

The big conclusion from my reading project is that attempts to specify functions for each emotion have slowed progress. Emotions make more sense when viewed as special modes of operation that increase ability to cope with certain *situations*.[48] Emotions are analogous to computer programs that adjust many aspects of the organism to efficiently cope with specific situations and tasks.[49,50]

What *Are* Emotions?

The question has been contentious for centuries. In his lovely textbook about emotions, the psychologist Robert Plutchik listed twenty-one different definitions, culled from hundreds of proposals.[51] Every year, new articles and books propose more. At the 2013 Society for Personality and Social Psychology meeting, the session on emotions was titled "What Is an Emotion?" You would think that by now almost everyone would agree on a definition, but different experts emphasize different aspects of emotions, so debates go on and on.

An evolutionary perspective suggests a simple definition of emotions based on the forces that shaped them: *Emotions are specialized states that adjust physiology, cognition, subjective experience, facial expressions, and behavior in ways that increase the ability to meet the adaptive challenges of situations that have recurred over the evolutionary history of a species.*[52]

Different emotions are like the musical styles programmed into electronic keyboards. Each style sets a combination of instruments, rhythms, chords, and timbre appropriate for a certain kind of music. If the keyboard is set to "classical," sonorous tones moan with plenty of echo. Set it for "salsa," and bright horns carry the melody over a lively drumbeat. Set it for "jazz," and the sound will be a bit different from salsa but very different from classical. Each mode adjusts many aspects to make sounds that are distinctive but that overlap in various ways with others. Just like fear, anger, love, and awe.

The natural next question is how many emotions exist. Lists of "basic emotions" go back as far as recorded writing. Research in the late twentieth century by Paul Ekman, Carroll Izard, Robert Plutchik, Silvan Tomkins, and others gave the question new legs.[53,54,55,56] They asked people to make lists of emotions, and then they looked for those that are common to many lists. Increasingly sophisticated methods and cross-cultural studies confirmed consistent recognition of some emotions, such as fear, joy, sadness, and anger.[57,58,59] However, every researcher offers a slightly different list, with the number of basic emotions ranging from three to seventeen.

Emotions are separate to the extent that they have been differentiated from ancestral emotions to cope with a related but somewhat different situation. This makes arguments about the number of basic emotions unnecessary. Each emotion has a "prototype," that is, characteristics that describe an exemplar at the center of a cloud of somewhat varying responses.[60] Those clouds have overlapping blurry boundaries.

An imaginary tree illustrates the evolution of the emotions, with interwoven boughs of different but overlapping emotions.[61] It is not the nice neat package scientists have been looking for, but it offers an evolutionary framework that can address some important questions. For instance, emotions are either positive or negative because only situations with threats or opportunities influence fitness. Positive emotions encourage organisms to seek out and stay in situations that offer opportunities to do things that are good for their genes. Negative emotions motivate avoidance of and escape from situations that involve threat or loss.

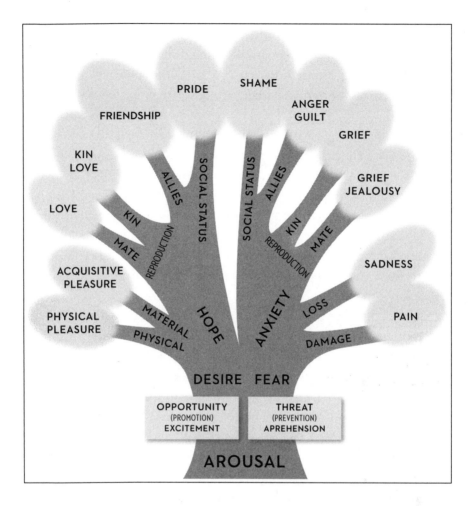

A Phylogeny of Emotions

The utility of an emotion depends entirely on the situation. In the face of threats or losses, anxiety and sadness are useful, but happy relaxation is worse than useless. When opportunities emerge, desire and enthusiasm are useful, but worry and sadness are harmful. The advantage goes not to individuals who are constantly anxious, sad, or joyful but to those who experience anxiety when loss is threatened, sadness after a loss, and enthusiasm and joy in the face of opportunity and success.

If only all situations were so simple. For humans trying to navigate inordinately complex social networks, almost every situation involves conflicting opportunities, risks, gains, and losses, with vast complexity and uncertainty. What do you do when you get an offer of a large grant to pursue your research from a politically tainted source? Or if you find out that a close friend's spouse is having an affair? Our emotions fuel mental machinations at all hours, especially at night, when we would rather be sleeping.

People sometimes assume that subjective feeling is the essence of emotion, but feeling is only one aspect. Sometimes it is missing.[62,63] I have seen some patients, mostly men, who reported fatigue, weight loss, sleep problems, and lack of initiative but no sadness or hopelessness. They had depression, but I missed the diagnosis repeatedly until I finally realized that subjective experience is only one aspect of depression. Once free from the idea that emotions always involve subjective feelings, it becomes possible to trace the heritage of emotions back to the origins of behavior regulation—all the way back.

Bacteria don't have feelings, but they certainly do have different states that turn on when needed.[64] The most dramatic shift occurs when their world dries up. A switch flips, and happily swimming bacteria transform into tiny, sturdy spores. Even in stable environments, bacteria demonstrate amazing abilities to adapt to changing circumstances.[65] High temperatures induce the synthesis of protective heat shock proteins. Food concentrations higher than they were a half second previously induce counterclockwise rotation of flagellar tails, making them swim straight ahead toward the food. If the concentration declines, the flagella reverse direction, creating a tangle that tumbles the organism in random directions.[66] When conditions again look better than they did a half second previously, straight swimming resumes.[67,68,69] That is how bacteria navigate to places in your body where they can grow happily.

A one-second memory and a switch that turns tumbling to forward swimming and back are all it takes for bacteria to swim toward food and away from danger. Doesn't life feel like that sometimes? You are cruising along, and then suddenly the path ahead looks dark and barren and you find yourself tumbling without a plan or direction. It feels awful, but trying out random directions is better than persisting in efforts that lead nowhere or worse.

Emotions and Culture

The labeling, expression, and experience of emotions differ dramatically in different cultures. Even the word *emotion* has no exact translation in many languages. The closest German word, *Gefühl*, combines the meanings of emotion and physical sensation. Samoan and French speakers have words that describe "having a feeling" but no word that includes feelings, thoughts, and physical sensations. Germans recognize bittersweet longing as *Sehnsucht*, but other cultures have no word for such a longing, and lacking the word may make the experience less common. Disgust seems universal, but no Polish word corresponds exactly. Japanese readily recognize *amae*, a feeling of dependency like what an infant feels toward its mother, but no comparable word exists in English, perhaps because that kind of relationship is less common in the West.

Culture influences emotions, just as it influences body weight, blood pressure, and most everything else.[70] Culture influences what emotions people recognize, the words they use to describe them, the kinds of situations that arouse them, and to some extent what emotions are experienced. However, the *capacity* to feel emotions is a product of natural selection that we share with one another, and to some extent with other species.

Several scientists have traveled to distant cultures to find out if emotional facial expressions are universal. Psychologist and leading emotion researcher Carroll Izard took thirty-two photographs of faces to eight cultures and found that people everywhere recognized all but a few emotional expressions accurately.[71] A German researcher, Irenäus Eibl-Eibesfeldt, got similar results from his extensive studies.[72] Another leading emotion expert, Paul Ekman, conducted similar studies that found cross-cultural consistency in the ability to recognize facial expressions of anger, disgust, fear, joy, sadness, and surprise but considerable variation in the ability to recognize expressions of contempt and other emotions.[73]

These studies have spurred a generation of controversy, with praise met by criticism,[74] rejoinders, and replies to the rejoinders.[75] They are swords in debates about nature and nurture. Such controversies make emotion research seem like a jungle of untamed science; however, like the lost medieval cities in Cambodia revealed by ground-penetrating radar, emotions have a consistent structure underneath all the overgrowth.

The Polish philosopher and linguist Anna Wierzbicka, now living in Australia, addressed these questions with profound clarity and depth.[76] She began by demonstrating large cultural differences in words for emotions, deftly destroying the notion that universal basic emotions could ever be described by a handful of English words. She went on, however, to show that all humans share what she calls universal "semantic primitives," concepts such as "big—small," and, notably, the concept of "feeling." The concept of emotion in English is culture bound, but the experience of feeling is universal, as are a few emotions, including fear, joy, sadness, and shame.

Wierzbicka concluded that each emotion corresponds to a specific *situation*, and most of the situations are remarkably universal. She developed a sophisticated but complicated system to define the situations that correspond to each emotion, such as being betrayed by a supposed friend. Her system shows that beneath cultural differences, emotions are consistent responses to situations, and the universality of some situations has shaped universal emotions.

The old dichotomy of biology versus culture is fading, replaced by a more sophisticated view of how they influence each other. Lisa Feldman Barrett's work exemplifies this advance by describing a "psychological construction" view of emotions that is positioned between appraisal theories and social construction theories.[77,78] Her work recognizes that the basic ingredients of emotions are shaped by natural selection and shared with other animals but emphasizes that this does not mean that emotions are each separate with dedicated brain circuits and a fixed pattern of expression. Instead, they are overlapping states that interweave with one another and cognition and perception influenced by culture to get the job done.[79] This is progress entirely consistent with the recognition of evolved organic complexity.

Are Emotions Ignoble?

A stream of thought that goes back to philosophers in ancient Greece views emotions as maladaptive interlopers that undermine human reason. In *Phaedrus*, Plato viewed human lives as chariots pulled by two horses. The one representing reason is "noble . . . upright, and cleanly made." The other, emotion, is "ignoble . . . a crooked lumbering animal . . . the mate of insolence and pride, shag-eared and deaf, hardly yielding to whip and spur."[80] Leave it to a philosopher to take sides with reason and disparage emotion.

More than two thousand years after Plato wrote, I received an email invitation to a lecture entitled "Unbridled Passions." The metaphor endures for good reasons. In states of passion, we may accuse a lover, attack a boss, insult a friend, or have sex with someone entirely inappropriate. Emotionally inspired actions often arouse regret. Emotions also cause useless suffering. Baseless fears keep bird phobics from picnics, flying phobics from wonderful trips, and agoraphobics trapped in the house for years. Unjustified feelings of guilt and unworthiness burden many lives, especially those of people who tend to be more moral than average. Envy, rage, and jealousy wreck the lives of many others. Between maladaptive actions, unwarranted suffering, and causing social conflicts, a lot of emotion seems ignoble and useless. Why did natural selection leave us with so much useless, painful emotion? An answer requires understanding why we care so much about our goals and how emotions help us to reach them.

Our ancestors encountered situations in which emotions were useful. A few are specific physical situations aroused by specific physical cues. Falling, the sight of blood, a looming shadow, and sudden loud noises all indicate possible danger, so they connect to fear directly, or they get connected very readily by learning.[81,82,83,84] However, more subtle situations also shape emotions, especially those that arise in the course of pursuing goals.

Organisms try to get sex, power, and resources and to avoid danger and loss. Pursuing these goals gives rise to a set of defined situations. Each one poses different adaptive challenges that shape a different emotional state. Opportunity arouses enthusiasm. Success arouses joy. Threat arouses anxiety. Loss arouses sadness. I was delighted to find that the four situations that arise in goal pursuit map so neatly to four emotions. Philosopher friends Allan Gibbard and Peter Railton pointed out that this is a very old idea: Plato recognized four closely related basic emotions: hope, fear, joy, and sadness.[85] Moreover, they noted, variations on this four-part scheme were central to most theories of emotions in ancient Greece and again in Europe since the Middle Ages. It can be expanded by separating physical from social situations and by adding the emotions aroused by alternative outcomes, disappointment when pursuit of an opportunity fails, and relief when a threat is avoided.

EMOTIONS FOR SITUATIONS THAT ARISE IN GOAL PURSUIT

		BEFORE	AFTER	ALTERNATIVE OUTCOME
OPPORTUNITY	PHYSICAL	Desire	Pleasure	Disappointment
	SOCIAL	Excitement	Joy	
THREAT	PHYSICAL	Fear	Pain	Relief
	SOCIAL	Anxiety	Sadness	

The word *goal* is completely inadequate to describe the diversity of human pursuits. Some goals are long term, such as raising happy children, while others are instantaneous, such as trying to convince your conversation partner that your joke was less offensive than it really was. For simplicity, I use the word *goal* to mean anything that someone is trying to get, find, become, lose, escape, or avoid. Psychologists have used many other descriptors, including mission, life task, enterprise, aim, purpose, objective, or pursuit of personal meaning or possible selves. Each of those terms connects to its own rich literature that explores emotions and goal pursuit.[86,87,88,89,90,91,92,93] Psychologists know all about how goal pursuit influences emotions. Psychiatrists, not so much.

Turning Emotions On

How does the brain know when to turn on an emotion? As already mentioned, some cues, such as looming shadows and sudden noises, race along special brain pathways to get fear up and running fast, as Alfred Hitchcock knew so well. Other cues arouse emotions only after learning. A buzzing noise that initially arouses only mild interest will evoke terror after being paired with a shock a few times, as Ivan Pavlov demonstrated to the vexation of his dogs. A light that has no effect at first will stimulate copious salivation after being paired with food a few times, as dog owners observe when a proffered biscuit results in saliva dripping on the carpet. Extra saliva in the seconds just before food arrives must give a selective advantage big enough to keep the classical conditioning mechanism intact.

Rewards and punishments also cause emotional learning. Memories of excruciating embarrassment the morning after you put a lampshade on your head at a party should arouse uncomfortable emotions that inhibit any impulse to do it again at tonight's party—unless, that is, your anxiety again floats away on a tide of tequila.

Humans share these learning capacities with other creatures, but we also have an extraordinary special ability. Our minds make models of the world and project alternative futures across months and years.[94,95,96] The outcomes of different possible actions play out in our minds. As we plan, fantasize, dream, and imagine, emotions nudge us toward some paths and away from others. What would marriage with the exciting person be like? What about the stable, boring one? The mind generates fantasies infused with emotions that direct us toward plans that will benefit our genes—and perhaps us as well.

Thanks to this ability to use internal models to predict alternative futures, we can pursue larger goals over longer time scales than any other species can. Our strategies often involve complex social relationships and difficult decisions. Decisions about whether to give up on big projects that are failing are especially tough. Is it worth living yet another year with the exciting one who won't commit? What about trying out for the basketball team again this year? Is there any point in applying for a promotion? Is it worth continuing to restore that 1955 Thunderbird without an engine?

What about continuing the search for genes that cause schizophrenia? We are pulled constantly by the demands of multiple different projects and conflicting strategies. The anthropologist Robin Dunbar argues convincingly that this explains why we have large brains.[97]

While some goals are universal, many are not. Human values and identities are gloriously diverse, so predicting what emotion will be aroused by new information requires knowing an individual's values, goals, projects, and strategies. The big news in emotions research is that emotions arise from the "appraisals" people make about the personal significance of information.[98,99,100] That tiny pink spot on a positive pregnancy test may induce tears of despair in a teenager or tears of joy in a woman who has been trying to get pregnant for years.

This is a world beyond crude stimulus-response models. It involves not only subtle social learning and information processing but also an individual's interpretation of the meaning of information for ability to make progress toward personal goals using his or her idiosyncratic strategies. People value health, money, status, and attractive partners to vastly different degrees. Some people mainly care about money; others care only about love or being good. Not only do values differ, but people also use diverse social strategies. One person seeks to gain social influence by being generous, another by being the life of the party, another by making threats. The first two will avoid revealing selfishness, while the third person will avoid revealing sympathy. Goals differ even in the same individual over time, so the same information may arouse very different emotions. For instance, that tiny pink spot.

An evolutionary view of emotions is sometimes thought to imply a rigid impersonal view of human behavior. However, far from assuming that everyone is identical, an evolutionary perspective encourages giving close attention to the hopes, dreams, fears, and manifold peculiarities of diverse individuals.

Regulating Emotion

Some people are extremely emotional, while others hardly react no matter what happens. Such extremes are laid bare in certain marriages. A couple came for help because of conflicts throughout their twenty years of unhappiness together. He manages a local bank branch. She is a graphic artist. He found her exciting from the time they first met in the college library on a Friday night. He says, "She was gorgeous and exciting. She got me out of my shell. But she won't listen to reason." She says, "I had a couple of drinks. My plan was to seduce a business student, but look what I got—a calculator!" Together they often make good decisions, but they don't much enjoy the process or each other. The futures they imagined proved poor predictors. The self-deceptions induced by romantic infatuation are exhilarating, but they benefit our genes more than our selves.

Some people worry for days about the meaning of a raised eyebrow that may have just been a twitch; others hardly notice direct insults. Some people are thrilled by small opportunities; others hardly shift in their chairs at a windfall. Both extremes have costs. People prone to intense emotions experience enthusiasms that shift their efforts from one unfinished project to another and demoralization that blinds them to new opportunities. People who hardly experience emotion neither take full advantage of opportunities nor fully protect themselves from threats. Why such a wide range of responsiveness? A good guess is that people across the range have generally had similar Darwinian fitness. There is no one normal genome. There is no one normal personality.

We all struggle to get relief from painful emotions. They are painful for a reason: to motivate efforts to change, escape, and avoid such situations. But changing or escaping a bad situation is not always possible. When it isn't possible to help an addicted child or a dying spouse, useless terrible feelings arise. Even in everyday life, useless feelings plague us. Controlling them is an understandable goal. Scores of books and articles suggest strategies for emotional regulation.[101] Most emphasize changing habits of thought or changing the meaning of the situation. Some try to dampen emotions directly by exercise, distraction, meditation, or psychotropic drugs. Some encourage trying to change the situation despite the costs.

Then there is the most common and effective strategy: just wait. The situation changes. The emotional fog clears. Anger fades. Becoming a paraplegic is terrible, and winning the lottery is wonderful, but one's overall level of subjective well-being tends to revert toward the level before the accident or big win.[102] We spend our lives chasing carrots and fleeing from possible calamities. We feel great when we succeed and terrible when we fail—for a while. Then the "psychological immune system" kicks in and helps us bounce back from disappointment much faster than we anticipated.[103] This may be because, like levels of emotionality, the average set point for subjective well-being may not influence fitness much. What matters is the ability to respond appropriately when circumstances change.

Emotional Disorders

An evolutionary perspective on normal emotions is the essential but mostly missing foundation for making sense of abnormal emotions. Every bodily response can go awry. The two obvious ways are too little response or too much. People who never cough have a serious disorder, as do those who cough for no reason. Deficient immune response results in infection; excessive response causes inflammatory and autoimmune diseases. People who lack the capacity to feel pain die young; those with chronic pain sometimes wish they had.

Research on emotional disorders has focused on negative emotions, mostly anxiety and low mood. The new field of positive psychology brings needed attention to deficits of positive emotions.[104] The tendency to focus on excess negative emotions and deficient positive emotions is readily explained by the pleasure principle: we want to get pleasure and avoid pain. But this neglects two other important kinds of emotional disorders.

Positive emotion can be excessive.[105,106,107,108,109] The extreme version is the serious and sometimes fatal abnormal state of mania. Some people in its grip are euphoric, but others are swept up in the uncontrollable pursuit of grandiose goals that generate a pressure cooker of mixed subjective states. Milder versions of unjustified positive emotion are great for those who experience them, but some perky people can be insufferable, while others blithely ignore social cues that make others wish they would be more sensitive.

Negative emotions can be deficient. Few complain, but these are serious diseases. Hypophobia, insufficient anxiety, can be fatal. Lack of jealousy reduces reproductive success. Lack of sadness can result in doing the same stupid things over and over.

Positive psychology and negative psychology get all the attention. An evolutionary perspective highlights the neglect of "diagonal psychology," that is, excess positive emotions and deficient negative emotions. Excesses and deficiencies of anxiety, low mood, embarrassment, disgust, surprise, guilt, pride, envy, jealousy, and love all deserve attention.

DIAGONAL PSYCHOLOGY

	NEGATIVE EMOTIONS	POSITIVE EMOTIONS
EXCESSES	Excessive negative emotions	**Excessive positive emotions**
DEFICIENCIES	**Deficient negative emotions**	Deficient positive emotions

Excesses and deficiencies are only the most obvious kinds of emotional abnormalities. Responses can also be too quick, too slow, too enduring, or in response to the wrong cues. A quick temper is a problem, but so is a slow one or a tendency to hold grudges or taking offense for no reason. Anger can be useful if it is aroused by the right cues at the right rate to the right intensity for the right duration, but it can go awry in many ways.

An evolutionary framework will eventually help us find new kinds of treatment for emotional problems, but it has practical implications even now. Emotions have meaning. We should try to understand their messages. They are usually trying to get us to do or stop doing something. Sometimes they are wise and we should heed them.[110,111,112,113,114,115] But not always. Sometimes they push us to do things that help our genes but harm us. Sometimes they arise from our distorted views of the world. Sometimes they come from brain abnormalities. Considering all the possibilities provides a framework for making wise decisions. We can often do that for ourselves, but an expert's advice can be invaluable.

Emotion experts who think like mechanics diagnose what is wrong and recommend a treatment that is likely to work. They tend to blame one kind of cause and provide treatment for that cause, whether crooked thinking or brain pathology. Emotion experts with an evolutionary perspective take an engineer's point of view. They recognize the utility of emotions and the historical and design constraints that make us all vulnerable to emotional problems. This encourages consideration of multiple causes and possible treatments. Instead of assuming that positive emotion is good and negative emotion is bad, experts with an evolutionary perspective can analyze the appropriateness of an emotion for the situation. Instead of assuming that the emotion regulation mechanism is awry, they can assess whether the severity of the symptoms is proportional to the situation. Instead of assuming that normally aroused symptoms are good for the individual, they recognize the possibility that an emotion is advancing the interests of genes at a cost to the individual. Instead of lumping together factors that arouse emotions as "stress," they can dig in to do the hard work of trying to understand the origins of an individual's problems. In short, they can think and act like physicians.

CHAPTER 5

ANXIETY AND SMOKE DETECTORS

*Whoever has learned to be anxious in the right way has
learned the ultimate.*

—Søren Kierkegaard,
The Concept of Anxiety, 1844[1]

I was standing on a boulder at the edge of the Pacific at Point Reyes, just
north of San Francisco, reveling in glorious sun, wind, and salt spray from
waves just a foot or two high. A sign read, "Danger! Sneaker waves. Do
not go out on rocks," but I saw no big waves headed toward my rock
on that lovely day. Then, in an instant, frigid water was up to my thighs,
dragging me off my suddenly slippery perch. I was lucky that my momentary fear deficiency wasn't fatal. Seaside jaunts still arouse a vivid
memory, with anxiety that motivates avoidance.

Those who experience only a thrill after a wave nearly sweeps them out
to sea are likely, at some point, never to be seen again. Others have the
opposite problem: they experience so much anxiety that they never go near
the ocean. Playing on the beach is no fun if you think a tsunami could arrive
any minute. For people with anxiety disorders, mere hints of danger arouse
sweating, tension, fast pulse, pounding heart, panicky feelings, and flight.

When Martha came to our clinic, it was the first time she had left the
house in years. Her husband did all the grocery shopping, and she bought
her clothes by mail order, in increasingly large sizes.

Sam was a capable carpenter, but if he sat with other workers at lunch, he got too anxious to eat. They wondered if he thought he was too good for them, so when he did say something, they were ready with ridicule that amplified his anxiety.

Julie also could not eat with others, but her fear was of choking. So she ate alone at home, blending her food to a thick liquid.

Mel loved the out-of-doors. He jogged every day until he became preoccupied by the fear that he would contract West Nile fever from a mosquito bite. After that he rarely left the house, and he slathered his skin with insect repellent when he had to go out.

Bill feared he would catch HIV, not from having sex but from using a public restroom. He knew that could not actually happen, but he never drove more than an hour from home, and he hadn't taken a vacation for years.

And then there was Marilyn, who was frightened of birds. She wanted treatment because her husband had invited her to go with him to London, but she was horrified by a mental image of being enveloped in a flock of pigeons.

I treated these patients and hundreds more with anxiety disorders. It is hard for many people to grasp just how devastating anxiety can be. Some people think that anxiety disorders are "just nervousness." That's a bit like saying that paraplegia is "difficulty walking." Serious anxiety is much more common than it seems. Just as you don't let others know about your fears, others conceal theirs, making many who suffer with anxiety think that they are the only ones. If only that were true.

Across a lifetime, approximately 30 percent of people have an anxiety disorder that qualifies for a formal diagnosis,[2] and some people with less anxiety nonetheless need help. For instance, the criteria for social anxiety are set so that only about 12 percent of the population gets the diagnosis,[3] but those criteria are arbitrary. The proportion of people who are afraid of giving public presentations, for example, is closer to 50 percent, and many are glad for help.

From Spiders and Snakes to the First Anxiety Clinic

As a medical student on my first research project, it was my job to get the snakes and spiders and to draw the blood. A new treatment for phobias called "exposure therapy" was just coming into its own in the late 1970s. It was a product of behavioral psychology studies that suggested that phobias could be extinguished if the patient stayed close to the snake or spider despite the terrible anxiety. My research mentor, George Curtis, had the inspired idea that this provided a remarkable opportunity to discover, with no ethical compromises, how intense anxiety influenced hormones.

Our volunteer phobia sufferers were eager at the start and grateful at the end, but in the middle, they were terrified. Each came for five sessions of three hours each. In order to study stress hormones at their peak, we started three hours after the midpoint of sleep, about 6 a.m. for most people.[4,5] That meant I had to go to the pet shop the night before to borrow a snake, spider, mouse, or bird. Our overnight animal guests didn't please my girlfriend, but she put up with them. The pet shop was hesitant until, to our surprise and their delight, a cured patient came in to buy a tarantula, the first of many such purchases. I got very good at drawing blood.

The project provoked anxiety in us as well as our patients. My psycho-analytic supervisors explained phobias as products of libido displaced from its original source because of unconscious defenses. They said behavioral treatment would cause new symptoms, the way popping one dent out of a Ping-Pong ball causes a new one. They got me worried, but it happened only once; a man with multiple phobias became more generally anxious after his bird phobia improved. Scores of others got fast relief from phobias that had crippled them for decades.

The treatment was simple. For the woman with a bird phobia, we brought a caged pigeon into the room and encouraged her to get as close to it as possible. After a few minutes of crying and trembling with the bird at the door of the room, she asked us to take it away. We did. We then asked if the anxiety was the same at the end of those minutes as it had been at the start. "No," she said, "it went down from ninety-five to ninety." We asked if she wanted to get better faster with more intense anxiety or get better slower with less. She chose fast, so we brought the pigeon back into the room without the cage and held it in front of her, moving it closer whenever she gave the okay.

Like many patients in the midst of exposure therapy, she demonstrated extraordinary courage. Her pulse was 130, she was sweating, trembling, and so frightened she could hardly talk, but she kept reaching out toward the pigeon. Her anxiety decreased to 80, then 70, then 50, at which point she suddenly relaxed and said, "I wonder why I didn't do this a long time ago." By the end of the session, she had her hand on the bird, which now was as anxious as she was. A month later, she was proud to report having had a happy lunch with the pigeons in Trafalgar Square. We were thrilled to see how effective treatment could be.

The experience of exposure therapy is intense for therapists as well as for patients. Doing it well takes a special combination of confidence, cajoling, sympathy, and patience. At first it seemed too stressful and even cruel to ask patients to endure such intense anxiety, but as we saw fast cures, our confidence grew and transferred to our patients. Many said the treatment was like surgery whose pain was worth it.

I was amazed not only by how well exposure treatment works but also by the patterns of improvement. Sometimes the anxiety gradually subsided, as you would expect if the treatment was reversing previous conditioning. Equally often, however, anxiety would plummet suddenly in the midst of an intense session. One minute a patient would be sweating and trying not to scream while looking at a boa constrictor. The next minute she would be saying, "I'm not sure why I've ever been afraid of these things. They're actually kind of cute. My anxiety is down to forty. Can I hold it now?"

There were other surprises. One woman with a snake phobia was trying hard to reach out and touch the snake when she suddenly said, "Oh, my God, I just remembered how this all began." She said that when she was six years old, her father had seen a snake on the road and stopped the car. He had chopped the snake into pieces with a shovel, put them in a jar, and given it to her to hold between her legs. The psychoanalysts who supervised my psychotherapy treatments were delighted to hear about a case that seemed to confirm Freud's theories, but they refused to believe that she had overcome her fears in two hours of exposure therapy, instead of two years of psychotherapy.

Then there was the time we heard screams coming from a room where a woman was reading a magazine during a control session. She had seen a tiny insect, a silverfish, crawling up a wall in our not-perfectly-hygienic laboratory. When she calmed down, she explained. When she was seven years old, she had been diagnosed with polio, whisked out the back door of the doctor's office, and put into a hospital room alone, where she had lain for weeks, paralyzed and terrified by visions of insects crawling on the wall next to her face.

Treating phobias firsthand provides insights that just talking with patients doesn't reveal. Behavior therapy is far more complicated and interesting than mechanically extinguishing a conditioned response. In some patients, it uncovered remarkable memories, and the patterns by which patients improved varied enormously.

Word about the availability of fast, effective treatment got out, and the phone started ringing. Far more people wanted help than we could treat. Many were desperate. We saw students who couldn't finish high school because of fear of being called on in class. We treated a corporate vice president who had lost his job because of fear of flying. I made a house call for a woman who had not left her small trailer for years. A stockbroker with an elevator phobia had to leave early for work so he could walk up the twenty stories to his office. His aerobic condition was superb, but he was tired of climbing and of making excuses to clients about why he couldn't ride the elevator.

Our research project soon expanded to become one of the first clinics specializing in anxiety disorders. It was gratifying to be able to provide relief for so many people who had not gotten help elsewhere. But what caused these disorders? And why did so many people have fears of snakes and spiders, while so few feared sneezes and unsafe sex? A big question gradually came into focus.

Why Does Anxiety Exist at All?

The general answer is obvious enough: individuals with a capacity for anxiety are more likely to escape from dangerous situations now and to avoid them in the future. After long conversations with the anxiety maven Isaac Marks, we recognized that there should be disorders of deficient as well as excess anxiety, as is the case for every other protective response.[6,7] Excessive immune responses cause much disease, but immune deficiencies can be fatal. Scores of articles report the harm caused by anxiety, but hardly any describe its benefits. When I was on the circuit lecturing about anxiety disorders, I asked every audience if anyone knew of studies showing the benefits of anxiety. Many thought I was daft, but finally someone suggested I look at an article about fear of heights by the New Zealand researcher Richie Poulton.

The prevailing theory was that people develop a fear of heights after a bad fall. That seemed intuitively obvious, but no one had ever proved it. Poulton identified a group of children who had been injured in a fall between ages five and nine and compared them to those who had had no similar injury.[8] At age eighteen, a severe fear of heights was present in 2 percent of those who had had a fall in childhood but 7 percent of those who had not. That was the opposite of the prediction! If mild as well as severe fears were included, the difference was even more dramatic. Fear of heights was seven times *less* common in eighteen-year-olds who had experienced a fall in childhood.[9] In retrospect, the explanation is simple: children who had too little fear to protect them against falls in childhood still had too little fear at age eighteen.

I began looking for other cases of hypophobia. We all know reckless people who lack the usual fear of dangerous animals, social criticism, driving fast, taking drugs, and death-defying stunts. At California ski resorts, young daredevils ski down (actually, jump off) slopes (actually, cliffs) that others fear. These men—they are nearly all men—are admired for their skill and courage, especially by women. Every year, several die.

I vividly recall a professional motorcycle racer who asked for my help. The night before a big race, he would vomit everything he ate, and he couldn't sleep. This began shortly after a friend had been killed in a race. Each year, he said, two or three other riders on the circuit were killed or severely injured. He had been in several wrecks but had no permanent damage so far. He denied feeling fear but reported that in addition to vomiting the day before each race, his heart rate went up, he sweated, he felt short of breath, and his muscles tightened up. He wanted a drug that would stop his symptoms. As a pro with many advertising endorsements, his income depended on it. When I told him I thought his anxiety was protecting him, he listened politely. When I told him it would be dangerous for him to take a drug to reduce his anxiety, he got angry and left. I don't know if he is still alive.

Hypophobia is serious and potentially fatal but underrecognized and rarely treated. Hypophobics don't come to anxiety clinics. Instead, they are found in experimental aircraft, on creative frontiers, and on the front lines of battlegrounds and political movements. They are also found in prisons, hospitals, unemployment lines, bankruptcy courts, and morgues. Pharmaceutical companies have not rushed to provide treatment for hypophobia, but several drugs would likely be effective. One might even be acceptable to a few people—yohimbine reportedly also causes intense orgasms. Starting a clinic for hypophobics could improve health and prevent injuries, but it doesn't seem like a good business proposition.

As I got more serious about understanding why anxiety exists, I began to see more connections. The panic attacks described by my patients seemed essentially the same as the "fight-or-flight response," a phenomenon first named by the great physiologist Walter Cannon in his seminal 1939 book, *The Wisdom of the Body*.[10] He noted that high heart rate, shortness of breath, sweating, freezing, and flight are all useful responses in the face of life-threatening danger. That was exactly what I was seeing in my patients. But was it really the same thing?

One evening as I pulled into my driveway at dusk after a long day in clinic, a rabbit froze motionless in the headlight's glare. It made me think. I had never heard my panic patients describe freezing, but then I had never asked them. The next day I did. My first patient said, "Oh, yes, sometimes I am so paralyzed that I wonder if I will ever move again." I asked all my panic patients for the next few weeks; about half reported feeling paralyzed for a moment as their panic attacks began. An evolutionary perspective opened my eyes to something I should have seen years before.

Why Is Anxiety So Often Excessive?

The Smoke Detector Principle explains a lot of useless anxiety. As mentioned in chapter 3, systems that regulate protective responses such as vomiting and pain turn the response on whenever the benefits are greater than the costs, even if that means false alarms. The costs of such responses tend to be low compared to the benefits of avoiding danger. So when danger may or may not be present, the small cost of a response ensures protection against a much larger harm. That is why we put up with false alarms from smoke detectors. It is why we can safely use medications to block responses such as vomiting and pain. And it is why useless anxiety is so common.

The Smoke Detector Principle is based on signal detection theory, used by electrical engineers to decide whether a click on a telephone line is a genuine signal or just noise.[11] The correct decision depends on the ratio of signals to noise, the costs of a false alarm, and the costs and benefits of an alarm when the danger is actually present. In a city where car theft is common, a sensitive car alarm system is worthwhile despite the false alarms, but in a safer locale it would be just a nuisance.

Panic disorder is caused by false alarms in the emergency response system. The system has been honed to speed escape when life-threatening danger may be present. You are thirsty on the ancient African savanna and a watering hole is just ahead, but you hear a noise in the grass. It could be a lion, or it might just be a monkey. Should you flee? It depends on the costs. Assume that fleeing in panic costs 100 calories. Not fleeing costs nothing if it is only a monkey, but if the noise was made by a lion, the cost is 100,000 calories—about how much energy a lion would get from having you for lunch!

Louder sounds are more likely to be caused by a lion. How loud does the sound need to be before you flee? Do the math. The cost of not fleeing if the lion is present is 1,000 times greater than the cost of a panic attack, so the optimal strategy is to run like hell whenever the sound is loud enough to indicate a lion is present with a probability greater than 1/1,000. This means that 999 times out of 1,000 you will flee unnecessarily. However, 1 time out of 1,000, fleeing will save your life.

Realizing that individual episodes of panic are often normal but useless helped both me and my patients to understand the problem better. The idea is not new. The philosopher Blaise Pascal used similar logic to argue that it is rational to believe in God; the cost is low, but failing to believe might result in burning in Hell for all eternity.[12] Adding a little math and evolutionary theory to Pascal's insight helps to explain why useless emotional suffering is so common. It can also help doctors to make good decisions about when it is safe to prescribe drugs that block normal responses such as pain, fever, cough, and anxiety, which are often not needed in the individual instance.[13,14,15]

Phobias

Snake and spider phobias are common. So are fears of bridges, heights, elevators, and airplanes. Fear of speaking in public is yet more common. Agoraphobia is characterized by fear of leaving the house and fear of open places. However, we never saw patients who complained about excess fear of books, trees, flowers, or butterflies. And we only rarely saw fears of many dangerous things, such as knives, electrical wires, bottles of pills, chemicals, or motorcycles. Why? This is an evolutionary question.

When Isaac Marks and I worked together for a summer on the question, we tried to figure out if different anxiety disorders corresponded to different kinds of dangerous situations. As the table below shows, they do.[16]

ANXIETY DISORDER	SITUATION/DANGER
Phobia of small animals	Possible damage by the animal
Fear of heights	Injury from falling
Panic attacks	Attack by a predator or human
Agoraphobia	Attack by a predator or human
Social anxiety	Loss of social standing
Hypochondriasis	Sickness
Fear of being unattractive	Social rejection
Fear of needles and fainting	Injury/bleeding

A few fears are built-in automatic responses,[17] but most common fears are not exactly innate. Fear of snakes, for instance, is not built in, but the brain is prewired to learn it fast, as shown by lovely experiments conducted by psychologist Susan Mineka and her colleagues in the 1970s. Young laboratory-raised monkeys reach blithely across a toy snake to get a treat. However, watching a single video of another monkey withdrawing in fright from the same toy snake created an enduring fear. Watching another monkey apparently withdrawing in fear from a flower created no similar fear.[18] The brain is prepared to learn to fear to some cues much faster than to others.

This is social learning of the most useful sort. Instead of a system that responds to only a few rigid cues, natural selection shaped a system that uses information from other individuals. Such fears can be transmitted from generation to generation. For instance, blackbirds were trained to fear a harmless honeyeater bird by showing them a doctored video. They transmitted that useless fear to six other birds in sequence.[19] Parents who fear spiders, snakes, or public restrooms can similarly transmit their fears to their children.

We can learn to fear novel dangerous objects, such as electrical sockets, drugs, and knives, but such learning is slow because those cues have no prewired connection to fear. The dangers of driving offer a telling and tragic example. Driving a car is the riskiest thing young people do. It is the single largest cause of death and devastating permanent injury. Nearly a quarter of all deaths in 2014 of people aged fifteen to twenty-four were due to motor vehicle accidents.[20] Worldwide, that is about three thousand per day.[21] Driver's education classes emphasize the risks of driving fast and of drinking while driving, but they don't generate nearly enough caution to provide reliable protection.

Panic Disorder

Panic attacks often come out of the blue. The first one may strike while reading a book, watching television, or waiting for a plane to take off. With no warning, the heart starts pounding, muscles tense, and the victim feels short of breath, a sense of impending doom, chest tightness, and a desperate urge to get away. Most people think they are having a heart attack or stroke, so they go to an emergency room, where they are given all kinds of tests. Far too many healthy young people get coronary arteriograms because their physicians missed the diagnosis of panic disorder.

Many of our patients reported being told in the ER, "We can't find any specific heart problem, but you should be very careful and come back immediately if things get worse." Such advice is the perfect way to transform an ordinary anxiety attack into a debilitating panic disorder. The patient begins monitoring for hints that the same kind of episode might be starting again. Soon enough, whether because of mowing the lawn or having an argument, the heart rate increases and the person feels short of breath. These symptoms arouse fear that an attack is beginning, causing a higher heart rate and more shortness of breath that spirals mild anxiety into a full-blown panic attack.

Some research attributes panic attacks to flaws in stress regulation mechanisms. A quick spurt of corticotropin-releasing hormone (CRH) from a brain center called the hypothalamus causes physiological arousal that nearly matches the experience of panic.[22] CRH excites cells in the locus coeruleus, so named because it is a blue-colored spot in a lower part of the brain. It contains 80 percent of the neurons that contain noradrenaline.[23] Electrical stimulation of the locus coeruleus causes symptoms like those of a typical panic attack. Some researchers suspect that panic attacks are caused by an abnormality in CRH or the locus coeruleus. Some may be, but usually the locus coeruleus is activated by signals from far higher in the brain.

The capacity for having a panic attack is nearly universal. Questionnaire studies find that most adults can recall experiencing paniclike episodes. Panic attacks induce a consistent constellation of symptoms including sweating, rapid pulse, shortness of breath, muscle tension, tunnel vision, acute hearing, fear of fainting, and a desperate urge to flee. As noted already, Walter Cannon recognized the utility of these responses in the face of danger. For our ancestors, that would most often have been in the presence of a predator or hostile human. This all seems abstract, but imagine kneeling by a pool to get water for your family and spotting a crouching lion on the far bank. Our ancestors were not all the same. Some experienced awe at the lion's strength or no response at all. They became lion lunch. Others dropped everything and fled to the nearest tree. They survived to live another day, and their genes survive in us.

I did a house call for a woman who had not left her trailer for years. Even putting one foot on the stairs to the outside caused terror. It took a few months, medications, and help from relatives, but she was finally able to get out and about again. People with her disorder, agoraphobia, experience intense fear when they leave their homes. They also fear wide-open spaces and enclosed places. That is an odd combination. If you are afraid of wide-open spaces, why also be afraid of enclosed places?

Most agoraphobia is a complication of panic attacks, and agoraphobics often experience panic symptoms when they leave the house. When they do go out, they stay close to home and close to trusted friends. All kinds of explanations have been proposed for the association of agoraphobia with panic disorder. Neuroscientists have looked at brain regions that might influence both. Freud was convinced that fear of being out on the street was a result of unconscious sexual impulses to become a streetwalker. That wasn't as daft as it now seems. Most of his patients did have wishes for more and better sex, and women alone on the street do encounter sexual opportunities. But there is an easier explanation for the association of agoraphobia with panic attacks.

Imagine you are a hunter-gatherer who narrowly escaped a lion yesterday. What would be smart to do today? Stay in camp if you can. If you must go out, don't go far and don't go alone. Avoid wide-open spaces and enclosed spaces, where you would be especially vulnerable to a predator. If any sign of danger arises, flee to home and safety as fast as you can. As the behavioral ecologists Steven Lima and Lawrence Dill put it, "Few failures . . . are as unforgiving as failure to avoid a predator; being killed greatly decreases future fitness."[24]

Most patients with panic disorder have never encountered a lion or anything else especially dangerous. Their attacks are false alarms in an otherwise useful system. These false alarms motivate more monitoring, causing increased arousal and increased system sensitivity in a vicious cycle that makes further attacks more likely.

For years, I explained to panic patients that they did not have heart disease or epilepsy, they were experiencing panic attacks, and they needed psychiatric treatment, not more medical evaluation. After listening politely, many said something like, "But, Doctor, it is not mental, it is physical. When an attack comes, I can feel my heart pounding, and I get short of breath. Do you know of a good cardiologist?"

My emerging evolutionary understanding changed my approach.[25] I began telling patients that the symptoms of panic are useful for escaping life-threatening danger and that panic attacks are false alarms, like the shrieking of a smoke detector when the toast burns. On hearing this, about a quarter of my patients said something like, "Thanks, Doctor, that makes sense. That's all I need to know. If I need more help, I will give you a call."

The rest needed further treatment. Behavior therapy works well for most cases of panic disorder, but medications are also effective. Antidepressants, taken consistently for a few weeks, stop panic attacks for most patients. However, many continue to have "miniattacks" in which they feel a panic attack coming on, but, like a stifled sneeze, it never quite goes all the way. Some patients worry that the medication is "just covering up my symptoms so they will come back when I stop the pills." They appreciate learning why this is uncommon; the body adjusts the sensitivity of the anxiety system depending on how dangerous the environment is. Several months without panic attacks make the system less sensitive, so future attacks are less likely, even after medication is stopped.

Posttraumatic Stress Disorder

People who come close to death are often changed in ways that make ordinary life impossible. Most people who live in safe neighborhoods and who have never experienced combat cannot even imagine the terror of watching a friend being blown to pieces. The stories of some patients are traumatic even to hear. A man crawled out of a burning car as it exploded with his friends inside. A woman was kidnapped, raped, stabbed, and left for dead. A woman working alone in a laundry had her arm trapped between the hot metal blades of the pants press for fifteen horrifying minutes.

Such close encounters with death change people forever. Many constantly relive the traumatic experience in nightmares and flashbacks. Some feel overwhelmed by fear every minute of their lives. Tiny cues—a distant helicopter, a slammed door, a stranger approaching—arouse fear as intense as the actual danger. To try to avoid such cues and the terror they provoke, some people live in a basement, move to a rural area, or avoid going out. Others feel numb, as if all emotions are dead, except for sudden outbreaks of rage or panic.

Researchers have tried to identify the individual differences that make some people more vulnerable than others. Michigan State University psychologist Naomi Breslau and her collaborators conducted a study on 1,007 members of a health maintenance organization in Detroit.[26,27] Thirty-nine percent of them had been exposed to traumatic events, and 24 percent of those developed PTSD. Those who developed PTSD after the trauma were more likely to have had early separation from parents, a family history of anxiety, or preexisting anxiety or depression.

The researchers then did something remarkable: they studied the same population again three years later. Nineteen percent had experienced a new traumatic event during the period, and 11 percent of those had developed PTSD. The strongest predictor of developing PTSD was a history of past exposure to traumatic events, and traumatic events were more likely to happen to people who had previously experienced something terrible. Such terrible events were more likely to happen to people with a tendency to neuroticism and extroversion, so those most vulnerable to bad feelings were also the most likely to experience trauma.[28] Breslau and colleagues reviewed this and many other studies to find out who is most vulnerable to developing PTSD after a trauma. The strongest factor was lack of social support, followed by experiencing neglect or trauma in childhood.[29]

Are enduring changes after trauma useful or just a screw-up in the system? I doubt that PTSD is a useful adaptation in general. However, following the Smoke Detector Principle, it is easy to see how extreme defensive responses could be aroused normally by cues only distantly similar to those associated with a life-threatening situation. After nearly losing your life, general increased arousal is likely to be worthwhile despite its large costs. Hair-trigger startle responses can be useful, as can extreme fear when exposed to cues that indicate even a 1 in 1,000 chance that potentially fatal danger is present. People with PTSD know perfectly well that they are not still on a battlefield, but their bodies and minds respond as if they were. A book by Australian researcher Chris Cantor reviewed the evidence about whether this extraordinary hypersensitivity is just an abnormality or part of a useful adaptation with a terrible price of extreme false alarms, but it is hard to draw a firm conclusion.[30]

Generalized Anxiety Disorder

Generalized anxiety disorder (GAD) is about as far as you can get from PTSD and still have an anxiety disorder. Instead of symptoms tightly connected to a very specific event or danger, GAD consists of diverse worries and physical symptoms of anxiety. "Worry" doesn't sound too serious, until you actually talk with people who suffer from GAD. To estimate its severity I ask, "What percent of your mental life is devoted to worry?" For many patients the response is "More than ninety percent, that's all I think about."

A typical patient with GAD worries about money, storms, health, children, and the security of employment and marriage. Things that most people would brush off become festering preoccupations. "I am only sixty-two. What happens if my company goes broke and I lose my insurance and I get sick before I am eligible for Medicare?" "What if my daughter plays in the backyard and a deer jumps the fence and she gets a tick bite and gets Lyme disease and I don't notice the rash?" Their mental lives are a continual stream of "What if?" potential catastrophes. They also experience physical symptoms, especially muscle tension, fatigue, trembling, sweating, and bowel symptoms. Such symptoms themselves are a fine focus for worry.

The danger-monitoring system is set to a hair trigger in people with GAD. Their minds fill with dire fantasies. Pride and pleasure as a daughter sets off for prom night are displaced by visions of accidents or pregnancy. Instead of time to relax in those few extra minutes when a spouse arrives home late, there is only worry about accidents or heart attacks.

A fascinating recent finding is that genetic tendencies to GAD overlap strongly with those for depression.[31] The specific responsible alleles have not been found, but relatives of people with GAD have an increased risk of both GAD and depression, and relatives of people with depression have an increased risk of depression and GAD. Both disorders reflect a state of caution in the face of adversity. Both may escalate because of vicious cycles instigated by evolved systems that make the systems more responsive after bad things happen.[32]

Many other psychiatric problems can also be viewed as excessive protective responses. Eating disorders arise from a desperate fear of obesity. Pathological jealousy arises from a fear that a partner will leave or be unfaithful. Paranoia arises from fears that others are plotting against you. Spending the right amount of energy on protection is wise, but many of us spend far too much, the Smoke Detector Principle notwithstanding.

What Should We Do Differently?

Understanding the evolutionary origins and functions of anxiety does not suggest a special evolutionary kind of treatment, but it nonetheless transforms treatment. In my early years of practice, I sympathized with my anxiety patients for having a disease. No matter how carefully I phrased it, that made many feel weak or flawed. When I instead began emphasizing that anxiety is a useful response that often goes overboard, many patients reported feeling normalized and empowered.

Women are twice as likely as men to have an anxiety disorder. Many explanations have been proposed based on hormones, brain mechanisms, and social forces, all of which suggest that there is something wrong with women. An evolutionary perspective flips the analysis on its head: women on average have about the right amount of anxiety for their own welfare; men have the right amount to maximize transmission of their genes, at a huge risk to their health.

Arguments about whether panic disorder, GAD, and social anxiety disorder are fundamentally the same or different are unnecessary; all are anxiety subtypes, each partially differentiated from ancestral precursor states to cope with dangers in different kinds of situations. Instead of seeking special explanations for why some people have more than one anxiety disorder, the association of multiple kinds of anxiety types makes sense in light of their common evolutionary origins. Instead of assuming that anxiety is always excessive, an evolutionary view calls attention to the Smoke Detector Principle and the need for research on hypophobia.

An evolutionary view also encourages setting aside abstract debates about whether anxiety disorders are mostly physical or mostly psychological and turning attention instead to a personalized assessment of all possible causes of an individual's anxiety. Some patients have lifelong problems similar to those of their relatives. Others have no family history and no problems with anxiety, until some life event sets off a disorder. An evolutionary perspective also helps clinicians and patients put aside the misguided notion that treatment choices should be guided by beliefs about causes. Problems that arise mainly from genetic or physiological causes often respond well to psychological treatments. Problems induced by life situations often benefit from medications.

An evolutionary perspective also illuminates how treatments work. Antianxiety drugs do not correct a neurotransmitter deficit; they disrupt the anxiety system, just as aspirin disrupts fever and pain systems. Behavior therapy also changes the brain. It acts via mechanisms that evolved to adjust anxiety responses as environments become less or more dangerous. These mechanisms do not just reverse conditioning. Instead, exposure therapy creates new inhibitory impulses from the frontal lobes that descend and prevent anxiety signals from getting to consciousness.[33] This is why stress can revive old unrelated fears. Pavlov conditioned dogs to fear a sound and then conditioned them to eliminate the fear. But after a flood nearly drowned the dogs in their cages, many showed a return of their fear.[34]

Positive feedback spirals escalate anxiety. Repeated exposure to danger indicates that the anxiety system is not providing sufficient protection, so the system adjusts to become more sensitive. This poses the risk of positive feedback. Daniel Nettle and Melissa Bateson, biologists at the University of Newcastle, have proposed a special version of the Smoke Detector Principle that describes this capacity for adjusting responses.[35] As noted already, such self-adjusting systems are vulnerable to dysregulation. Monitoring for symptoms of panic makes it more likely that minor physiological changes will escalate to a full-blown panic attack.

Fearless individuals are often admired, but their challenges are small compared to the gritty resolve many anxiety patients demonstrate by giving a talk, going to the dentist, flying on a plane, leaving the house, or coming for anxiety treatment. Treatment can reduce their suffering, and evolutionarily informed treatment can do that faster. In the meanwhile, people with anxiety disorders deserve recognition for their courage and daily determination to live full lives despite their symptoms.

CHAPTER 6

LOW MOOD AND THE ART OF GIVING UP

Pain or suffering of any kind, if long continued, causes depression and lessens the power of action; yet is well adapted to make a creature guard itself against any great or sudden evil.

—Charles Darwin, *On the Origin of Species,* 1887[1]

If at first you don't succeed, try, try again. Then quit. No point in being a damned fool about it.

—Attributed to W. C. Fields

A young man came to our clinic for treatment of moderately severe depression. He had lost interest in most everything, was sleeping poorly and losing weight, and said he was a failure and that his future was hopeless. He attributed his failing grades in community college to his poor sleep and depression. His father was a mason; his mother was a teacher. There was no family history of depression, and he did not have problems with drugs, alcohol, or medical conditions. He easily qualified for a diagnosis of major depression. We started him on an antidepressant and cognitive behavioral therapy.

A month later the psychiatry resident treating him said there was no improvement and asked me to see him again. He said that he was about to be expelled from school but his girlfriend would leave him if that happened. I asked about his girlfriend. He said that she was beautiful and brilliant and he would do anything to stay with her. She was still in high school but would graduate soon. I asked about her future plans. "She's going to go to this college out east, Vassar, maybe you have heard of it." "Um, yes, I've heard of it."

What a dilemma! He hated school but had to continue to keep his girlfriend. But he must have known, on some level, that the relationship was unlikely to continue after she left the state for an extremely high-status college. I asked, "What do you think will happen when she moves out east?" He said he had thought about that, and, though it might be difficult, he loved her and was committed to making the relationship work. I said that sometimes it was hard to have a relationship with someone who was far away. He became pensive and said he did not always feel like he fit in with her crowd, but they loved each other. Toward the end of the interview, I asked if he had previously dated other women or if he was thinking of dating other women. He said definitely not.

A few months later the resident asked me to see him again. He was transformed. From a somber, slouching, slow, and soft-speaking disheveled man looking at the floor, he now was enthusiastic and well groomed. He looked me in the eye and said he thought he didn't need more treatment. We reviewed his symptoms; they were mostly gone. When asked what had happened to make the transformation, he said, "Maybe the drugs worked or something." However, he had stopped his medications weeks previously. I then asked, "How is school?" "No problem now. I decided to go to work with my dad instead." "How are things with your girlfriend?" "Great," he said. "We have lots of fun, it's really good." It was now summer, so I asked, "Is she still headed off to Vassar in September?" He replied, "Oh, you mean *that* girlfriend! She was too uppity. My new girlfriend likes to do all the same kind of things I do. She's great."

The Missing Question

Mood disorders pose perhaps the most urgent and frustrating medical problem facing our species. Depression causes more years lived with disability than any other disease.[2] Suicide is a leading cause of death, increasing by 24 percent from 1999 through 2014 in the United States.[3] Prevention and treatment of heart disease and cancer are increasingly effective, but the rates of depression and suicide have stayed the same or increased, despite decades of intensive research and treatment efforts. Most of the efforts attack depression head-on. They define it, diagnose it, and try to find causes and cures. But the process of revising the *DSM* diagnosis of depression revealed deep disagreements about a fundamental question: How can pathological depression be distinguished from ordinary low mood?

Jerry Wakefield and his colleagues raised the question with their suggestion that the diagnosis of depression should be excluded not only in the two months after loss of a loved one, as specified in *DSM-IV*, but also after other equally devastating losses. As noted in chapter 3, the authors of *DSM-5* not only failed to adopt the suggestion, they eliminated the exclusion for bereavement.[4] So now someone who has five or more depression symptoms for more than two weeks can be diagnosed with major depression even if he or she is in a medical intensive care unit after an auto accident that killed a son or daughter. To most people, that seems ridiculous. Newspapers published impassioned editorials. The blogosphere exploded with opinions. Scientists addressed the problem by studying the differences and similarities among depression, grief, and responses to other losses. However, those studies did little to resolve the debate. Some emphasized the risks of failing to recognize and treat serious depression in the bereaved. Others saw the risk of medicalizing and overtreating ordinary grief. Between these positions is a major gap in our knowledge.

Everyone agrees that some symptoms of depression are normal for a time after a loss. Everyone also agrees that extreme symptoms of depression are obviously abnormal. But disagreement about how to distinguish normal low mood from abnormal depression is intense and enduring. When so many smart people disagree, something is usually missing. What is missing from debates about depression is knowledge about the origins, functions, and regulation of normal low mood.

Trying to understand pathological depression without recognizing the evolutionary origins and utility of normal low mood is like trying to understand chronic pain without recognizing the causes and utility of normal pain. Pain is useful. Physical pain protects against tissue damage. It gets organisms to escape from situations that are damaging tissues and avoid them in the future. Mental pain stops behaviors that are causing social damage or wasting energy. Mental and physical pain can be equally excruciating, even in situations where they are useful. But both are also prone to excess expression when they are not useful, causing chronic pain and pathological depression.

The challenge of deciding if depression symptoms are normal or abnormal is mirrored by the challenge of deciding if physical pain is a product of tissue pathology or an abnormality in the pain system. Pain from a broken leg or a tumor pressing on the spinal cord is obviously normal. However, when no specific cause can be found, doctors consider the possibility that the pain system is abnormal. As a consultation psychiatrist, I was asked to address the question for many medical and surgical patients.

For physical pain, such decisions can be difficult, but finding a tumor or a source of inflammation settles the issue. For mental pain, the challenge is vastly harder because the cause is in the motivational structure of a person's inner life. Specific life events, such as loss of a loved one, are the closest we can get to a specific cause of pain of the sort that surgeons can find. But ongoing life situations also cause low mood and depression.

When is low mood normal, and when is it abnormal? No amount of knowledge about mood mechanisms can answer the question. An answer requires understanding the origins and adaptive significance of mood. It requires knowing how the capacity for normal mood variation gives selective advantages, the situations in which high and low mood can be useful, and how mood is regulated. It requires recognizing that many mood changes are normal but not useful. This knowledge is the essential but mostly missing foundation for understanding mood disorders and for discovering why mood regulation mechanisms are so vulnerable to failure.

A Few Definitions

Much confusion arises because words describing mood states are used in different ways. *Mood* usually refers to a long-term pervasive state, akin to climate, while *affect* is the expression of a current emotional state, more like the weather. However, there is no sharp boundary among mood, affect, and emotion, and the terms *mood disorders* and *affective disorders* are used interchangeably. I will use the word *mood* here to refer to the dimension that ranges from depression to low mood to high mood to mania. The word *depression* is now so closely associated with pathology that I will use *low mood* to describe symptoms of mild depression, without any implication of pathology or normality.

High mood is a pleasurable state of enthusiasm, energy, and optimistic activity usually associated with situations where activity is likely to pay off grandly. It is closely related to joy, the short-term pleasure from getting what has been desired, and happiness, the enduring state that can persist if most desires can be satisfied. Low mood is the painful state characterized by demoralization, low energy, pessimism, risk avoidance, and social withdrawal that is aroused by certain situations, especially those in which efforts to reach a goal are failing. Sadness can feel very similar to low mood, but it results from specific losses; it often does not include the pervasive lack of motivation that can characterize low mood and depression. Grief is the special kind of sadness caused by death of a loved one or other major loss. Tomes have been written to distinguish these and other mood states, but because emotions are products of evolution, not design, they overlap in untidy ways that defy exact description.

LOW MOOD	HIGH MOOD
Pessimism	Optimism
Risk avoidance	Risk taking
Inhibition	Initiative
Low energy	High energy
Social withdrawal	Social engagement
Quiet	Talkative
Slow thinking	Fast thinking
Unimaginative	Creative
Submissive	Dominant
Lack of confidence	Confidence
Low self-esteem	High self-esteem
Analytic thinking	Subjective thinking
Expecting criticism	Expecting praise

How Can Low Mood Be Useful?

Much confusion about depression results from the human tendency to think that specific things must have specific functions. Things we make, such as spears and baskets, have specific functions. So do parts of the body such as the eye and the thumb. It therefore seems natural to ask "What is the function of low mood?" For emotions, however, that is the wrong question. A better question is "In what *situations* do low mood and high mood give selective advantages?" However, most ideas about the utility of mood have been framed as possible functions, so we must start there.

One possibility is that even ordinary mood variations are not useful. They could arise from glitches, having as little utility as epileptic seizures or tremors. There are good reasons for thinking that this is incorrect. Syndromes that arise from defects in the body, such as epilepsy or tremor, happen to only some people, but nearly everyone has the capacity for mood. We all have a system that adjusts mood up or down depending on what is happening. Such regulation systems can be shaped only for useful responses. Pain, fever, vomiting, anxiety, and low mood turn on when they are needed. This does not mean that every instance is useful; false alarms can be normal. But it does mean that such systems need to be understood in terms of how and when they are useful.

The London psychoanalyst John Bowlby was one of the first to propose evolutionary functions for low mood. Thanks to conversations with the German ethologist Konrad Lorenz and the English biologist Robert Hinde, he turned an evolutionary eye toward the behaviors of babies separated from their mothers.[5] After a short separation, some reconnected with the mother quickly, others acted distant, and a few acted angry. A longer separation led to a reliable sequence: initial wails of protest, followed by silent rocking and huddling in a ball that looks for all the world like an adult in a state of despair.[6,7]

Bowlby saw that crying motivated mothers to retrieve their infants. He also saw that extended crying would waste energy and attract predators, so if the mother did not return soon, inconspicuous withdrawal would be more useful. These ideas developed into attachment theory,[8] which provides the foundation for understanding mother-infant bonding and the pathologies that result when it goes awry. Bowlby deserves recognition as a founder of evolutionary psychiatry for his insight that attachment evolved because it increases the fitness of both mother and baby.

More explicitly evolutionary analyses in recent decades have challenged the idea that only secure attachment is normal. In some situations, babies who use avoidant or anxious attachment styles may motivate their mothers to provide more care.[9,10,11] If regular smiling and cooing don't work, it may work better to scream indefinitely when she leaves or to give her the cold shoulder when she returns.

George Engel, the psychiatrist at the University of Rochester who coined the term *biopsychosocial model*, proposed a function for depression that is related to attachment. He suggested that a lost young monkey could conserve calories and avoid attracting predators by staying quiet in one place. He called this "conservation-withdrawal," noted its resemblance to depression, and emphasized the similarity of depression to hibernation.[12,13]

Aubrey Lewis, a founder of the Institute of Psychiatry in London, believed that depression could signal the need for help.[14] The idea was advanced further by David Hamburg, the former chair of psychiatry at Stanford University.[15] Some evolutionary psychologists give the idea a cynical twist by suggesting that depression symptoms, and especially suicide threats, are strategies to manipulate others into providing help. Edward Hagen has suggested that postpartum depression is a specific adaptation shaped to blackmail relatives into providing help.[16,17] He views the symptoms as a passive threat to abandon the infant and finds support for this view in evidence that postpartum depression is more likely when the husband is unsupportive, resources are scarce, or the baby needs extra care. Depression and suicide threats certainly can be manipulations. However, there is little evidence that depression is a reliable response in most mothers in such situations, and it is not at all clear that those who express more depression get more help from otherwise unhelpful relatives. Also, the theory does not fit well with prior research by psychologist James Coyne showing that depression elicits caring, helpful responses only briefly from relatives; after that they tend to withdraw.[18]

The Canadian psychologist Denys deCatanzaro suggested the even more disturbing idea that suicide can benefit an individual's genes.[19] If an individual in a harsh environment has little chance of future reproduction, suicide could free up food and resources that relatives could use to have children who would carry some of the individual's genes into future generations. This would be the ultimate example of selection shaping a trait to benefit genes at the expense of the individual. But the idea, while creative, is almost certainly wrong. Even in harsh environments, suicide is by no means routine. Even sick elderly people who can't reproduce are often desperate to live longer. Also, why bother killing yourself? Why not just wander off or stop eating?

British psychiatrist John Price recognized an important function of depression symptoms based on his close observations of chickens.[20] Chickens that lose a fight and descend in the pecking order withdraw from social engagement and act submissive, thereby reducing further attacks by chickens higher in the hierarchy. Price went on to study the same phenomenon in vervet monkeys.[21] They live in small groups containing a few males and a few females. The alpha male, who gets essentially all the matings, has bright blue testicles. Until, that is, he loses a fight with another male. Then he huddles into a ball, rocks, withdraws, and acts depressed as his testicles turn a dusky gray. Price interprets these changes as signals of "involuntary yielding."[22,23] By signaling that he is not a threat, the loser escapes attacks by the new dominant male. Better to yield, and signal yielding, than to be attacked.

Price worked with psychiatrists Leon Sloman and Russell Gardner to apply these ideas in the clinic.[24] They observed that many depressive episodes are precipitated by failure to accept a loss in a status competition. They view low mood as a normal response to losing a competition and depression as the result of continuing useless status striving, a situation aptly described as "failure to yield." Other researchers, especially the British psychologist Paul Gilbert and his colleagues, have developed these ideas further.[25] They interpret diverse stressful life events as a loss of status, and they observe that many patients recover when they give up an unwinnable status competition.

The anthropologist John Hartung independently proposed an interesting variation, with the intriguing designation of "deceiving down." He notes that being subordinate to someone with lesser abilities is a perilous situation. The natural inclination to show one's stuff will be perceived as a threat, likely resulting in an attack or even expulsion from the group.

The solution? Deceive down; that is, deceptively conceal your abilities.[26] The best way to do that is to convince yourself that you are less worthy and able than you are, a pattern similar to the neurotic inhibition and self-sabotaging that Freud attributed to castration anxiety.

Further support for the connection between status losses and depression comes from the extraordinary data gathered by the British epidemiologists George Brown and Tirril Harris.[27] In their detailed studies of women in north London, they found that 80 percent of the women who developed depression had experienced a recent life event that met their careful definition of "severe." Of all women who had experienced severe life events, only 22 percent developed depression; however this rate is twenty-two times higher than the 1 percent of women who do not experience such an event. Of the women who had experienced a severe life event, 78 percent did not develop depression during the next year, leading to new studies of "resilience."[28] This careful research provides superb evidence for the role of life events causing depression. Scores of newer studies confirm and extend the role of life events in causing depression.[29,30,31,32,33,34,35,36,37]

Some events are much more likely to precipitate depression than others. In the Brown and Harris study, an episode of depression occurred after 75 percent of events characterized by "humiliation or entrapment" but only 20 percent of loss events and 5 percent of danger events.[38] These data support Price's theory nicely, especially if humiliation or entrapment is assumed to involve status conflicts. Describing specific life situations vastly increases predictive power compared to generic measures of life events or "stress."

The involuntary yielding hypothesis seems correct for many cases of depression I have treated. Myriads of spouses limit their achievements, and even their view of their own abilities, to preserve their marriages. The deceiving-down social strategy prevents attacks by those with more power, at the price of depressive symptoms. An ambitious young lawyer I treated did not use deceiving down; he gave a brilliant presentation that upstaged an ineffective senior partner—who subsequently proved to be very effective at derogating the work of the young upstart, who was soon depressed.

The function of signaling yielding to prevent attack can be reframed in terms of the situation in which it is useful: loss of a status competition. This allows consideration of other ways in which low mood might be useful in that situation: reassessing social strategies, considering possible alternative groups, investing more in selected potential allies, or withdrawing socially until a better time.

Even when reframed as a response to a situation, however, the theory remains specific to one domain—social resources—and one aspect of that domain—social position in a hierarchy. Fighting an unwinnable status contest is one subtype of the more general situation of failing to make progress in the pursuit of any goal. After a status loss, signaling submission stops attacks by those with more power. What about failing in other efforts? Is preventing attacks after a status loss the main function of depression symptoms?

My experience with patients suggests not. Even within the domain of social status, depression symptoms do things other than signaling submission, such as motivating consideration of alternative strategies and new alliances. Also, while about half of my patients with depression seem to be trapped pursuing unreachable goals, many of those goals are not about social position. Is unrequited love a pursuit of a status goal? What about trying to find effective treatment for a child with cancer?

Debate won't answer such questions; we need data about what events and situations give rise to which symptoms of depression. Billions of dollars have been spent in the search for brain abnormalities in people with depression and millions investigating the role of "stress." It is a great scientific embarrassment and tragedy that funding agencies have not allocated the resources needed to discover exactly what kinds of life events and situations cause exactly which depression symptoms.[39,40,41]

Increased thinking about one's problems is characteristic of low mood. The thinking is often actually rumination. The problem goes around and around in the mind without ever reaching a solution, like a wad of grass that a cow chews, swallows, regurgitates, and chews again. One of my former colleagues, the psychologist Susan Nolen-Hoeksema, viewed rumination as a maladaptive cognitive pattern that is central to depression and best stopped if at all possible.[42] In an astounding but tragic bit of luck, she gathered data on depression and tendencies to ruminate just before the 1989 Loma Prieta earthquake in California. Interviewing the same subjects again after the earthquake revealed that those who had a tendency to ruminate were more likely to have become depressed, even when other predictors of vulnerability to depression were controlled.[43]

In a widely discussed 2009 article in *Psychological Review*, biologist Paul Andrews and psychiatrist J. Anderson Thomson, Jr., proposed nearly the opposite view.[44] They argued that rumination helps to solve major life problems. In their view, depression withdraws interest from action and outer life to free up time and mental energy for ruminating to solve the problem. This article extended a related proposal Andrews and biologist Paul Watson had made in a 2002 article, that depression evolved to serve the function of "social navigation."[45] In a firm critique of these ideas, the Newcastle University evolutionary psychologist Daniel Nettle pointed out that there is little evidence that rumination solves social problems, or that depression speeds finding solutions.[46] The Norwegian evolutionary clinical psychologist Leif Kennair concurs, and I agree with their critique.[47]

Nonetheless, social withdrawal and thinking a lot can be useful when one encounters a dead end in life. I greatly admire a 1989 book by the Swedish psychoanalyst Emmy Gut entitled *Productive and Unproductive Depression: Its Functions and Failures*.[48] Using vivid case studies based on historical figures, she argued that depressive withdrawal and intense cogitation can improve coping when major life problems require a major change but can also leave some people stuck in unproductive depression. Major life failures may motivate allocating enormous effort into finding new strategies. However, as Gut, Nettle, Nolen-Hoeksema, and others note, rumination and withdrawal are not reliably optimal responses to such situations.

The functions summarized in the previous paragraphs are some of the most compelling that have been proposed to explain low mood and depression. Framing these functions as alternatives has motivated much useless debate; all may be relevant. However, their significance and relationships to one another become clearer when the frame shifts from their functions to the situations in which they can be useful.

Mood Adjusts to Cope with Changing Propitiousness

Most behavior is in pursuit of a goal. Some efforts are attempts to get something, others to escape or prevent something. Either way, an individual is usually trying to make progress toward some goal. High and low moods are aroused by situations that arise during goal pursuit. What situations?

A generic but useful answer is: *high and low moods were shaped to cope with propitious and unpropitious situations.*[49] A propitious situation is a favorable one in which a small investment gives a reliably big payoff. If a herd of mastodons is coming down the valley, exuberant pursuit will likely be worth the effort and risks. If your job is selling new cars, extra effort in a boom year will pay off. In an unpropitious situation, efforts are likely to be wasted. If no mastodons have been sighted for months, expeditions to look for them will likely waste time and energy. Trying to sell cars during an economic downturn is not as fruitless, but it is no fun.

Individuals whose mood rises in propitious situations can take full advantage of opportunities. Individuals whose mood goes down in unpropitious situations can avoid risks and wasted effort and can shift to different strategies or different goals. The capacity to vary mood with changes in propitiousness gives a selective advantage.

The story gets more interesting fast. When times are good and likely to stay that way, there is no need for exuberant effort now. If mastodons come by every day, seeing a herd is no reason to get excited. If your crop can be harvested anytime, relax. But if mastodon sightings are rare, intense effort now will be worth it. It seems paradoxical, but intense high mood is valuable mainly for short-lived opportunities. Low mood is more useful for temporary unpropitious situations than indefinite bad times. People who experience sudden big losses improve with time, but the distortions of depression often make that impossible to see.

Life's Three Decisions

Making three decisions well is all it takes to maximize fitness. The challenge of picking wild raspberries illustrates how mood helps to make these decisions well. First, how much energy should go into your efforts at the current bush? Should you pick berries as fast as you can or at a leisurely pace? Second, when should you quit? Is it better to keep picking berries from this bush or to stop and look for another one? Finally, when it is time to do something else, what should you do next? Gather another kind of food, do something else, or go home?

Our lives are sequences of such decisions on varying time scales. Should

I keep editing this paragraph or move on to the next one? Should I keep writing or take a break for lunch? Should I keep trying to write this book or give up and take up golf? My writing is slowing and my enthusiasm is waning, so now is a good time for lunch.

There, that's better. A brief break refocuses attention to a slight variation on the central question: Why are people who lack the capacity for mood at a disadvantage? Mood variation does not have to exist. We could go about our days in a steady state, neither enthused by unexpectedly finding a tree laden with ripe fruit nor discouraged by walking for hours to find a tree empty. We would experience neither the excitement at smiling, steady eye contact from the most attractive person in the room nor the deflation upon realizing that the invitation was intended for someone else. Without a capacity for mood, neither winning the lottery nor going bankrupt would influence levels of energy, enthusiasm, risk taking, initiative, or optimism. How best to pick berries offers a model for much else in life, even intensely personal decisions such as deciding whether to continue in a job or a marriage.[50]

Berry Picking and Mood

If you have ever spent an afternoon picking wild raspberries, you have experienced the emotional changes that guide foraging. Finding a bush laden with ripe fruit arouses a tiny thrill. With joyful enthusiasm, you pull off berries in handfuls, some of which are so delectable they never make it to the bucket. As the bush gets depleted, the berries come more slowly, then slower yet. Enthusiasm wanes. Finally, you are reaching through prickles to try to get that one last deformed berry. Your motivation for picking from this bush is gone, and a good thing, too. It is senseless to try to get every berry from every bush. However, jumping too quickly from bush to bush is also unwise. How long should you stay at each bush to get the most berries per hour? The problem may seem abstract, but making such decisions well is crucial to the fitness of nearly every animal.[51]

The mathematical behavioral ecologist Eric Charnov came up with an elegant solution, one that illuminates much about mood in everyday life.[52] To keep things simple, assume that it always takes the same amount of time to find a new bush (Search Time on the graph). When you find a bush, berries come fast at first, then slower and slower yet; that is why the curved line is steep at first, then slowly levels off. You can stop picking at any time along that curve. The longer you stay, the more berries you get from that bush, but to get the most berries per hour, you need to stop and go looking for the next bush at just the right time.

The best time to stop is at the point that gets you the most berries per hour. The number of berries is the height (the dotted vertical lines), and the time is the width (Search Time plus Picking Time), so you will get the most berries per hour if you stop at the point where the line with the steepest slope (the solid one) just touches the top of the curve. If you leave sooner (the lower dashed line), or stay longer (the higher dashed line), you will get fewer berries in an hour.

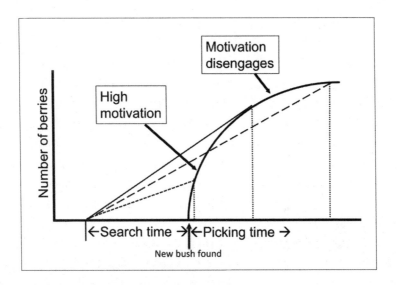

The Marginal Value Theorem

Charnov called this the Marginal Value Theorem, because all the action is at that spot "on the margin" where the rate of getting berries at the current bush dips below the number of berries you can get per hour by moving to a new bush. The core idea is simple but profound. You don't have to do calculus to get the right answer, you just need to follow your emotions. To maximize the number of berries you get in a day, go looking for a new bush whenever you lose interest in the current bush. Thanks to your emotions having been programmed by natural selection, that will generally be the point at which the rate of berries coming from the current bush slows to the average number per minute across many bushes. This decision-making mechanism is built into the brains of nearly every organism. Ladybird beetles, honeybees, lizards, chipmunks, chimpanzees, and humans all make such foraging decisions well. No calculation is needed; motivation flags at the optimal time to make a switch.

The decision about when it is best to quit one kind of activity and do something different follows the same principle. If bushes and berries are so sparse that you are spending more calories each hour wandering about than you are getting from picking berries, the best thing to do is to quit. Even if berries are plentiful, there comes a time when quitting is best, because if you already have a thousand, picking more means lugging a heavy bucket and spending whole days in the kitchen making more jam than you can eat in a year. Well before that point, motivation turns negative and sensible people head home.

The Marginal Value Theorem sets the rhythm of our days. We start an activity with gusto, stay with it awhile, then lose interest and move on to something else. How long we stay depends on the start-up cost, which is equivalent to the cost of finding a new berry bush, how the payoffs decline with time, and the payoffs of available alternatives. To read a book, for instance, you need to find the book, settle into a chair, turn on a light, and start reading. If you jump up to do something else after just a few minutes, you will never read much.

People with attention-deficit/hyperactivity disorder (ADHD) know this all too well. Their motivation for the current task fades fast, and new opportunities glow brightly, like neon invitations. They shift quickly from one activity to another, rarely getting much accomplished. It would be interesting to study how people with ADHD forage for berries. I bet they quit each bush too quickly. However, staying too long is also unwise. People who persist excessively also deserve a diagnosis: attention surplus disorder.[53] Interestingly, drugs used to treat ADHD increase dopamine, the same substance released in the brain in response to rewards. Increasing dopamine may make the brain respond as if more berries are coming per minute from the current bush, encouraging persisting at the current task.

When to Quit All Activity

When to quit all activity and go home—or never to go out in the first place—is a related decision that brings us closer to low mood and depression. The general answer is simple: when you are spending more calories each minute than you can get from any possible activity, it is best to go home and wait for a better time.

Bumblebees gather pollen and nectar every minute on warm summer days. As evening comes, cooler air makes flying more costly, and flowers close and become harder to find. At some point in the gathering dusk, it is best to go home. Bumblebees make this decision superbly.[54] Their ancestors who quit too soon or persisted too long got fewer calories per day and so had fewer baby bumblebees. For a rabbit, the principle is the same, although the cost of staying out too long is more dramatic: becoming dinner for a fox. For all species, when the expected costs are greater than benefits for any possible activity, the best thing to do is . . . nothing. Don't just do something, stand there! Find someplace safe and wait for a better time. This analysis gets us closer to low mood and depression.

Some animals go into a dramatic conservation state nightly. The stripe-faced dunnart is a mouselike Australian marsupial that lives in desolate deserts where food is scarce and temperatures fluctuate widely. It can't get enough calories in a day to keep its body warm through cold winter nights. So its metabolism slows after dark, dropping its body temperature 20 degrees in a bout of minihibernation.[55] Sometimes the best strategy is doing even less than nothing.

Other animals must make life-and-death decisions in which taking big risks is best. In a classic experiment, the behavioral ecologist Thomas Caraco and his colleagues let juncos learn that they could find seeds at two bird feeders. Both gave the same average number of seeds per visit, but one gave a tiny consistent payout every time, while the other gave a payout that varied widely. In ordinary temperatures, the birds preferred the sure-thing low-payout feeder. But when the temperature decreased below the point that made survival through the night unlikely on the calories provided by the consistent but low-payoff feeder, they switched. Instead of freezing to death for certain, they took a risky bet that offered some chance of survival, like otherwise doomed prison camp inmates who run for the fences despite guards with guns.[56]

Harsh times require difficult high-risk decisions. My grandmother was born in February 1884 on a small island off the coast of Norway. On the day of her christening, her father sighted a swirl of fish offshore. A heaven-sent gift for extra mouths to feed in a lean winter? He and his partner rowed out despite the waves. They hoisted their nets again and again, until the boat was full. Should they persist or go home? The fish were still there, and they might not come back, so the men also filled a spare dinghy, connected to their boat by a chain. The wind rose, the dinghy flipped, the chain could not be cut, and both boats went down. My great-grandmother was helpless onshore, holding her newborn daughter as her husband drowned. Optimism and boldness are often worthwhile, but occasionally they are fatal. The perils of risk-taking in a harsh environment may help to explain why my great-grandfather's surviving descendants have tendencies to anxiety and pessimism.

Making decisions about foraging or fishing remains central to the lives of many people, but most of us now pursue long-term social goals in complex webs of relationships that confront us with difficult decisions about whether to continue big efforts that may be futile. Some competitions offer huge payoffs for a few winners and years of useless efforts for everyone else. Making it as a professional football player is fabulous, but 999 out of 1,000 who try will fail. The rewards for even successful novelists pale by comparison, but even more people try writing fiction. Career pursuits offer easy examples, but mood also guides more personal goals: trying to lose weight, find a job, get along with a cranky boss or spouse, or cope with everyday life despite crippling arthritis. Progress speeds and slows, and mood rises and falls, as we pursue the projects that make up our lives.

This brings us back to the crucial question posed by the Marginal Value Theorem: When is it best to give up on a major life goal? Early in my career, I always encouraged patients to keep trying, keep trying, don't let your depression symptoms fool you into thinking you can't succeed. Often that was good advice. Some applicants get into medical school the fourth time they apply. Some singers land a gig with the Grand Ole Opry after their fifth year in Nashville. But more become increasingly despondent as failure follows failure. Sometimes a five-year engagement turns into marriage. Sometimes staying another year in LA trying to break into film pays off. But not often.

Sober experience combined with my growing evolutionary perspective to encourage respecting the meaning of my patients' moods. As often as not, their symptoms seemed to arise from a deep recognition that some major life project was never going to work. She was glad he wanted to live with her, but it looks increasingly like he will never agree to get married. The boss is nice now and then and hints at promotions, but nothing will ever come of it. Hopes for cancer cures get aroused, but all treatments so far have failed. He has stayed off booze for two weeks, but a dozen previous vows to stay on the wagon have all ended in binges. Low mood is not always an emanation from a disordered brain; it can be a normal response to pursuing an unreachable goal.

Animal Models

The standard way to tell if a drug will be an effective antidepressant is to see if it makes an animal persist in useless efforts. The Porsolt test measures how long a rat or mouse swims when dropped in a beaker of water.[57] Rats on Prozac or another antidepressant swim longer. Because the test works to identify antidepressant drugs, it is the basis of more than four thousand scientific articles, with new ones being published at a rate of one per day. Persisting seems like a good thing, and many of those articles describe cessation of swimming as a sign of low mood or despair. But stopping swimming does not mean giving up and drowning, it just means switching to a different strategy: floating with the nose just out of the water. Rats switch to this strategy at about the right time. Those on drugs that make them swim longer are more likely to get exhausted and drown.[58]

Learned helplessness is another animal model that presumes persistence is good. The psychologist Martin Seligman put dogs in a box with two compartments separated by a partition. Dogs that received a shock learned quickly to jump to the other side to escape. But dogs previously exposed to shock they could not avoid did not jump over even when they could.

This "learned helplessness" is thought to be a good model of depression.[59] As is the case for swimming rats, however, the dogs may only look dumb. There are no electrical shocks in the wild, but there are other dogs ready to inflict pain again if necessary to maintain their dominant position.

Other Situations in Which Low Mood Is Useful

I emphasized the situation of pursuing an unreachable goal in my 2000 article "Is Depression an Adaptation?"[60] In retrospect, my view was too narrow. Low mood can give advantages in several other situations. Striving for social status often creates unreachable goals, but chronic low mood can also be useful for those stuck in a subordinate position. I saw scores of depressed women who had small children, no job, no relatives nearby, and an abusive husband. We tried hard to get them into a shelter, but few would go, and few returned for continuing treatment. If depression diagnoses were based on causes, "depression in someone who has no way to escape an abusive spouse" would be a common mental disorder.

While the focus has been on social situations, physical situations also influence mood. Three are especially salient: starvation, seasonal weather changes, and infection.

The Minnesota Starvation Experiment conducted on World War II conscientious objector volunteers provided dramatic evidence of emotional changes. All subjects were initially healthy and emotionally stable. They agreed to go on diets that reduced their body weight by 25 percent. By the time they got to that body weight, most were fatigued, depressed, and hopeless, spending most of their days thinking about food.[61,62] Such caloric deprivation occurred at times for our ancestors, and it continues in many parts of the world. In such situations, it is wise to avoid vigorous competitive activities.

Lack of sunlight makes many people feel down, and seasonal affective disorder is common. It's hard to say whether low mood in the gloom is an adaptation or a by-product of other mechanisms, but when activity is likely to be dangerous or unrewarding, low mood will be useful.[63,64,65]

Have you ever awakened with new symptoms of a cold and felt like there was not much point in doing anything? The syndrome was named *sickness behavior* by the ethologist Benjamin Hart in the 1980s.[66,67] He described its possible evolutionary benefits, including conserving energy to fight infection, and avoiding predators and conflicts when not in top form. Many studies document depression symptoms during infection.[68] Especially dramatic are severe cases of depression precipitated by treatment with interferon, a natural chemical that gears up the body's immune response. Nearly 30 percent of patients receiving interferon treatment for hepatitis C get serious depression symptoms, not just fatigue but also feelings of hopelessness and worthlessness.[69] This demonstrates that immune responses can cause clinical depression and suggests that some aspects of low mood may be useful when fighting infection.[70]

Fatigue and lack of initiative make sense during infection, but why have terrible feelings of guilt and inadequacy? These symptoms could be by-products of a crude system. A related possibility is that some systems that regulate goal pursuit evolved from preexisting systems for coping with infection. Or perhaps infections in ancestral environments caused only fatigue, and full-fledged depression occurs mainly in people with modern immune systems that are hyperactive because of excess nutrition or disrupted microbiomes.

The bottom line is that infection is yet another situation that arouses low mood. This does not mean that all depression is a product of immune systems. However, if natural selection co-opted aspects of the immune system to create the systems that regulate mood, that would help explain the strong association of depression with inflammatory diseases such as atherosclerosis.[71,72,73,74]

What Good Is High Mood?

High mood has been neglected. It seems so obviously wonderful and useful that its adaptive significance has only recently been studied. It fits nicely as the converse of low mood, a suite of responses useful in propitious situations, especially those likely to be temporary. People whose motivation and energy rev up in response to opportunity get a selective advantage compared to those who simply carry on at the same old rate. High mood includes not just increased energy but also flares of creativity, risk taking, and eagerness to take on new initiatives. As Shakespeare put it, "There is a tide in the affairs of men, which taken at the flood, leads on to fortune."[75]

Barbara Fredrickson, a former colleague at the University of Michigan, proposed that the benefits of high mood come from tendencies to "broaden and build." Her experiments, and those of others who followed her lead, demonstrate that high mood creates a more expansive view of the world and a greater likelihood of taking new initiatives.[76] These changes are just the ticket to taking advantages of opportunities. However, framing them as functions leads to neglect of other aspects of positive mood and other subtypes that are useful in different domains. For instance, people newly in love feel spectacularly happy. They're motivated to do anything and everything for the beloved, actions likely to pay off with a relationship and probably sex and offspring.[77] Similarly, in the world of status competition, being newly appointed to a high position is exhilarating, motivating new initiatives and alliances likely to have grand payoffs. It is good to take advantage of such opportunities early, before competition from others grows.

A Model

Physiologists investigate what organs are for by cutting them out and watching what goes wrong. Take out the thyroid gland, and the resulting hypothyroidism reveals what thyroid hormone is good for. But there is no way to excise mood. Research on people who do not experience much emotion (alexithymia) is relevant, but it is unclear if people with alexithymia really lack emotional responses or if they suppress awareness of emotions.[78]

I created a simple computer model to see if a tendency to variable mood would be a better strategy than just carrying on without mood variations. It opened my eyes to things I had not imagined. The model is a game in which three different strategies compete by making different amounts of investment on each of 100 moves. Each starts with 100 resource units.

The "Moodless" strategy invests 10 units each time. The "Moderate" strategy invests 10 percent of its resources on each turn. The "Moody" strategy invests 15 percent of its resources if the previous move gave a payoff and 5 percent if it gave a loss. The payoff for each move is based on a combination of a random number and the payoff on the previous move, so there is some predictability. The average payoff is 1 percent, but on any move the entire investment could be lost or as much as doubled.

It is great fun watching the game run. One click sets off 100 moves, and four lines crawl across the computer screen, one for each of the three strategies and one to indicate the payoffs at each move. Every run of the game turns out different thanks to tiny variations in the random factors.

What strategy wins? It depends on the environment. Usually all three strategies come out about the same. When payoffs are moderately predictable, Moody tends to win because it takes advantage of good times

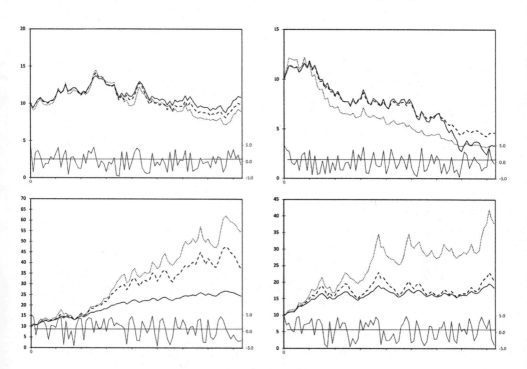

Four Runs of the Mood Model

Four runs of the mood model illustrate how chance variations in payoffs result in vastly different outcomes for the three strategies: Moody (dotted), Moderate (dashed), and Moodless (solid). The thin line at the bottom indicates how payoffs vary at each different move in the game.

and avoids risk in bad times. As payoffs become less predictable, however, the Moody strategy does worse and worse because it often risks a lot and loses a lot.

Other outcomes were unexpected, just what you hope for from a computer model. The illustration shows the results of running the game four times with identical formulas and starting values. Like the famous hypothetical example of a butterfly flapping its wings in Brazil setting off a hurricane in Florida,[79] slight variations in the random numbers result in wildly different outcomes. Usually all three strategies give similar results. Sometimes no strategy does very well. When there is a big winner or loser, however, it is usually Moody.

The results from this simple model may help to explain why mood regulation mechanisms vary so much from individual to individual. Minor environmental perturbations can result in drastically different payoffs for different mood regulation mechanisms, even when everything else stays the same. No one system reliably wins; much depends on chance.

When he was a graduate student in my laboratory, Eric Jackson took this much further. He programmed a computer to do 10,000 runs of the game to find out how much mood variability is best. His main conclusion is simple: when rewards vary widely and are somewhat predictable, the optimal strategy is to vary your investments substantially depending on recent payoffs—that is, use the Moody strategy. When rewards are unpredictable, however, more stable strategies win and the Moody strategy goes extinct quickly.

Psychologists Knew It All Along

The idea that mood tracks propitiousness was inspired by my studies of animal foraging, but it is not new. Psychologist friends pointed me to many articles that described the phenomenon in detail. Eric Klinger, a University of Minnesota psychologist, laid out the central ideas especially clearly in 1975.[80] When people are making progress toward their main life goals, they feel fine. Obstacles provoke frustration, often observed as anger and aggression. Inability to make progress toward a goal causes demoralization and temporary withdrawal. Prolonged failure of a strategy leads to more severe demoralization and attempts to find alternatives. When extended efforts fail to find a new route to the goal, intense low mood disengages motivation from the goal. When the unreachable goal is truly given up, low mood is replaced by temporary sadness aroused by the loss, and the person moves on to pursue other more reachable goals. Sometimes, however, the goal is something the person cannot give up, such as finding a job or a partner or a cure for a fatal condition. In such a situation, people can get trapped pursuing an unreachable goal, and ordinary low mood escalates into severe depression. Every clinician should read Klinger's work.

Others have extended these ideas and studied related phenomena. The German psychologist Jutta Heckhausen, now in California, studied a group of childless middle-aged women who were still hoping to have a baby. As they approached menopause, their emotional distress became more and more intense. But after menopause those who gave up their hope for pregnancy lost their depression symptoms.[81] The irony is deep: hope is often at the root of depression.

The Canadian psychologist Carsten Wrosch followed up with related studies on parents trying to get help for their children with cancer. The parents who were most set on their goals were more prone to depression.[82] Those with a greater ability to shift or give up their goals tended to experience less depression.[83]

American psychologists Charles Carver and Michael Scheier conducted a series of studies about how the exigencies of goal pursuit influence mood.[84] They found that mood is influenced most not by success or failure but by rate of progress toward a goal.[85] Faster-than-expected progress bumps mood up, slower-than-expected progress pushes mood down. This is not as obvious as it might seem. Many people think that mood reflects what a person has. This is an illusion, as illustrated by the many rich, healthy, admired people who are nonetheless despondent. People strive to get things, expecting happiness, but it doesn't work for long. Mood is only modestly influenced by what a person has and only briefly influenced by success or failure. Baseline mood is remarkably stable for most people, and variations reflect mainly the rate of progress toward a goal.[86,87]

Bad Situations, Low Motivation, and Feeling Bad

When progress toward a major life goal is slowing or stopped, low mood symptoms disengage motivation and induce waiting and considering alternative strategies; then, if no alternative seems viable, giving up on a goal. But is low motivation really the best response in such situations? It avoids wasting energy on fruitless efforts, but if a life strategy is failing, why mope alone in your room? Risk taking and enthusiasm would seem more likely to lead to a successful new strategy. Why don't life's reverses shift cognition to an optimistic view of self, the world, and the future to energize a shift to a more useful project?

Sometimes they do. Some people come home after losing a job and quickly realize they have been freed from what would have been decades of drudgery. After a divorce, initial despair is often followed by realizing that better relationships are possible. Even giving up on a failing scientific research project can be exhilarating if it opens new opportunities to conduct more interesting studies. Lines from Tony Hoagland's poem "Disappointment" capture the moment when "he didn't get the job,— / or her father died before she told him / that one, most important thing— / and everything got still. . . . You don't have to pursue anything ever again / It's over / You're free."[88]

Many benefits of an optimistic view of life are obvious, such as avoiding depression and its associated health risks.[89] Compared to pessimists, optimists are half as likely to die of a heart attack.[90] Their rose-colored glasses make optimists persist happily without the hesitations that plague others. This can, however, lead to the "Concorde Effect," the mistake of continuing to sink effort into a hopeless cause. If you walked for hours to get to a hunting place and no game animals show up in the first hour, it is probably worth staying longer but not for days. Making good decisions about when to move on is crucial. Persistence and optimism pay off for most life projects. The costs of finding a new job or partner are huge. Usually it is better just to carry on despite problems, oblivious to possible alternatives, with hopes that things will eventually get better. They usually do.

At some point, however, carrying on is a mistake. If an effort is never likely to succeed, cold-eyed objective assessment becomes necessary. Dozens of studies show that low mood makes people more realistic, a phenomenon called *depressive realism*.[91] People generally are unjustifiably optimistic.[92] When asked to press a button to control a light that flashes at random times, most subjects think their presses control the flashes. Depressed subjects, by contrast, soon recognize their helplessness. Depressive realism has been documented in many cultures.[93] Using sad stories or films to induce low mood shifts people's assessments of themselves and the future toward greater accuracy,[94,95,96] although the effect may be smaller than once thought.[97]

When a major life goal is slipping away despite major efforts, low mood dispels optimistic illusions and promotes objective consideration of alternatives. The shift is often painful. I have talked with many patients who thought that their marriages could recover, until a moment when suddenly all hope fell away, as if their rose-colored lenses had suddenly gone dark. However, the lenses of depression are not just gray; they distort reality so people can't see opportunities that others find obvious. Some unemployed people believe that they will never get another job. Some recently divorced people believe that they are inherently unlovable. Frustrated researchers may believe that their careers are over. What gives?

Pessimism prevents hasty moves. If bad stretches in marriages, jobs, or even writing projects quickly aroused optimism about alternatives, we would move on quickly, oblivious to the costs of starting fresh. Negative views of the self and the future delay big changes, giving time for the original enterprise to bounce back. Sometimes it is best to pull up anchor and move to a different fishing spot, but extra consideration and hesitation are worthwhile if waves or weather make moving risky. The costs and risks of moving to a new city, job, or marriage are larger. I suspect that persistence in failing big life enterprises and accompanying low mood are proportional to the costs and risks of finding something better. But so far as I know, the idea has not been tested.

Finally, as we prepare to shift focus from ordinary low mood to mood disorders, it is worth asking why low mood feels so awful. Why doesn't the system respond to failing efforts by assessing the alternatives objectively and shifting to the next best one at the right time, without self-doubt, rumination, and psychic pain? Multiple explanations contribute, but I think the main one is the same as the explanation for why physical pain hurts. The suffering that accompanies nausea, vomiting, diarrhea, cough, fever, fatigue, pain, anxiety, and low mood motivates escape from a current bad situation and avoidance of future similar situations. Individuals who do not experience physical pain accumulate injuries and usually die by early adulthood. People who don't feel bad when pursuing unreachable goals spend their lives in contented useless efforts. More low mood might help their genes, but a clinic to boost low mood would be about as popular as a clinic to help people feel more anxious.

Solved?

While attributing specific functions to specific mood states is a mistake, the capacity for mood can be said to have a general function: mood reallocates investments of time, effort, resources, and risk taking to maximize Darwinian fitness in situations of varying propitiousness. High and low moods adjust cognition and behavior to cope with propitious and unpropitious situations.

This global summary makes a large tacit assumption: that mood is one thing. It certainly seems like one thing. We have a word for it, and most people readily recognize descriptions of low and high mood. But do the various parts of low and high mood always come together in consistent packages? Do enthusiasm, risk taking, fast thinking, and optimism always arise in synchrony? Does low self-esteem always come along with pessimism, fearfulness, and low energy?

The different aspects of low mood arise together in the same way as the different symptoms of a cold. They are closely associated but in patterns that differ depending on the specifics of the problem. Matthew Keller took on the risky project of looking to see if different kinds of problems aroused different depression symptoms. Three different studies confirmed his hypothesis. In particular, loss of a partner aroused crying, emotional pain, and a desire for social support, while a failing effort caused pessimism, fatigue, and lack of ability to experience pleasure.[98] Another former student, Eiko Fried, took this to the next level with a series of studies showing that the common practice of measuring depression severity by summing up the number and intensity of symptoms tosses out the most interesting and important variations. Analyzing individual symptoms may provide data that help demonstrate the effectiveness of antidepressant drugs and help find the brain mechanisms that go awry in serious depression.[99]

Relieving Mental Pain

Finally, a caution about a common but dangerous bit of illogic. On learning that low mood can be useful, some people conclude that it therefore should not be treated. This mistake is like the one that arose when anesthesia was first invented: some doctors refused to use it, even during surgery, because, they said, pain is normal. We must not let new understanding of the utility of low mood interfere with our efforts to relieve mental pain.

People come for treatment because they are suffering. Whether pain is physical or mental, finding and eliminating the cause provides the best solution. Sometimes low mood should be respected as normal and useful to help adjust a person's motivation and life directions. However, often the situation can't be changed. The loss of a friend, continuing abuse, inability to get a job, trying every night to help a child get off drugs, finding no relief from chronic pain—those are good reasons, but the resulting bad feelings are harmful even if they are normal. In other situations, low mood can be normal and useful for a person's genes but harmful for the person. Sometimes it is normal but useless in the specific instance because of the Smoke Detector Principle. Sometimes it is normal but useless because we live in social environments so different from those we evolved in. And sometimes low mood is caused by abnormalities in the mood regulation system. Considering all the possibilities allows clinicians and patients to take the same medical approach to low mood that they would for physical pain. Try to find the cause and fix it, but always do what you can to relieve suffering.

CHAPTER 7

BAD FEELINGS FOR NO GOOD REASON: WHEN THE MOODOSTAT FAILS

Sadness is to depression what normal growth is to cancer.

—Lewis Wolpert,
Malignant Sadness: The Anatomy of Depression[1]

If any could desire what he is incapable of possessing, despair must be his eternal lot.

—William Blake,
"There Is No Natural Religion," 1788

Ordinary low mood is like the pain caused by a broken leg. Abnormal depression is like chronic pain caused by a defective pain regulation mechanism. Mania is like an engine without a governor. Mood disorders result when the moodostat fails.

I had just met my new patient, a professor in his early sixties. He sat up in his hospital bed, looked out the window, and spoke painfully slowly. "It looks like the smoke is clearing."

"What smoke is that?" I asked. He replied, "It's all gone now, isn't it, the whole city, all burned. But you can still smell it."

There had been no fire, the city was fine, and no one else could smell smoke. He went on slowly, "I would help, but I have nothing now. I can't pay for being here. I should leave. I'll probably have to go to prison."

His wife spoke up. "He has been talking like this for weeks, but no matter how many times I tell him that we have a retirement account, he keeps saying that all our money is gone and it doesn't matter because he will die soon." His psychotic depression gave him delusions of poverty, olfactory hallucinations, and visions of imaginary catastrophes. He got better, but it took several weeks of electroconvulsive therapy.

The police are more familiar with mania. I was on call the evening they were called to a fine dining restaurant because a woman in her early thirties was gyrating unsteadily on a tabletop, taking off her clothes, and singing garbled ditties at the top of her voice. She said she was the dancer for the evening's entertainment, but that fancy boring restaurant never scheduled entertainment. She started yelling and fighting as the police took her down from the table. In the emergency room, she talked a mile a minute, shouting incoherent phrases about winning a television dance contest and wanting to give a preview for her fans. She was not drunk or on drugs. A review of her hospital record showed five previous admissions for manic episodes. A friend said she had stopped her medications two weeks previously "to prepare for the dance contest."

There is nothing normal or useful about psychotic depression or mania. Both are serious diseases that result from broken mood regulation mechanisms. Discovering why those mechanisms fail in some individuals is a huge, well-funded enterprise that is making slow progress. Its accomplishments and limitations were on display at the mood disorders conference I attended at a posh resort hotel, where three hundred psychiatrists heard elegant talks summarizing the latest research findings.

The meeting opened with reports about depression prevalence so appalling it was hard to know whether to get motivated or get out of the room. On any given day, 350 million people suffer from a mood disorder that makes them miserable, unable to work, and, all too often, unable to go on living.[2] In the United States alone, depression costs the economy $210 billion, about three times as much as all food supplement programs. A powerful editorial in *Nature* with the title "If Depression Were Cancer" noted that the $400 million the US National Institutes of Health invests each year in depression research is less than 10 percent of the amount allocated to cancer research.[3,4] Mood disorders pose a gigantic public health crisis that requires urgent efforts to find the causes and better treatments.

The experts at the conference summarized the results of hundreds of studies about how the brain influences mood and how drugs influence the brain. The science was spectacular, but the takeaway message was, in a word, depressing. Despite the wonderful research, no specific brain or genetic abnormality that causes depression has been found. Studies of treatment were equally sophisticated but only a bit more optimistic. Most patients get some benefit, but many are "treatment resistant" or experience intolerable side effects. Only a minority of patients gets enduring complete relief.

Some new findings were surprising and solid advances. For depression that is a part of bipolar disorder, it is now clear that the usual antidepressants don't work but other drugs do. In other good news, some new antidepressants may have fewer sexual side effects than older drugs. Overall, the conference demonstrated the amazing progress in understanding the brain mechanisms that influence mood and the slow progress in finding causes and better treatments. The participants came away better prepared to provide optimal treatment for their patients.

During one particularly technical talk just before lunch, my mind drifted to the Sherlock Holmes story in which the crucial clue was a dog that didn't bark in the night. Why did my mind drift there? Was something missing?

At lunch I asked other psychiatrists why they thought the capacity for low mood existed at all. Their answers were miles away from biology. "Depression is what makes us human." "Depression is essential for relationships to be meaningful." "I never even thought of that. Does there have to be a reason?" "Depression is a brain disorder, there is nothing useful about it."

When I suggested that there must be some reason evolution shaped a capacity for mood, their comments ranged from the shocking to the perplexing. "Hasn't evolution been disproven?" "I think it is learning and culture, not biology." "That sounds like one of those just-so stories." "Mood is caused by chemical imbalances, not evolution." Hearing those comments from friendly, well-educated doctors forced me to recognize that psychiatrists were not even thinking about the utility of mood, much less its evolutionary origins.

By the end of the day, I felt hopeless, frustrated, inadequate, lonely, anxious, fatigued, and pessimistic. My brain had changed. Was it the spontaneous onset of an episode of depression? Did a day with no exercise and too high a ratio of cookies to sunshine create a chemical imbalance? Or were my symptoms caused by being forced to recognize that my years of effort to get psychiatrists to think about the evolution of mood had come to nothing?

If my symptoms had persisted for two weeks, I would have qualified for a diagnosis of major depression. Fortunately, on the second day of the conference I sat next to a friend, Cynthia Stonnington, who leads the psychiatry department at the Mayo Clinic in Arizona. Her whispers and timely arched eyebrows suggested that I was not the only one who noticed that something was missing. We skipped the drug company–sponsored lunch and found a sunny patio, where we tried to figure out what bothered us about the morning's presentations.

We soon realized that the experts had focused exclusively on what is wrong with some individuals that make them vulnerable to depression. They never mentioned how life situations influence mood in everyone. They had mentioned "stress" in the abstract, but no one talked about patients trapped in abusive marriages or dead-end jobs. No one described treating a parent who feels hopeless, exhausted, fearful, and depressed because of the inability to help a psychotic teenage child who screams and threatens mayhem at random times in the night. No one mentioned the despair of an addict begging for a tenth try at detox or a patient who has just heard that a cancer has recurred.

The focus had been entirely on characteristics of the person. Life situations had been ignored. I recalled the first principle of social psychology, laid out by the field's founder, Kurt Lewin, in a simple formula: $B = f(P, E)$: **B**ehavior is a function of a **P**erson in his or her **E**nvironment. Characteristics of a person—things like genes and personality—stay the same.[5] Environments change. Both must be considered together for a full explanation.

As noted in the chapter about diagnosis, humans are prone to the fundamental attribution error, blaming characteristics of individuals and neglecting the effects of environments and situations.[6,7] Once you recognize it, you can see that the error is everywhere. If someone takes a cup of coffee from a shared pot without contributing to the donations jar, it is easy to label the person "dishonest" without considering that the person might have put in five dollars yesterday. If an acquaintance walks by without greeting you, it is easy to assume that the person is an oblivious jerk, although the person might be on the way to chemotherapy. If someone is downcast, it is easy to attribute the state to a pessimistic personality. In a conversation with a colleague with a private practice about psychotherapists who were having affairs, I suggested that it might be because people especially interested in sex might be likely to become therapists. He replied, "Therapists are no different from anyone else. It is having a private office. It makes having affairs so easy, there is no resisting. Get a private office, you will see."

A Scholar's Depression

The morning after the conference, I was dejectedly browsing *The Atlantic*, where I came across an article by the famous child psychologist Alison Gopnik entitled "How an 18th-Century Philosopher Helped Solve My Midlife Crisis."[8] Like many a "midlife crisis," hers was actually a classic episode of depression. Her symptoms were set off by the end of her twenty-year marriage, her children leaving home, and moving to lonely new lodgings. Soon she was convinced that she would never again accomplish anything significant. Her symptoms seemed to justify that conclusion: she was spending hours each day crying and could not work. She knew she needed help, but she was not a compliant patient. "My doctors prescribed Prozac, yoga, and meditation. I hated Prozac. I was terrible at yoga. But meditation seemed to help, and it was interesting, at least. In fact, researching meditation seemed to help as much as actually doing it. Where did it come from? Why did it work?"

Being an academic, she turned to David Hume, the eighteenth-century Scottish philosopher who is remembered for his penetrating insights into the subjectivity of human experience, the impossibility of ever satisfying our desires, and his good humor despite all. His was not, however, a carefree life. At age twenty-three he fell apart, convinced, like Gopnik, that he would never again accomplish anything. However, in the subsequent three years, he wrote *A Treatise of Human Nature*, now recognized as one of the great books in Western philosophy—an inspiring role model for a depressed ambitious academic three centuries later.[9]

As she read Hume, Gopnik thought she detected a whiff of Buddhism in his attitudes toward desire. She followed the scent like the bloodhound scholar she is. I was fascinated because Buddhist ideas have so much to say about how desire causes depression.[10,11,12] Did anyone in Europe even know about Buddhism in the early 1700s? Gopnik discovered a Jesuit missionary, Ippolito Desideri, who had studied Buddhism at a monastery in Tibet from 1716 to 1721. He completed his book on the topic in 1728, a year after returning to Europe. The church did not allow publication of books about competing religions, so Hume probably never saw a copy. However, Gopnik discovered a remarkable coincidence. Desideri had spent time at the monastery in La Flèche, a small town south of Paris. David Hume lived in that same town eight years later and talked with the monks there as he was writing his *Treatise.*

Gopnik soon met a man who shared her passion for investigating this mystery and fell in love with him. Her depression vanished. Was this a spontaneous remission? Or was it new love, a new social network, new career opportunities, and perhaps a new recognition that desires are illusions that can never be satisfied?

Her account was deeply moving. She described without flinching how her terrible depression had been set off by major life enterprises coming to dead ends. She did not, like some other famous authors, minimize and conceal the roles of personal conflicts and losses by attributing her symptoms to the spontaneous onset of a brain disease. Instead, she went into darkness and came out with new understanding and purpose.

Her disorder was serious and might have benefited from more aggressive treatment. If she had been my patient, I would have tried to convince her to continue her antidepressants. Also, I would not have taken her explanation at face value. She may have minimized family history or previous symptoms. Depression could have contributed to the end of her marriage and career obstacles. But her description of her descent and recovery nonetheless helped me to transcend my own despair and dig in again to the challenge of figuring out why mood exists at all. The effort will be worthwhile if it encourages others to help construct a framework that will allow us to make sense of mood disorders in the context of normal mood. But first it is essential to ask why so many smart doctors don't see why understanding the origins and functions of normal mood is essential for understanding mood disorders.

The Fundamental Error

Current psychiatric research on depression exemplifies the fundamental attribution error. It is as serious as it is common. I was assigned to complete a rating scale on a young woman who was hospitalized for depression. Partway through the interview she said, "It all started when I got raped." I found no reference to the rape in her chart, so I asked her doctor if he knew about it. He said, "Yes, but not everyone who gets raped gets depressed." That is like saying that not everyone who smokes cigarettes gets lung cancer.

Treating symptoms without paying attention to what is arousing them is not unique to psychiatry. VSAD is also common in the rest of medicine. Doctors sometimes use drugs to relieve pain, vomiting, cough, and fever without knowing the cause. However, most doctors who treat cough look carefully for asthma, heart failure, pneumonia, and other problems that arouse the normal cough reflex. They consider the possibility that the cough regulation system has run amok only as a last-ditch explanation. Experts who treat abdominal pain look for irritable bowel syndrome, Crohn's disease, cancer, ulcers, and other problems that arouse pain, along with the possibility that the pain regulation system might be awry. But the experts at the mood disorders conference said nothing about how to look for life situations that cause mood changes. They viewed symptoms as diseases.

There are good reasons why the VSAD fallacy is more common for emotional disorders. The problems that cause cough and abdominal pain are tangible. You can see pneumonia on an X-ray and ulcers via a gastroscope. The situations that influence mood are often invisible. Depression symptoms rise like a vapor from invisible gaps between desires and expectations. As if that were not challenge enough, different individuals have different desires, different ways of coping with frustration and failure, and different ways of avoiding unpleasant ideas and emotions. The nun who is upset by "unclean thoughts." The executive passed over for a crucial promotion. The father whose child is using heroin. All are trying to cope with major failures, but the situations are vastly different.

Measures of stress and checklists of life events don't begin to describe the specific life situations that influence mood. Sometimes even a long conversation is not enough. I spent an hour talking with a middle-aged woman to try to find out what had set off her depression but got nowhere. She denied losses, frustrations, marital problems, substance abuse, and other usual causes. But as she put her hand on the door handle to leave she said, "You know, I remember the exact moment my depression began." "When was that?" I asked. "It was six months ago. I was just leaving the house, and the phone rang. It was my boyfriend from high school. I hadn't heard from him in years. We just said hi, nothing else. It wasn't any big deal. But it started that night."

During our next visit, I asked in detail about her marriage and her previous boyfriend, but she said everything was fine. Maybe she had decided to avoid thinking about what could have been. Maybe her unconscious mind had suppressed thoughts about possible alternative paths her life could have taken. Maybe it was a coincidence and her depression had a spontaneous onset that she attributed to the phone call. If only there were some kind of "lifeoscope" that could reveal life problems the way a gastroscope shows an ulcer.

Why Is Psychiatry Out of the Loop?

VSAD is the main obstacle to progress in understanding mood disorders. Physiologists study the evolutionary origins and utility of special states such as fever and stress. Behavioral biologists and psychologists have conducted scores of studies describing the situations that influence mood and how mood variation influences thinking and behavior. In psychiatry, however, VSAD remains the norm.

Why? Some blame industry money and the rewards it provides to those who promote slogans that promote drug treatments, such as "It's a brain disease." I am less cynical. Many neuroscientists and psychiatrists have good reasons for thinking that mood problems are usually caused by brain abnormalities. One big one is that most of the serious disorders they see in clinic really are products of abnormal brains. Bipolar disorder, for instance, is an inherited brain disease in which mania and depression arise and fade in cycles that are often unrelated to changing life situations. Other patients have episodes of serious depression that come and go for no apparent reason. Some people are born with a tendency to constant low mood or extreme emotional reactions to even mild events. In such cases, excessive symptoms from a broken regulation mechanism really are the disease.

Also, many patients wrongly attribute their symptoms to life events. I recall a woman who insisted that current work stress caused her depression, but probing revealed that she had had symptoms most of her life, as had her siblings and parents. In many cases of marital problems I treated, a mood disorder seemed to be more a cause than a result of relationship problems.

However, the opposite error is equally common: some patients blame their brains to avoid acknowledging a life problem. I recall a young woman who wanted an antidepressant prescription for what she said was "obviously a chemical imbalance" because it had begun the same month she started a new job that had doubled her income. It took extensive discussion to discover that she had spent the previous decade trying to make it as a graphic artist. Taking a job as an assistant stockbroker marked the end of her dream. I saw so many patients who misattributed their symptoms either to life events or to brain abnormalities that I found myself becoming skeptical whenever a patient expressed strong opinions about causes.

It is also easy to miss important life problems. When an unfamiliar doctor asks, "Have you experienced any stress recently?" many patients give a noncommittal answer to avoid a potentially upsetting and likely useless conversation about abuse, illicit affairs, gambling losses, or problems coping with a sick child. Some carefully conceal the source of the problem. A severely depressed man with a solid family and a good job was not improving after a month of weekly treatment sessions. Then, in the middle of a session, he started sobbing. When he was finally able to talk, he revealed a heart-rending story about how his closest relationship had for years been with a secret lover who had died suddenly. He couldn't even attend the funeral and had not been able to talk with anyone about his grief.

A fourth reason for glossing over life situations is that learning the details doesn't always help. Problems with easy solutions get solved. Those that cause major mood problems are usually tough or impossible to solve. A man was constantly berated and belittled by his wife's wealthy and powerful parents, to whom she was devoted. He could not imagine leaving his wife and children, and all efforts to improve the behavior of his in-laws failed. Minimizing contact with them helped some, recognizing the inaccuracy of their criticisms helped a bit more, and antidepressants took the edge off, but he remained depressed, trapped in a bad situation, looking forward, with only some guilt, to the demise of his aged in-laws.

On top of all these reasons, the very idea that low mood can be useful seems ludicrous. Sadness occurs after a loss has already happened, so it seems as if it's too late to be useful. The pessimism, lassitude, social withdrawal, and low self-esteem of depression interfere with the ability to cope.

What proportion of cases is caused mostly by situations, what proportion is caused mostly by characteristics of the person, and what proportion by interactions between the two? A rough answer comes from the original classic study of depression by Aubrey Lewis, the chair of the Institute of Psychiatry in London during the middle of the twentieth century. He analyzed detailed notes on sixty-one of his patients with severe depression and concluded that in about a third the onset of depression was unconnected to any life event, another third had a vulnerability to depression that had magnified the effect of a negative experience, and the final third had depression caused by a specific event such as a death or divorce.[13] Scores of more sophisticated studies have confirmed his basic finding.[14,15,16,17] The vast majority of first episodes of serious depression are precipitated by a bad life event, but third or fourth episodes of depression are more likely to arise in the absence of any specific event.[18,19,20] Such episodes unconnected to life events were previously called "endogenous depression," in contrast to cases of "exogenous depression" that had a precipitant.[21,22] However, the symptom patterns and responses to treatment turned out to be very similar, so the distinction was dropped, further encouraging VSAD.

Symptom patterns can help to separate depression that is a response to an event and depression that is part of a larger and longer pattern. Jerome Wakefield and Mark Schmitz looked at how often depression recurred for different groups.[23] Patients with uncomplicated depression (symptoms lasting less than two months and not including suicidal thoughts, psychosis, feelings of worthlessness, or moving slowly) were no more likely than anyone else to have depression later. The authors concluded that such cases of normal sadness are very different from cases of severe depression characterized as "melancholia," which often have repeated autonomous episodes.

How Many Ways Can Mood Fail?

Recognizing the utility of normal mood changes makes it possible to apply the same framework that doctors use to understand other disorders. Dozens of mechanisms adjust the body to changing situations. Sweating and shivering cope with changing temperatures. Anxiety rises in response to threats. Blood pressure increases with threats and exercise and decreases with calm and rest. What is normal depends on the situation. A blood pressure reading of 170/110 is abnormal at rest but useful and normal during exercise. Whether high or low mood is normal depends on the situation.

Regulation systems can fail in at least six ways. Distinguishing them is crucial for understanding them.

SIX WAYS THAT REGULATION SYSTEMS CAN FAIL

1. Baseline is too low.

2. Baseline is too high.

3. Response is deficient.

4. Response is excessive.

5. Response is aroused by inappropriate cues.

6. Response is independent of cues.

Low or high baseline levels are common problems. People with low blood pressure are more likely to faint than to win an athletic competition. People with chronic low mood (*dysthymia* is the technical term) are bundles of misery who accomplish little and often seek help. People with high blood pressure are likely to have a stroke or a heart attack. People with chronic high mood (hypomania) accomplish a lot and don't seek help; their disorder is rarely recognized, except by exasperated family members and coworkers.

Even if baseline levels are normal, responses can be deficient. If your blood pressure does not increase when you stand up, you are likely to faint. If your mood never changes, something is wrong. Lack of low mood is rarely recognized except when people are unmoved by events that would shake others. In our study of bereavement, a remarkable number of people reported no grief symptoms after the death of their spouse, but no diagnosis applies to them.[24,25] Deficiencies of high mood are finally getting more attention thanks to positive psychology.

Excessive responses are more obvious. Exercise makes blood pressure go sky-high in some people; they are likely to develop chronic hypertension and its complications. Excessive emotional response to minor events is also common. I recall a woman crying intensely while reporting that she had discovered a quart of sour milk in her refrigerator, blaming herself for what she saw as an abject failure. This could have been just depression, but a few minutes later, she was rhapsodic about her son getting into a band. Patients with borderline personality disorder are especially prone to extreme mood changes. A partner's facial twitch or tone of voice can trigger rage or sobbing.

Inappropriate responses are a different kind of problem. Seeing blood or a needle makes blood pressure plunge in some people; I learned not to draw blood from patients sitting on a high examination table after one fainted and fell off. Television dramas are intended to arouse emotions, but my patient who was still upset days after watching an episode of *The Brady Bunch* had a serious problem.

Finally, broken regulation mechanisms can cause apparently spontaneous changes. Sudden blood pressure spikes or plunges can occur for no discoverable reason. Severe bouts of mania or depression can cycle on their own, unconnected with any life events.

Why Mood Regulation Systems Are Fragile

Mood regulation systems are vulnerable to failure for the same evolutionary reasons as other bodily systems. Sometimes the failure is only apparent. Sometimes it is because of living in a modern environment. Sometimes it reflects trade-offs or the limits of what natural selection can do. Each deserves consideration.

The Smoke Detector Principle explains some normal but nonetheless excessive mood responses. Low mood conserves calories and avoids risk; high mood is expensive and can be dangerous. When outcomes are hard to predict, erring on the side of low mood may provide advantages, especially in harsh environments. Recognizing that misery may be useless even when it is normal is a foundation for making wise treatment decisions.

Some mood changes benefit our genes at our expense. Our desires for the perfect partner and great sex provide great pleasure when they can be satisfied, but for many people they cause chronic grinding frustration. Desperate striving for high status and wealth gives big payoffs for a few but wrecks life for many.

I treated, or tried to treat, many depressed VIPs, mostly corporate vice presidents and deans. The core problem for many was overweening ambition that left them perpetually unsatisfied despite their substantial accomplishments. Recognizing that such desires can't be satisfied could relieve immense suffering.[26] However, our ancestors who found it easy to ignore such desires had fewer children, so we have brains that push us to strive in ways that benefit our genes.

Plato warned that pursuing pleasure leads to unhappiness. The Buddha taught that desires can never be satisfied. Every religion provides advice about how to get off the hedonic treadmill, leaving its emotional baggage behind. However, such advice is like advice about diets: correct, well-meaning, plentiful, and, for good evolutionary reasons, well-nigh impossible to actually follow.

The Perils of Modern Environments

Abundant food we can't resist explains atherosclerosis, obesity, and high blood pressure, but modern social environments provide plenty of other novel temptations and hassles. Hunter-gatherers never tried to get into the NBA. They did not stay up late on Twitter. They never had to cope with bureaucracies. They didn't ruminate about whether to have children. They never spent months preparing for divorce court. They did, however, get depressed.

For two decades, I asked anthropologist colleagues about rates of depression in the cultures they studied. Kim Hill is an anthropologist who spent many years with the Ache, a tribe living in the Amazon jungle. Each year when he returned, I asked him how much depression he had seen. Each year he told me he had seen almost none, despite the prevalence of infected wisdom teeth, tuberculosis, and other health problems that might make anyone miserable.

Finally, about the tenth time I asked him, the answer was different. His group had started a medical clinic. They were amazed to hear about problems they had never suspected. Many people came to the clinic complaining of pessimism, hopelessness, lack of interest, lack of appetite, poor sleep, poor digestion, and just not feeling like doing much of anything. I was especially intrigued to hear his observation that whoever became chief of the tribe was likely to show up in the clinic within a few months with symptoms of anxiety and depression.

The differences between our environments and those of our ancestors are getting larger, faster and faster. There is some evidence that mood disorders may be more common in modern environments.[27] However, carefully conducted studies find no increase in major depression rates in recent decades.[28] It can nonetheless appear as if we are in an epidemic. Drug advertising and reduced stigma make depression a common conversation topic. Publicity campaigns emphasize the prevalence of depression. Rates of low mood in the normal range have been increasing even if serious depression has not. Finally, a quirk of memory distorts perceptions. A large questionnaire study found that younger people reported many more depression episodes than older people and concluded that depression rates must be rising fast.[29] It seems more likely, however, that memories of depression fade with time.[30,31]

The tendency to forget bad times can also make depression rates seem lower than they really are. The current prevalence rate for depression in the United States is about 9 percent.[32] Across 148 surveys around the world, the average prevalence of any mood disorder was 5.4 percent each year and 9.6 percent for lifetime estimates.[33] However, asking young people about symptoms every few months paints a different picture. A large study of Wisconsin women found that 24 percent of women and 15 percent of men had experienced major depression or dysthymia before age twenty.[34] Of women followed yearly from ages seventeen to twenty-two, 47 percent had one or more episodes of major depression.[35] Among college students the rate is about 30 percent in a given year.[36]

While depression rates tend to be stable across decades in a given culture, they vary widely by country. Lifetime rates range from 1.5 percent in Taiwan to 19 percent in Beirut.[37] Another study found rates ranging from 3 percent in Japan to 17 percent in the United States.[38] Why such huge differences? That is the most important unanswered question for mood disorders research.[39] If we could get the rate in every culture down to the 1 to 3 percent rates in Taiwan and Japan, that would reduce depression more than all treatment efforts put together. Differences in family stability and support are likely important. Differences in values and expectations for success and competition influence mood. Differences in diet, drug use, social structure, and shared beliefs are all likely relevant. Some combination of factors must account for the huge differences in depression rates. Discovering what those are should be a research priority.

Modern media make life more interesting, but they also encourage social comparisons that cause dissatisfaction.[40,41] Vivid stories about other people's fame and wealth spur ambitions that few can satisfy. Characters on television, whether *Downton Abbey* or *Keeping Up with the Kardashians*, are so extraordinarily attractive, successful, wealthy, and famous that the rest of us can't help but feel inadequate (or superior or contemptuous). Even the actors and actresses can't live up to the expectations aroused by the characters they play.

Media exposure generates dissatisfaction, not only with ourselves but with our friends and partners, who rarely measure up to alternatives we see in the media. Dozens of studies show that mood plummets when people compare themselves to others who have more than they do.[42,43,44] Even browsing Facebook posts of friends, inevitably biased toward the positive, tends to make people feel worse about themselves and their lives.[45,46] Despite the documented ability of social media exposure to cause dissatisfaction, there is little evidence that the use of social media is increasing rates of pathological depression. However, the pursuit of grand goals may be relevant.

The biggest rewards in mass societies go to those who pursue grand goals single-mindedly. This usually requires an unbalanced life. In many fields, the price of trying to get into the big leagues is neglect of self, health, partner, children, and friends. The predictable problems provide fodder for television shows that exploit the problems of the famous to provide schadenfreude for the masses. Magazines about celebrities are equal parts veneration of superachievers and consolation for the rest of us. Every issue offers advice for getting rich, thin, attractive, and famous, followed by advice about how to cope with feelings of inadequacy, anxiety, and low self-esteem.

Physical aspects of modern life also increase vulnerability to mood disorders. Electricity provides light and entertainment that disrupt sleep. Increased inflammation due to obesity[47] or high levels of omega-6 fatty acids[48] may also increase depression. Lack of exercise may account for some depression in modern societies,[49,50] and increased exercise can relieve symptoms a bit on average.[51]

One week before I was scheduled to leave for an extended sabbatical, I saw a new patient who was desperate. She had experienced chronic severe suicidal depression for ten years and had gotten no relief from behavior therapy, cognitive therapy, psychoanalysis, and many medications. She said she would do anything. I said, "Anything?" She replied, "Yes, anything." I told her to join a gym and spend at least one hour every day working out to the maximum of her endurance on a treadmill, followed by a long walk outdoors. I was not hopeful, but it was the only untried option. A few months into my sabbatical I got an email message saying that she had called the front desk at the clinic, asking them to let me know that she was symptom-free and immensely grateful.

What Natural Selection Can't Do

Mood regulation mechanisms seem prone to failure even in natural environments. One possible explanation is that there are some things selection can't do, such as prevent all genetic mutations. Perhaps mood disorders exist because mutations happen and they are only slowly purged from the gene pool. About a third of the variation in depression vulnerability is accounted for by genetic variations. The siblings and children of people with major depression are 2.8 times more likely to get the disease. Over a lifetime, that means the average risk of about 10 percent in the United States increases to about 30 percent for those whose close relatives have had depression. Nearly all of that increase is from shared genes; what family you are raised in has remarkably little influence.[52]

This evidence for inheritance has spurred a huge search for the genetic culprits. Studies in the first years of the twenty-first century identified many suspects, but subsequent studies exonerated every one. The arrival of cheap DNA sequencing changed everything. Hopes for answers were raised by a mega-analysis that pooled data from nine studies. It analyzed more than 1.2 million genetic locations in 9,240 people with a history of major depression and 9,519 controls. However, the results, published in 2013, found that not one of those 1.2 million sites reliably predicted who would get depressed.[53] The authors of the report pleaded for larger studies on more homogeneous populations.

A subsequent study looked for genetic variations in a genetically homogeneous group of more than 10,000 women of Han Chinese descent, half of whom had major depressive disorder. It identified two locations on chromosome 10 that predicted rates of depression. However, together they explained less than 1 percent of the variation.[54] A further analysis of the data provided a remarkable finding: larger chromosomes had more locations influencing depression; the correlation was 60 percent.[55] This suggests that depression is caused not by a few alleles on a few chromosomes but by thousands spread relatively evenly over the entire genome.

A yet larger study of more than 300,000 people used self-report data on depression and genetic data from the consumer genome-scanning company 23andMe. Published in 2016, it identified seventeen locations that are associated with tiny increases in the risk for depression. However, the two locations found in the study of Chinese women were not among them.

It is harder to measure depression than blood pressure or diabetes. Could that account for why these studies have not found specific alleles with large effects? Probably not. Type 2 diabetes and high blood pressure are also highly heritable, but they also have no common alleles with substantial effects.[56] The same is true for something easy to measure, height. Ninety percent of height variation is caused by genetic variation, but there are no "height genes" with large effects. A 2008 study of 13,665 individuals found twenty genetic variants that each influence height by two to six millimeters, but taken together they explained only 3 percent of the genetic variation.[57] All the genetic information from about 25,000 people explained about 4 percent of height variation. A sample of 130,000 people explained only 10 percent. To explain half of the genetic variation in height required combining seventy-nine studies with a quarter of a million people.[58] Variations in thousands of genes influence height, diabetes, blood pressure, and depression, but their individual effects are minuscule. It makes no sense to call them abnormal. The hope that most cases of major depression are a disease that results from abnormal genes is misplaced. A new approach is needed.

Cybernetics

Everything is cyber this or cyber that these days, but cybernetics is a specific scientific approach described by Norbert Wiener in his brilliant 1948 book, *Cybernetics; or Control and Communication in the Animal and the Machine*.[59] It describes how feedback mechanisms stabilize things such as blood pressure and mood and the dire results when stabilization fails. It includes a profound chapter on mental disorders caused by feedback dysregulation.

Positive feedback is nice from your boss, but in cybernetics it refers to something different: vicious cycles, things like snowballs rolling downhill and runaway trucks. The founder of cognitive therapy, Aaron Beck, and a few other depression experts have noted that positive feedback loops can make depression worse,[60] but much work remains to investigate the actual mechanisms. Positive feedback cycles worsen depression. People respond to low mood by going home, closing the door, getting in bed, and not answering the telephone and email. Out of contact, they soon conclude that no one cares about them. Poor nutrition and lack of exercise cause more depression and more isolation, creating a downward spiral.

It is intriguing to consider whether this spiral is more likely in modern societies. Way back when, people got hungry and had to go out to find food. That meant seeing friends and getting exercise. Today, therapy that encourages active involvement in life despite lack of interest can initiate a virtuous cycle in which activity improves mood, which initiates more activity in an upward spiral to recovery.[61,62]

Having one depressive episode may make future ones more likely. This is called "kindling," because it is similar to how small pieces of wood can ignite a larger blaze.[63] It is related to the observation that epileptic seizures are set off more easily after previous seizures. For depression, life events precipitate most first episodes, but the role of events declines with each subsequent episode, until they seem to come on for no reason.[64,65] This observation is sometimes explained by suggesting that depression damages the brain in ways that make more episodes likely.

Kindling could also be explained by a mechanism that adapts organisms to unfavorable environments. Just as multiple episodes of intense anxiety indicate a dangerous environment in which anxiety is especially useful, multiple failures may reflect an unpropitious social environment in which low mood is more useful. The mechanism that adjusts depression so it becomes more likely after bad times may be a feature, not a flaw.[66,67] However, other explanations are possible. Depression episodes damage a person's social network. Obstacles to major life goals that cause depression may persist after the symptoms lift, making more episodes likely. Such persisting problems may not show up on a checklist of life events, making some depression episodes appear to come out of the blue, when in fact they arise from continuing problems. The person's spouse is still abusing alcohol. The mother-in-law remains in the house, as critical as ever. A beloved child still won't return phone calls.

Bipolar Disorder

Bipolar depression is different from regular depression, and mania is very different from happiness.[68] Bipolar disorder results from a fundamental failure of the mood regulation system. The normal system shifts mood higher and lower as situations change, then returns mood to the individual's set point. We strive mightily to get a new job or house or spouse in the belief that it will finally bring enduring happiness. It works temporarily, and then mood reverts to its previous level. Like a thermostat, the moodostat keeps mood close to a set point.

People with bipolar disorder have a broken moodostat. When they encounter a new opportunity, their mood goes up, but it does not come back down. Instead, increasing energy, ambition, risk taking, and optimism create imagined future successes that fuel still greater energy toward still more grandiose goals, in a process of runaway positive feedback that peaks in manic excitement that can be fatal, just from physiological exhaustion. Usually just before that point, some kind of overload switch turns motivation off suddenly and completely, sending elation plunging into depression that also feeds on itself, stabilizing mood at a negative extreme for weeks or months. It is as if the thermostat is missing, replaced by a switch with only two positions: full-bore high mood or motivation completely turned off.

Modern thermostats do not turn on the furnace when the temperature gets below a certain point and turn it off again once the temperature again reaches the set point. That would result in wide swings of temperature because the temperature continues to go down while the furnace is getting going and heat keeps pouring out for a time after the temperature gets back up to the set point. To avoid these swings, thermostats have an "anticipator" that turns the furnace on or off a few minutes before the set point is reached. If the anticipator breaks, temperature swings are extreme. Could a broken anticipator mechanism explain why some people have wide mood swings? That could explain wider-than-usual oscillations, called cyclothymia, but not why the system gets stuck in high or low mood.

Engineers who design control systems recognize what they call "bistable systems" that switch fast between two extreme states, never stopping in the middle.[69,70] The best example is a light switch. It's either on or it's off, never in between. Many biological systems are bistable. For example, once the mechanism that initiates bacterial spore formation turns on, it goes all the way; stopping partway through the process would be fatal. The evolution of two sexes is another example. The advantages go to individuals who make either large eggs that last quite a while or millions of tiny sperm that can swim fast. Medium-size gametes that can swim at a medium speed are less likely to succeed, so most species have two sexes.[71] The interesting thing about bistable systems is that they require positive feedback to work. Once the system deviates a bit from the middle, positive feedback pushes it all the way to the extreme, just like a light switch. This is a lot like bipolar disorder.[72]

Why would natural selection have left mood regulation mechanisms especially vulnerable to dysregulation? To expand a speculation mentioned previously, I wonder if vulnerability to mood disorders is related to the fitness benefits of pursuing big goals. Mechanisms that motivate ambitious striving may be selected because they offer occasional big payoffs to a few people. This hypothesis predicts that many people will make big efforts to reach big goals despite experiencing many failures. The ability to disengage from a failing enterprise seems to be missing in many people with bipolar disorder. When ordinary low mood is not available to disengage failing efforts, positive mood escalates into ever-more-intense efforts that eventually collapse into serious depression.

The fitness advantages of ambition may help to explain vulnerability to depression and mood swings. Ambition is not just for recognition and money; the craving to be appreciated can be equally strong. Accomplishments generate satisfaction that often seems to inflate ambitions that are already magnified by modern mass media and well-meaning encouragement from parents and mentors. William James captured the problem in a succinct formula: Self-esteem = Success/pretentions.[73]

In the midst of an episode, bipolar patients think their extreme moods are rational. I have seen many examples.

A sculptor was certain that hundreds of students would flock to her studio to learn her new methods. She had already sunk her life savings into a lease and was furious that the bank wouldn't give her the loan she needed to furnish the studio.

An entrepreneur woke in the night with the revelation that an empty storefront could be transformed into the first of a new chain of fine restaurants. He bought a Mercedes to take celebrities from the airport to the restaurant, but as a series of chef candidates turned him down, he became increasingly agitated and frustrated.

A professor was certain that his brilliant new method could predict the stock market. Despite his wife's objections, he remortgaged the house to get cash. He blamed the ensuing big losses on competitors, who he said had stolen his formula and manipulated the market.

Obstacles and slowed progress toward a goal normally shift mood lower to conserve effort and reconsider options. In mania, this system does not kick in; instead, impending failure sets off yet more intense efforts to reach yet grander goals. Persistence in the face of adversity is widely praised, but it can lead to spectacular failures. Such failures convince many patients that they are worthless and have no possible future. The sculptor went to bed and would not get out, saying she was a fraud, she had no talent, and she would become a bag lady. The entrepreneur lost his car to the bank and ruminated about his inability to get any job. The professor was admitted to the hospital and crashed into depression a few days later. People who have bipolar disorder have broken mood regulation mechanisms, and losses sustained during episodes can make the objective situation bleak.

It would be nice if bipolar disorder were one specific disease, but it has blurry edges and many subtypes. Type I, with serious episodes of both depression and mania, occurs in about 1 percent of populations worldwide. However, expanding the spectrum of bipolar disorders to include more mild versions of mania brings the rate up to 5 percent.[74] Of patients with a diagnosis of major depressive disorder, 31 percent have had mild symptoms of mania as well.[75]

Bipolar episodes come at unpredictable times, last for durations of weeks to months, and then depart. Patients experience mania about 10 percent of the time, depression about 40 percent, and neutral moods about 50 percent of the time.[76] The most problematic cases experience both depression and mania at the same time, in what is called a "mixed state," making it clear that high and low mood are not just opposites on a single dimension; both can be present simultaneously.

Bad Genes?

Who gets bipolar disorder is explained almost entirely by genetic variations; they account for more than 80 percent of the variation in vulnerability. If your identical twin has bipolar disorder, your risk is 43 times higher than that of other people.[77] This strong effect suggests that it should be possible to find the responsible alleles. However, as is the case for so many other genetic diseases, no common alleles have a substantial influence on bipolar disorder.

That is so disappointing! However, the situation is not as bleak as the search for depression alleles. In some families plagued by bipolar disease, specific large chunks of DNA are missing or duplicated only in affected individuals.[78] Those chunks are all over the genome; however, tracking their functions gives hope of finding gene or brain networks crucial to causing the disorder.

Embracing the Reality of Organic Complexity

Finally, we return to thermostats and the moodostat. Attempts to understand mood disorders illustrate the human tendency to blame problems on a single cause. Blaming depression mainly on genetics or personality or life events makes it seem tractable. However, mood disorders result not just from multiple causes but from complex interactions among multiple causes that lead to symptoms via different routes in different individuals and even in the same individual at different times.

This complex reality is increasingly acknowledged. In a thoughtful article about the "dappled" causes of depression, the psychiatrist Kenneth Kendler lists eleven categories of causes ranging from genes to culture. He argues that "mutually re-enforcing dichotomies" such as mind/brain "have had a pernicious influence on our field" and do not explain research findings. "Instead, the causes of psychiatric illness are dappled, distributed widely across multiple categories. We should abandon Cartesian and computer-functionalism-based dichotomies as scientifically inadequate and an impediment to our ability to integrate the diverse information about psychiatric illness."[79]

Instead of asking what causes symptoms in some people, we can return to the question about why we all have somewhat unreliable mood regulation systems. I have emphasized the utility of high and low moods in propitious and unpropitious situations and how persisting in the pursuit of unreachable goals escalates low mood to clinical depression. However, this is just part of the picture. Sometimes there is no striving, just something missing in life.[80] Sometimes depression results from desire without hope. Our desires were shaped by natural selection. We can no more set them aside than we can decide to stop eating. A real solution to depression would require either changing society and providing opportunities for all or manipulating brains and minds to control desire. However, natural selection is way ahead of us. It has already created ways to control desire and dissatisfaction; repression and unconscious defenses are addressed in chapter 10.

How Does This Help?

Low mood is psychic pain. Depression is chronic psychic pain. This should guide how we evaluate and treat it. The first step is to try to figure out if something specific is arousing the pain. Investigation often reveals the inability to give up an unreachable goal. Many such problems are caused by "social traps," the title of an interesting book by my former colleagues John Cross and Melvin Guyer.[81] A student in her last year of graduate studies was $200,000 in debt, could not pay tuition or rent, and could not get more loans. A politician was being blackmailed by a former lover who demanded ever escalating sums to keep explicit photos private. An artist wanted to divorce her philandering husband, but that would have meant getting a job and giving up her studio. Social life often creates traps whose escape requires great sacrifices.

Have you ever walked through a bog, placing your feet carefully on tufts of grass that grow between the swampy parts, always looking for that next little tuft to make your way forward? There often comes a point where a slightly elevated bit begins to sink and your feet begin to get wet with stinking mud, but as you look around there is no route to high ground without going knee-deep into muck. Life has times like that. Patients with depression feel like they are sinking on a small tuft, fearful, often for good reason, of taking that first step into the muck. Leaving a job or marriage with no place else to go can make things worse. Much of the work of therapy is to help people get up the courage to make changes and to help them see other little tufts of grass on the way to higher ground.

Understanding low mood as a useful response and depression as excessive low mood suggests different approaches to treatment. Depression is caused by the situation, the view of the situation, and the brain. Treatment can change the situation, the view of the situation, and the brain. However, all three interact in tangled webs of causes, so addressing only one of them will miss many treatment possibilities.

This view has implications for understanding how antidepressants work. The idea that they normalize a "chemical imbalance" is appealing and helps to justify drug treatment, but there is no evidence for any specific chemical abnormality specific to depression. It seems more likely that antidepressants do for psychic pain what analgesics do for physical pain: they disrupt a normal response system. People have wondered how antidepressants with effects on different brain chemicals all can be effective. There is no mystery here. Aspirin, acetaminophen, ibuprofen, and morphine all act on somewhat different links in the pain regulation mechanism. Different antidepressants act on different links in the mood regulation system. The analogy goes further. Our strategies for relieving psychic pain are about as effective as our strategies for relieving physical pain—modestly to moderately effective, usually with side effects, often with risks on withdrawal, but still an enormous boon to humankind.

There may be a connection between the pursuit of unreachable goals and how antidepressants influence motivation. They often seem to disrupt the motivation system in ways that make everything seem less important. They calm grand ambitions and make pleasing others not quite so important. More than half of patients taking serotonin-influencing antidepressants experience decreased libido and/or delayed or absent orgasm.[82,83] It would be very interesting to learn if patients who experience a greater decline of sexual desire also experience more mood benefits.

I recall one professor who started an antidepressant in the spring and experienced an excellent remission from moderately severe depression. She returned in the fall to report that the stress of teaching was no longer a problem. In December, she returned to report that her mood was still fine but she was in danger of losing her job. She had become so free from concern that she had not graded any student papers or exams all term. She decided to stop her medication.

There are also implications for cognitive and behavioral therapy. Reframing the meaning of a situation is often the most powerful intervention.

Being abandoned by a spouse who departs without a word can be a source of weeping and hopelessness or a blessed opportunity to escape from an untrustworthy, cruel partner. New approaches to cognitive therapy "go meta" by trying to correct not just inaccurate thoughts about specific situations but inaccurate thoughts about the whole system of mood regulation and what is worth pursuing in life.[84] Some, such as the British psychologist Paul Gilbert, have written about ways to use evolutionarily sophisticated ideas to make such therapies more effective.[85,86,87]

What About the *Person?*

I have emphasized the Situation to counter the tendency of both psychological and neurological approaches to blame mental disorders on characteristics of the Person. However, people vary dramatically in their tendency to experience emotional disorders. Whether these differences are accounted for by innate factors or by experience has been the focus of interminable debates about "nature versus nurture." The nature side is fundamental to the neuroscience schema that dominates modern psychiatry and therefore has already received great emphasis. However, a huge body of literature describes how poor early rearing, especially neglect and abuse, can scar people for life.[88,89,90,91,92,93]

Thousands of therapists devote their careers to helping such people transcend such experiences, or at least cope with their effects. Such treatment can be remarkably effective. Early in my career I spent hours trying to discover what past experiences had shaped each patient's personality and vulnerability to problems. Sometimes transformative insights emerged. A patient who viewed her mother as superbly good came to recognize that her mother had steadily subtly undermined her. A patient who had blamed himself for his parents' divorce recognized that he had nothing to do with it. Another realized that guilt for sexual experiences with her father should belong to him, not her.

This book emphasizes the impact of current situations. The powerful influences of early experiences on vulnerability to mental problems are equally important, and much work is needed to discover the extent to which such influences are products of useful systems and the extent to which they are by-products. It will also be essential to learn the extent to which such effects are transmitted by neuroendocrine mechanisms, versus the beliefs they induce about others and the self. And, of course, early experiences interact with innate aspects of persons to make certain situations likely. Reviewing what we know and what we need to know about how early experiences influence mental problems is an important project whose scope is far beyond that of this book.

PART THREE

The Pleasures and Perils
of Social Life

CHAPTER 8

HOW TO UNDERSTAND AN
INDIVIDUAL HUMAN BEING

Perhaps the greatest problem faced by the academic social sciences is that what is measurable is often irrelevant, and what is truly relevant often cannot be measured.[1]

—George Vaillant, 2012

On Tuesdays in the 1990s, I experienced two different approaches to psychiatry in a disturbing but profoundly instructive way. I spent the mornings poring over spreadsheets of numbers at the Institute for Social Research. We had detailed data about age, sex, income, depression symptoms, and dozens of other measures from thousands of people. The goal was to use the numbers to predict who was depressed.

Big findings jumped out. Rates are higher for some groups than others. For instance, early in life, depression is twice as common for women than it is for men. Dozens of other factors had smaller influences: number of children; their ages; church attendance; body weight; race; losing a parent early in life; number of severe life events in the past year. The project offered fascinating statistical challenges, because every individual belonged to many different overlapping groups. For instance, people who had health problems were more likely to be older, single, taking medications, and unable to attend church; each of those factors influenced depression and one another, making it challenging to figure out what caused what.

At noon I walked a few blocks to the psychiatric clinic, where I spent the rest of the day treating individual patients and supervising the work of resident doctors. The shift was wrenching. Instead of neat mathematical generalizations about groups, I am suddenly there with Ms. H, a fifty-five-year-old heavy individual with dirty yellow-white hair, who is crying and hopeless, telling me, through sobs, that her husband killed himself because she hadn't taken his threats seriously, so she was planning to do the same to join him. Mr. J complains of skipped heartbeats whenever he sees his boss, who, he is convinced, wants to fire him. He says he has a heart condition, is depressed, and wants to get disability. Ms. K has been staying at home, not answering the telephone or doing much of anything ever since another woman was elected president of the gardening club after an election that was swung by a campaign of vicious gossip. And Ms. L, a thirty-five-year-old office manager in treatment for depression for ten years, is worse this month, almost certainly because she stopped taking her medication because it inhibits her orgasms and she is trying to date again. Or does her depression reflect her intuition that her new, already married lover might cause even more heartbreak than the previous one?

At the end of each clinic afternoon, the doctors, nurses, psychologists, and social workers met to discuss each case. We had the same data on our patients that I used in my morning statistical analyses. We knew each patient's sex, age, marital status, employment, health status, and more. Did we use those data to figure out the causes of an individual's depression? Never. Instead, we wove what each patient told us into stories that described how the individual had come to have this specific problem.

Consider the case notes on Ms. D.

Ms. D is a forty-five-year-old white married insurance agent. She is the mother of two teenagers; her husband is an engineer. She has always had a tendency to anxiety and mild negative mood, but the symptoms have become worse over the past six months, with crying episodes once or twice a week, usually in the evenings, for no specific reason she can identify. Her score on the Hamilton Depression Rating Scale is moderate, at 22. She has begun wakening at 4 a.m. several days a week; she is able to get back to sleep about half the time. Her appetite has increased, and she has gained

10 pounds. She feels fatigued most of the time. She is not suicidal, but she says she feels hopeless and lacks interest in her usual activities. She was active in a community group but has not participated for several months. Her mother also had chronic problems with anxiety, and her father was an alcoholic who may have been depressed at times. She recalls being criticized a lot by her mother, but she was never abused. Her health has been generally good, except for hypertension and episodes of chronic back pain for which no specific cause has been found. She says she drinks only occasionally. Medications include an antihypertensive, ibuprofen, and a PRN narcotic for pain. She uses Valium about three nights a week for sleep. Her husband is working two jobs to get money for the children's education. Her daughter is doing well in school, but Ms. D is worried about her son. He was arrested for underage drinking about six months ago, but he is on track to graduate from high school in June. Her diagnoses are major depression, marital and family problems, chronic pain, and possible substance abuse.

That brief case summary contains most of the facts that you would find in her medical record. But it does not say much about what set off her depression.

In response to more questions, she said her symptoms had worsened after a fight in which her husband had criticized her for "lying around all the time and not keeping track of the kids." When she began crying uncontrollably, he left the house, slamming the door. He called the next day to say he would be away on a business trip. She suspects that he might be seeing another woman but says she does not really want to know. Nonetheless, she ruminates all day about who her husband might be with, whether he will leave her, and what she will do if he does. She does not dare to confront him for fear that he will demand a divorce and blame her for their son's drinking in order to get custody.

Such heart-rending stories made my fancy statistical models seem cold and empty. Even the clinical summary in the medical chart often didn't quite get to the kernel of a person's problem. The stories we constructed in our team meetings did, but were they correct?

Tuesday nights I often went home with my head spinning, eager to pour a stiff drink. It was all so confusing. With my scientist hat on in the morning, I was discovering how groups of people with and without depression differed. When I put on my clinician's hat in the afternoon, all that went out the window as I joined my colleagues to weave the particularities of an individual's life into a story that would explain that person's depression. Neither approach was fully satisfying.

The Rector's Solution

Browsing online, I found a very old article that relieved my confusion. In May 1894, the philosopher Wilhelm Windelband gave the rector's welcome speech to inaugurate the 273rd year of the University of Strasbourg.[2] He skipped the bragging you usually hear from American university presidents about their institutions. He didn't even mention a sports team or thank generous donors. Instead, he gave a short talk that established and explained a profound distinction between two different kinds of explanation. One is based on general laws that are true in all times and instances; examples include the laws of gravity and economics. The other traces a history of specific events that explains how something specific came to be the way it is now; examples include the origins of our moon and the origins of the United States as a nation.

He gave those two kinds of explanations fancy names. Explanations based on general laws that are always true he called *nomothetic* (*nomos* refers to laws, *thetic* to a thesis). Explanations based on historical sequences that occur only once he called *idiographic* (*idio* refers to individual unique events, *graphic* to description). You can call them generalizations and narratives if you like, but nomothetic and idiographic are wonderful technical terms.

Tuesday mornings I had been doing nomothetic science without knowing it, trying to extract generalized laws about the causes of depression from masses of data about groups of people. Tuesday afternoons I used an idiographic approach to try to understand how a sequence of unique events resulted in an individual having these symptoms now. My confusion resulted from failing to realize that idiographic and nomothetic explanations are different beasts.

In 1899, Hugo Münsterberg introduced the distinction to the New World by featuring it in his presidential address to the American Psychological Association.[3] However, it got wide recognition only after the 1937 publication of the book *Personality* by his student Gordon Allport, the father of modern social psychology. Although he advocated integrating both approaches, Allport gained fame for advocating an idiographic "science of the individual." He wrote:

> Psychology has been striving to make of itself a completely nomothetic discipline. The idiographic sciences, such as history, biography and literature . . . endeavor to understand some *particular* event in nature or in society. A psychology of the individual would essentially be idiographic.[4]

Idiographic explanations are the foundation for much current work in the humanities, and they persist in psychology and sociology as "qualitative research." But individual narratives have faded to oblivion in psychiatry. They have not just faded; they have been aggressively purged, despite their persistence wherever clinicians gather to discuss cases. Many journals don't even allow publication of case studies. Idiographic explanations are the embarrassing wayward sibling of the far more successful nomothetic approach, with its objective definitions, quantifiable variables, repeatable experiments, statistical generalizations, and big grants.

Some clinicians skip asking about personal details. They check symptoms on a list, put patients into diagnostic categories, and then recommend whatever treatment has been shown to help patients with that diagnosis. This nomothetic approach saves time, effort, and the emotional entanglements that ensue from creating relationships with individuals. Fewer midnight phone calls. Other clinicians try to understand how each patient came to have his or her particular problem. Here are a few sample idiographic narratives that connect motives, strategies, and events to explain the depression of individuals.

Ms. W is a middle-aged woman with a strong family history of depression and a long history of dysthymia and generalized anxiety. Over the past six months, she has become depressed and lost interest in her job and in sex. Only her children are still important to her, but they have become increasingly demanding as she has become more withdrawn. Her husband does not know how to help her and has become more and more distant.

Ms. X has always been angry with her father, blaming him for leaving the family when she was young, resulting in her being raised by a mother who was often away working and who was depressed when she was at home. The patient continues to be angry at men in general and resentful and depressed when her husband's work requires weeklong trips.

Ms. Y has had problems with sleep resulting mostly from chronic pain but also from anxiety. About ten years ago she began using benzodiazepines for sleep, and she now cannot sleep well without them. Sometimes she adds a drink to her pill in the evening. She finds it hard to get up in the morning, and she is tired all day, sometimes getting in trouble for taking naps at work. Her husband berates her, saying she is not doing enough housework and is neglecting the children.

Ms. Z has always dedicated her life to her children, much to the consternation of her husband, who feels left out. This was satisfying to her for years, but as her children have gotten older, they have begun getting into trouble and refusing to talk to her about their problems. She has long been distant from her husband, but lack of closeness with her children makes her feel helpless and hopeless as she realizes that they are likely to get into serious trouble.

As you may well have guessed as you read those four narratives, they are all about the same person, Ms. D, whom we met at the start of this chapter. All five explanations are plausible. If presented at a case conference by a distinguished professor, each one could be convincing. This is a problem. A big problem. If we have no method for distinguishing true from false stories, we are not doing science. We have no such method. Now what?

One approach is to treat each narrative as a different hypothesis and see which one best matches the evidence. That leads to interesting discussions; however, no single story is completely correct, and each one highlights relevant factors. Can we throw them all into a pot and call it a complete explanation? No. Some factors are more important than others, and different stories propose different causal connections.

Idiographic explanations can be scientific; they are routine in astronomy and geology. Cosmology relies on the general laws of physics to explain stars and black holes in general, but to explain a specific blue dwarf or red giant star requires discovering the sequence of events in the development, decline, and death of a particular star. The laws of gravity are necessary to explain our moon, but they are not sufficient to explain how a particular moon came to exist. Ours could have been formed from consolidated dust or by a captured asteroid, but substantial evidence suggests that a Mars-sized mass (Thedia) grazed Earth about 4.5 billion years ago, knocking off a piece of our planet that eventually became our moon.[5]

Geology also routinely uses idiographic explanations. Explaining a valley requires applying the general laws of gravity, hydraulics, and climatology to a particular sequence of events in a particular place. Some valleys arise from glacial movement, others from erosion, and others from shifting continental plates. Each valley has its own explanation, sometimes involving several causes.

Alas, idiographic explanations are more problematic for psychology than for cosmology or geology. The laws of behavior are less specific than the laws of gravity, and manifold causes interact to create people who choose and shape their own environments. Some general laws are useful. The famous opening sentence of Jane Austen's *Pride and Prejudice* is often cited as an example: "It is a truth universally acknowledged, that a single man in possession of a good fortune, must be in want of a wife." But Bingley, that man in possession of a good fortune, could have been gay or a cad or a solitary scholar with no interest in finding a wife. A method of predicting an individual's emotions and behavior needs to incorporate the idiographic details of that individual into a nomothetic framework. There is no great way to do that, but an evolutionary perspective on emotions provides a good way. First, however, the standard approach.

Studying Life Stress

Most psychiatric research searches for nomothetic generalizations about why some people get sick while others don't. Stress is recognized as a precipitant, but the emphasis has been on what makes some people more vulnerable to stress: genes, brain chemistry, early rearing, traumatic experiences, personality, and habits of thinking. The flip side of this approach is to look at people who are "resilient," those who carry on despite dire experiences. The implication is that there is something wrong with vulnerable people and it would be good if we could find ways to make more people resilient. Either way, it is all about the Person. What about the Situation?

The role of situations in causing symptoms usually gets simplified to stress, and stress usually measured in terms of life events. This glosses over how an individual's appraisal of the meaning of events gives rise to symptoms, but it avoids messy problems. If you ask people what is causing anxiety or depression, you hear stories about abuse, abandonment, attacks, and all manner of adverse life events. How bad is bad enough to cause a problem? How do you count the events?

Psychiatrists Thomas Holmes and Richard Rahe initiated a new era in life events research in the 1960s. Their group had long followed the lead of Adolf Meyer, a founder of American psychiatry, by creating a life chart showing the dates of major life events and how they corresponded to symptoms. However, those data were hard to use in research. So they instead gave people a list of forty-three possible life events and asked them to check off the ones they had experienced. Just counting the number of events predicted who would get sick, even from infections.[6] By quantifying objective events, the Schedule of Recent Experiences led to rapid progress and hundreds of publications.

However, there is much more to an event than whether it happened or not. To get at the details, London researchers George Brown and Tirril Harris created the Life Events and Difficulties Scale.[7] It takes hours to administer, and learning to use it takes weeks. The results of each interview are transcribed and then coded by a team that did not see the patient. At the end of the process, each event is rated as "severe" or not. This painstaking method, applied to 458 women in London, led to solid conclusions. In addition to those presented in chapter 6, they showed that factors such as having support from a partner were strongly protective. It is wonderful research, but the instrument is unwieldy and rarely used.

Methods of measuring life stress have developed steadily since then,[8,9] but substantial challenges remain.[10] Long interviews are expensive, so most research uses checklists. However, the big problem is the very notion of "stress." The word fosters the notion that stress is one thing, a misconception that is magnified by the tendency to think that it can be measured by levels of stress hormones. Trying to collapse the problems in a person's motivational structure into a number measuring the severity of "stress" is like trying to collapse all brain changes into a single measure of "level of brain activity."

Some attention has been paid to the nature of stressors. For instance, events causing humiliation or entrapment are especially likely to cause depression, as noted already.[11,12] However, emotions don't arise from events; they arise from a person's appraisal of what events mean to his or her ability to reach personal goals.[13,14,15]

Evolution and Understanding Individuals

Some imagine that an evolutionary approach must emphasize generalizations about human nature, but it instead forces acknowledgment of diversity. There is no single normal genome, brain, or personality. Variation is intrinsic. Debates have raged for decades about evolution and human nature. Has selection shaped a common core that makes human nature a sensible idea? Or is the idea empty because people and the cultures that shape them vary so much?

The goals we pursue are universal: food, friends, sex, safety, status, and, most of all, offspring—healthy, happy offspring, on their way to reproducing themselves. However, people prioritize these goals differently and pursue them in diverse ways. John puts all his energy into getting fame and admiration and does not even date. Mary cares about her children far more than anything else. Jack spends most of his life's effort trying to make himself physically attractive. Sally wants mostly to get rich, and she is succeeding, at the cost of friends, family, love, and health. Donna works seventy hours a week, half at her job, the rest caring for her aging mother. Sam plays eighteen holes of golf each day and spends evenings talking about his games. Rachel is devoted to church mission work that she hopes will provide, for others, the peace and meaning her faith provides for her.

Most of us try to lead somewhat balanced lives, allocating our resources across many life enterprises in pursuit of many goals. There is never enough time and energy for everything, but we cope. In the psychiatry emergency room, however, you see many people in situations that are genuinely impossible. The kids are sick, their father abandoned the family, the car won't start, there is no money to repair it or get a babysitter, and the boss said last week that one more absence would be the end of the job. It is not just an event or stress that causes symptoms; it is a situation in which it is impossible to do what must be done. I recall trying to help a young couple with depression and marital problems. They both made minimum wage at the same grocery store, working alternate twelve-hour shifts so one of them could always be at home taking care of their three young children. They saw each other only coming and going and on occasional holidays, and their debts and frustrations mounted with each passing month.

Strategies for influencing other people differ as dramatically as values and goals. Peter controls his employees by constantly reminding them that they can be fired at any moment. Sally is beloved for her warmth and sense of humor. Dan negotiates everything and expects others to be as rational and dutiful as he is. Sam's threatening manner makes others wary of crossing him. Gertrude is friendly and congenial, but those who compete with her become the targets of sly gossip. Bill does not always pull his weight in a group, but his sense of humor makes him nonetheless welcome. Call it personality if you want to, but the diversity of how people influence others makes life interesting and studies of emotions difficult.

In addition to differences in values, goals, and personality, people have different responses to success and failure. Some attribute outcomes to their own efforts, which is fine when they are successful but paralyzing when they are not. Some routinely blame others. Others hardly acknowledge failure; they deny and carry on. Still others quit quickly and shift their efforts to something else.

Such diverse goals, strategies, and personalities make it difficult, at best, to predict a person's emotional state. The nomothetic approach measures dozens of things about groups of individuals and analyzes the numbers to try to predict who will feel what and when. The resulting generalizations don't predict what emotion a specific individual is likely to be experiencing now. Idiographic explanations are richer but unreliable. Psychotherapists listen to each patient for hours. Novelists craft words and plots for months.

The rest of us tell and listen to stories to try to make sense of our lives and those of others. Scientists studying emotions wonder what to do.

The Review of Social Systems

If you consult a doctor about a general symptom such as fatigue, she is likely to ask you a series of questions: Do you have a chronic cough? How is your digestion? Can you climb stairs easily? The questions may seem unrelated to your complaint, but your answers may point to a problem in your respiratory, gastrointestinal, or cardiovascular system. Your stomach pain may indicate a bleeding ulcer that is causing anemia that explains your fatigue. To identify such possible factors, doctors conduct what is called a "review of systems" by asking a standard set of about thirty questions. A review of systems is essential to avoid missing a possible cause.

A comparably systematic Review Of Social Systems (ROSS) is equally essential to identify the sources of emotional symptoms. However, what systems need to be reviewed? Different social systems don't have well-defined boundaries the way the liver and kidneys do. However, scientists who study animal behavior recognize several different kinds of resources organisms seek. Personal resources such as health, attractiveness, and abilities are essential (♟). Food, shelter, and material resources such as money (💲) are essential. Modern humans get those resources by working at jobs or other social roles (⚒). Efforts to find, impress, and care for mates require substantial effort (♥). So do efforts to help and protect offspring and other relatives (👪). Finally, having allies and roles with recognized status in a group (☺) are keys to Darwinian fitness. Six kinds of resources: ♟ 💲 ⚒ ♥ 👪 ☺.

Efforts to get one resource take time and effort away from getting others. Foraging far from home will result in more food but will compromise safety. Time caring for children is not available for working or impressing potential mates. Brains generally make good decisions about how to allocate effort even without sophisticated conscious thinking. All animals make such decisions, from aphids to zebras.

Emotions are one part of the decision-making system. What causes a particular emotion in a specific person can be hard to determine, but a systematic search is nonetheless essential. Dozens of questionnaires and structured interviews are available for gathering relevant information, but few of them attempt to capture the dynamics of how emotions emerge as humans pursue their idiosyncratic goals. Short questionnaires never get to specifics. Long interviews get reams of rich information, but they are impractical to administer and difficult to summarize.

What is needed is something like an Apgar score.[16] Virginia Apgar was an obstetrician who recognized the need for a simple system to record the condition of a newborn. Her name provides a convenient acronym for five categories of information: Appearance, Pulse, Grimace, Activity, and Respiration. Each is recorded as 0, 1, or 2 depending on the infant's condition. This simple score has proved invaluable in documenting an infant's condition and predicting outcomes.

The resources crucial for humans are the same as those for other organisms, with one addition: people have specialized social roles that others value and often pay for, that is, occupations. **SOCIAL** provides an acronym as memorable as **Apgar** to keep track of the resources that need to be considered when doing a ROSS.

REVIEW OF SOCIAL SYSTEMS

Social resources, including friends, groups, and social influence ☺

Occupation; this is often paid work, but many other social roles are also valued by others ⚒

Children and family, including relatives 👪

Income and sources of material resources 💲

Abilities, appearance, health, time, and other personal resources 👤

Love and sex in an intimate relationship ♥

An analysis of a person's motivational structure requires answers to several questions about each kind of resource. Do you have secure ways to get sufficient amounts of this resource? How important is this resource to you? Is there a gap between what you want and what you have? What are the main things you are trying to do, get, or prevent in this area? How are you going about your efforts? Any recent losses, gains, or other changes? Any big opportunities or threats on the horizon? Are you faced with difficult decisions about what to do in this area? Is there something important you are trying to accomplish that isn't working out? Overall, what is the outlook for your efforts in this area?

This kind of comprehensive assessment of a person's motivational structure is valuable. An even longer structured interview, of the sort that Eric Klinger has suggested, is valuable for research.[17] However, a full ROSS takes at least an hour. In keeping with the theme that time and energy are always limited, it isn't always possible to ask all these questions about each domain. For busy clinicians, something as short and simple as the Apgar score is essential.

The aim is to identify problems that may be causing symptoms. That requires determining, for each area of life, the adequacy of resource availability and the magnitude of problems. People with plenty of resources can have plenty of problems, so resources and problems need to be recorded separately. For instance, attractive young people who can certainly find a mate are sometimes reduced to mental tatters by ambivalence about whether to marry a current partner. People whose abilities, attractiveness, and general health are all fine now may nonetheless struggle because of fears about their future. I recall a brilliant scientist who came for treatment because he was paralyzed by fears of death. At age thirty-five, he was already a world expert on atherosclerosis, with tenure at a leading university and invitations to travel the world. What no one knew, however, was that his father and his siblings had all died before age forty from heart attacks. Then there are the millionaires whose gambling debts make it impossible to keep up with a mortgage, and the accomplished people in every field who are failures relative to their outsized expectations.

A numerical score like that of the Apgar can be useful for research, but I discourage summing resource scores in a general setting because it can be misleading and hurtful. It is bad enough that people rate the appearance of others on a scale of 1 to 10; using numbers to compare people's life resources is worse. However, recognizing the complex realities of individual motivational structures is essential for understanding the origins of symptoms. To get the needed information in a way that is gentle but efficient, here are some questions that I use, always adapted, of course, to the individual.

QUESTIONS FOR INQUIRING ABOUT THE SITUATION IN EACH LIFE DOMAIN

Social: Are there friends and groups that you spend time with? Do they appreciate you? Any big problems?

Occupation: How are things going in your job (or other major social role, such as parenting or volunteer work)? Is it satisfying? Is it secure?

Children and family: Do you have children? How are they doing? For adults who don't have children, I ask: Is that fine for you? Are there family members you keep in close touch with? How are they doing?

Income: How are things going financially? Is debt a problem?

Abilities and appearance: Do you have any major health problems or concerns about your appearance or abilities?

Love and sex: How are things going in your main relationship?

In addition to recording the person's access to each resource and the size of problems in each area, I also use one or two emotion words to summarize the overall situation for each area. It is fascinating and revealing to note that we have words so well suited to the diversity of situations that arise in pursuing goals.

EMOTIONAL STATES FOR THE SITUATIONS IN EACH DOMAIN

- **Excited** by new opportunities
- **Satisfied** and secure in this area for the most part
- **Hopeful** that future success will relieve current dissatisfactions
- **Dissatisfied** by the inability to accomplish goals in this area
- **Worried** about threatened losses
- **Sad** after losses
- **Confused** about what to do in this area
- **Frustrated** by obstacles that block progress toward goals
- **Demoralized** by slow or no progress toward important goals
- **Waiting** for a better time to pursue goals in this area
- **Accepting** of the inability to reach goals in this area
- **Trapped** in the pursuit of an unreachable goal
- **Disengaged** emotionally after failing to reach goals in this area
- **Uninterested** because goals in this area are not relevant now

As we discussed cases in clinic meetings, we sometimes used the ROSS to try to better understand people's life situations. It changed our views of many patients. Some with severe mental illness nonetheless had friends, jobs, relatives, income, abilities, and a stable partner. One woman with severe obsessive-compulsive disorder spent hours washing her hands each day. Her husband was frustrated with the time she wasted and the limits her symptoms imposed on their social life, but he was supportive in general. Despite her symptoms, she worked, took care of her children, and kept up with her friends. Such patients usually get better.

Others were in much worse situations. One desperately depressed young woman had severe multiple sclerosis. She was living alone in a small apartment on meager disability payments, unable to get around because she could not operate her wheelchair. She had no occupation, friends, relatives, groups, or places to go. Antidepressants don't help much for people in such straits.

The ROSS is not a substitute for validated instruments that measure symptoms or life events, and it does not elicit the same kind of rich information as a long clinical interview. It does, however, bring idiographic information into a nomothetic framework. The ROSS can be used to search for the causes of aversive emotions, the same way general physicians use a review of systems to search for possible causes of pain.

Methods like the ROSS that combine idiographic and nomothetic approaches[18,19] should predict treatment response and rates of relapse better than purely idiographic or purely nomothetic measures. Categories of motivational situations gleaned from the ROSS may help demonstrate the effectiveness of antidepressant drugs and could strengthen neuroscience studies. For instance, brain scans of people whose depression results from a recent loss may well be different from those whose depression results from pursuing an unreachable goal and may be different yet from those of people whose depression has been lifelong for no obvious reason. The benefits of an antidepressant may differ markedly for people whose depression results from pursuing an unreachable career goal as opposed to those who are bereaved or suffering from an infection. The cost to bring yet another modestly effective antidepressant to market is about $2 billion.[20] It would cost only about 1 percent of that amount to develop the ROSS to the point where it could be used to assess drug effectiveness and neuroscience findings for people in different life situations.

People in social traps with no way out are at high risk of suicide; using the ROSS to identify them could be lifesaving. A San Francisco social worker, Helen Herrick, organized a summer experience to encourage undergraduate students to consider mental health professions. I was one of the lucky participants. We all lived on the grounds of mental hospitals and were assigned to "observe as much as you can." The experience was transformative. It succeeded in convincing me to become a psychiatrist but forever prevented me from taking only a psychiatrist's point of view. Learning about Herrick's research with the families of Golden Gate Bridge suicide victims was also a huge influence. She initially took the nomothetic approach of trying to find the factors all victims had in common. But after hundreds of interviews she concluded that no generalization would ever be adequate. Some people jumped while drunk or showing off, others to inflict guilt. Some sought revenge, some to join a lost loved one, some because of anxiety, depression, or psychosis, others because of dementia or terminal cancer. She concluded that individuals need to be understood as individuals. She convinced me.

Data from the ROSS can be diagrammed to illustrate the flows of effort and resources in a person's life. For instance, the upper left box in the diagram below illustrates an ordinary complicated life, in which every kind of resource is contributing to every other kind of resource in a complex matrix. The upper right shows a workaholic who puts all energy and time into working and getting money. The lower left shows someone whose effort goes almost exclusively into taking care of children, with investment in occupation and finances only as a means to that end. Finally, the party animal spends most of life's effort trying to create status and

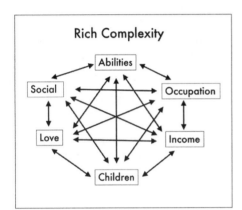
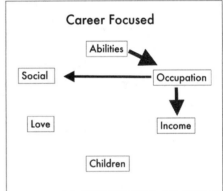
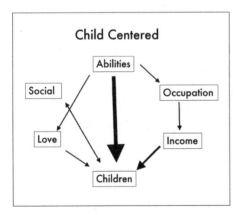
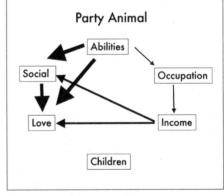

Some Patterns of Resource Allocation

relationships, mostly sexual relationships. These are all very different lives, with different events having very different influences on emotions.

Know Thy Patient—So What?

Back to the other half of the equation: What about the person? For about half of the patients I saw in clinic, their current life situations did not seem very relevant to their symptoms. Social anxiety, for many patients, was a lifelong problem that was not much influenced by events. Some people with depression have always had symptoms; others were fine until a specific trauma set everything off. Researchers and clinicians are fully aware that most problems arise when a potentially vulnerable person encounters a stressful situation. This is called a *stress diathesis model*, *diathesis* being a fancy word for "vulnerability."[21,22]

Sensitive types have emotional reactions that others would not. People who care enormously about their work have symptoms when there's a problem in that area, not so much when there's a problem in their marriages. The well-known psychologist and positive psychology researcher Edward Diener did a study to confirm this. He showed that changes in areas that are especially important to an individual have more influence on subjective well-being.[23]

Instead of attributing symptoms to stress or an event or characteristics of a person, an evolutionary view suggests an approach like that used in the rest of medicine. Joint pain, for example, can have many causes. It can result from repeated motions at work, abnormal posture at a desk, or some special exercise regimen. Other joint pain is caused by infection, rheumatoid arthritis, or lupus erythematosus. Doctors routinely investigate not just how "stress" on a joint and inflammation might arouse symptoms but the specific kinds of situations and mechanisms that cause pain in a specific joint in a specific individual.

Some life situations cause certain kinds of symptoms so reliably that they might well qualify as diagnostic categories. Parents of children with cancer. People whose spouses are having affairs. Single people with married sexual partners. People whose spouses are alcoholic, violent, or both. People experiencing sexual harassment. People accused of sexual harassment. Single parents with insufficient money or social support. People struggling with a chronic debilitating illness. Employees whose bosses demean them. When we talk with friends, and when clinicians talk about cases at team meetings, they rely on such categories. Conducting a ROSS offers an opportunity to measure such situations and analyze how they affect symptoms and treatment responses.

But these analyses are still far too simple. People have dramatically different personalities. They create the situations they find themselves in. The situations they find themselves in further create the person. Very often those situations are self-stabilizing. People who are resentful and angry provoke anger in those around them, confirming their view of the world. People who see good in everyone often find it, sometimes because they have created it. But trying to shift an individual's worldview is like trying to replace the girders in a high-rise building. No amount of logic or argument helps much. What works is experiencing a kind of relationship that is different from all previous ones. Sometimes that happens with love, sometimes in relationships at school or work. It can happen in good intensive psychotherapy, especially when patients begin to recognize how they create the situations that torment them. People can change in fundamental ways. Helping them do that is difficult but satisfying work.

CHAPTER 9

GUILT AND GRIEF:
THE PRICE OF GOODNESS AND LOVE

Nature, when she formed man for society, endowed him with an original desire to please, and an original aversion to offend his brethren.

—Adam Smith,
The Theory of Moral Sentiments, 1759[1]

Our capacities for morality and loving, trusting relationships are human traits as distinctive as language and extraordinary intelligence. We view warm, secure relationships as normal and natural, so explanatory efforts go mostly toward relationship problems. Clinicians attribute them to relationship dynamics and characteristics of individuals, including mental disorders that often wreck marriages and families. The focus, as in the rest of medicine, is on why things go wrong for some people.

By now you will anticipate the more fundamental questions an evolutionary view encourages: Why are humans social at all? Why do we feel it is so important to be a part of a group? Why do we care so much about what people think about us? How does the capacity to feel guilt give advantages? Why do we experience grief? Answers to these questions require turning the usual question on its head: How can the tendency to help others possibly provide a selective advantage? The mystery is not why some people have relationship problems; the mystery is how love and goodness are possible for organisms shaped to maximize Darwinian fitness.

For most of the twentieth century, biologists assumed that cooperative tendencies evolved because they were good for groups. Groups with more altruistic individuals grow faster than other groups, so it seemed obvious that this would select for cooperative tendencies. This naive view met its demise in 1966, when George Williams pointed out that especially altruistic individuals would have fewer offspring than others, so alleles for altruism would be selected out. Debate about the idea was mostly within biology until the 1976 publication of *The Selfish Gene* by Richard Dawkins[2] ignited an intellectual firestorm that still smolders.[3,4,5]

Many voiced outrage, accusing Dawkins of saying that altruism was not possible. Others were gleeful, finally seeing support for their cynical view of life. Reactions to the controversy provided examples of every possible psychodynamic defense.[6] The final paragraphs of Dawkins's book suggested that knowledge about selfish genes should allow us to better control ourselves and transcend our impulses, but that was overwhelmed by his metaphor of robots obeying the dictates of selfish genes.

The idea that our brains were shaped to get us to behave in the interests of our genes is deeply disturbing. On first grasping it, I lay awake for nights wondering if my moral impulses were just manipulations at the behest of my genes. The core idea seemed necessarily true, but it was at odds with the guilt, social sensitivity, and genuine goodness I thought I saw in patients, friends, and myself. Were my attempts to do good, in the clinic and elsewhere, just subtle ways my genes were getting me to advance their interests? Even guilt and moral passions appeared to be selfish, from a gene's point of view. It seemed as if Dawkins had found the evolutionary explanation for original sin.

This not an arcane academic issue. What people believe changes how they behave. At the peak of debates about selfish genes, I sat by a fireplace one evening with evolution-minded colleagues planning a project. Each said in turn without apology, "I will help, but only if it is to my personal advantage." The belief that we are selected for selfishness is a social corrosive. Its spread would make life more lonely and brutal than it already is. I fear that the idea may be spreading and that it may already have changed social reality.

Economists have taken this seriously; Matt Ridley and Robert Frank soon weighed in about the implications.[7,8] Frank found that taking an economics class decreased the willingness of students to contribute to public radio and to donate blood.[9]

In the clinic it is obvious that what patients believe about human nature influences their lives and problems. To get a quick take on personality, I use a one-question test: "Could you tell me how you view human nature?" The answer most encouraging for therapeutic success is "Most people can be good or bad; a lot depends on the situation." But the more common answers display the strong human tendency to judge most everything, including our whole species, as generally good or generally bad. Patients who say something like "Most people are pretty good; they try to do what is right," tend to be neurotic and to do well in treatment relationships. But those who say "Most people are out for themselves, but what else can you expect?" tend to have problems with close relationships.

Such beliefs are self-sustaining. People capable of trust pair up with similar others and are likely to have relationships that confirm their positive expectations. They shy away from cynical types. So, people who think that others are self-interested tend to have untrusting and often untrustworthy associates who confirm their views. I recall a dinner conversation about altruism at which the cynical distinguished visiting speaker said, "So, have any of you ever really experienced any altruistic behavior in your entire lives?" No one knew what to say.

People defend their worldviews. Those who believe people are basically bad discount the possibility of altruism and trusting relationships. In therapy, they may go to considerable effort to confirm their beliefs. "You are just doing it for the money" is a routine test. Midnight phone calls demanding a house call to prevent suicide take the challenge to another level.

Richard Alexander, the University of Michigan biologist who wrote one of the first books about the evolution of human morality,[10] reported trying to convince his mentor that he was altruistic by describing going out of his way to avoid stepping on a line of ants. His mentor responded, "It might have been, until you bragged about it."

Viewing social life as a product of self-interest is anathema for others. I have asked many religious people why they oppose teaching evolutionary biology. Their most common concern is that it will undermine motivations for moral behavior. There is little evidence for this. Nonreligious people are about as likely as religious people to get a divorce, go to prison, or otherwise violate social rules.[11,12,13] However, many people have told me that their ability to control their selfish impulses depends on their belief in God. If that works for them, why would anyone want to interfere?

George Williams was more disturbed by his own idea than most anyone else was. After spending years considering the implications, he came to the darkest possible conclusion: "Natural selection . . . can honestly be described as a process for maximizing short-sighted selfishness. . . . I account for morality as an accidental capability produced, in its boundless stupidity, by a biological process that is normally opposed to the expression of such a capability."[14] The irony is that George was an immensely moral man. He could have made a fuss to claim credit for the idea of kin selection based on a 1957 paper he wrote with his wife, Doris,[15] but he didn't. He was always generous in his work with me. But he saw no alternative to the logic that selection shapes behavior to maximize individual fitness.[16]

Despite weeks of discussion, George never convinced me of his view. Perhaps my cultural background makes me unable to accept an unpleasant truth. As the grandson of missionaries, with plenty of early exposure to churches, I have always assumed that most people have inherent strong moral capacities. Choosing a helping profession exposed me to many others who were motivated to do good. Working with patients who have anxiety disorders further shaped or distorted my view of human nature. Most such patients are inhibited, guilty, socially sensitive people who try hard to do what is right. Subsequent experiences have given me a more worldly view. I didn't know it was possible for someone to look you in the eye and make a commitment with no intention of keeping it. But like other people, I defend my core schemas, so I am more aware of moral behaviors and wishes to please others than examples of deception and selfishness. Others have had very different and less fortunate life experiences.

To try to resolve the conflict between theory and observations, I joined the throng of scientists searching for evolutionary explanations for cooperation and moral emotions. Many explanations have been proposed, and most authors advocate for one over the others. This quest for simplicity causes much unnecessary controversy when, as is the case here, several different explanations are all relevant. Fair warning: the following review of possible explanations concludes that many are important, and I will, like most everyone else, suggest that one is especially so.

First, a brief executive summary of the origins of cooperation. (1)

Benefits to groups of unrelated individuals cannot explain the evolution of extreme human social abilities. (2) Benefits to kin who share the same genes explain most altruistic behavior. (3) Much apparent cooperation among nonrelatives is just individuals doing things that help themselves and that also happen to help others. (4) Extensive cooperation among nonrelatives is explained mostly by reciprocial favor trading. (5) Reciprocity systems shape costly traits for establishing a good reputation. (6) The previous five explanations explain most social behavior in most organisms, but not quite all. They represent a spectacular fundamental advance in human knowledge even though they cannot fully explain human capacities for commitment and moral behavior. Important additional explanations are offered by cultural group selection, commitment, and social selection. First, however, a bit more about group selection.

Group Selection Redux

Some scholars argue that group selection works after all.[17] Classic group selection is the process that increases the frequency of alleles that induce behaviors that decrease an individual's fitness but that benefit a group of unrelated individuals. Groups with more individuals who are willing to sacrifice for the group grow faster than other groups do, so group selection is possible. However, alleles for such tendencies can persist only when three special circumstances are met: groups with more cooperative individuals must grow much faster than groups with fewer cooperative individuals; individuals with alleles for helping must reproduce only a little less than others in the group who do not have such alleles; and finally, exchanges of individuals between the groups must be limited, otherwise nonhelping individuals will move into the group and their alleles will displace the ones for helping.[18,19] These conditions rarely occur together. Group selection of this kind is weak and unable to explain costly traits. An essay by Steven Pinker explains why in crystal-clear detail.[20] However, most people, including some evolutionary psychiatrists, find group selection intuitively correct and emotionally appealing, so I will say a bit more about its limits before describing alternative explanations of our extraordinary capacities for cooperation and morality.

The consensus among scientists is that group selection among nonrelatives cannot explain human genetic tendencies that make morality possible, but controversies persist. In part this is because models of the evolution of cooperation can be framed equally well in terms of kin selection or group selection.[21,22] Most experts find kin selection far more useful;[23] however, a few famous scientists have argued that it is irrelevant.[24,25] I agree with the vast majority of scientists[26] who find kin selection a profoundly useful explanation.

Despite its intuitive appeal, examples of group selection are few. Some apparent examples mostly document its weakness. For instance, chickens in cages peck one another, causing injuries that slow their growth. Breeding chickens for a few generations using eggs from the cages with the least pecking shapes more cooperative chickens that grow faster.[27,28] This is real group selection. However, it is not natural selection. In fact, it illustrates that no such group selection happened to chickens previously. Except in very special circumstances, genetic tendencies that benefit the group are eliminated if they decrease the reproduction of individuals.

Sex ratios can be influenced by natural selection, and groups with almost all females grow twice as fast as those with one-half males—only females can have offspring, after all. But most sex ratios are close to fifty-fifty. The great geneticist Ronald Fisher explained why in his 1930 classic, *The Genetical Theory of Natural Selection.*[29] He asked what sex of offspring would maximize transmission of an individual's genes. In a group with almost all females, the average male offspring would have many times more offspring than the average female. In a group with almost all males, the average female would do better. Having offspring of whatever sex is in short supply maximizes an individual's genetic contributions to future generations, at a substantial cost to the rate of growth of the group.

Fisher's logic is illustrated by pub choices on a Saturday night. When looking for women partners, men don't go to a sports pub; the odds are terrible there. A pub with ladies' night is a much better bet. For women, the logic is reversed. The prevalence of fifty-fifty sex ratios demonstrates the dominance of individual selection relative to group selection.

Then there are forests. Magnificent towering tree trunks testify to the waste that results because selection maximizes the interests of genes instead of species. All available solar energy could be harvested by clusters of leaves close to the ground. Trees that cooperated could maximize energy collection without spending huge resources to grow tall trunks. However, each tree competes to get more sunlight than other trees. They even know when to compete harder. Light reflected from adjacent green leaves shifts many saplings into desperate competition mode, putting every ounce of effort into growing tall as fast as possible, at the risk of breakage. Even trees of the same species put most of their life's effort into competing to be higher than other trees. The exceptions are instructive. Aspen flourish in tight groves of modest height. You can guess why: they are all clones with the same genes, so there is no need to compete; they also cooperate to create dense shade in that keeps competitors in the dark.

The cells in our body are cooperative for the same reason: they all start off genetically identical, thanks to a process that strips DNA down to a single strand from each parent, one in the egg, one in the sperm. The cells in our bodies are like 40 trillion identical twins. Alleles can get into the next generation only by doing things that benefit the body as a whole. The exception proves the rules. When cells replicate without regard for the good of the whole, the result is cancer.[30] Natural selection has shaped powerful mechanisms to inhibit such rogue replication, including a mechanism called apoptosis that induces suicide in cells that are replicating out of control.

Cooperation Explained (Mostly)

As noted in chapter 3, William Hamilton's discovery of kin selection revolutionized our understanding of social behavior. When he came up with it, he wasn't a great biologist; he was a lonely graduate student who had spent years pondering how evolution could explain sterile honeybee workers, which die when they sting to protect the hive.[31] He proposed a doctoral thesis on the topic but was told that the project was unacceptable. So he submitted a manuscript describing his idea to a scientific journal.[32] The editor, John Maynard Smith, immediately recognized that Hamilton had solved a problem that had vexed biologists for decades. Maynard Smith quickly published his own article on the idea in the widely read journal *Nature*, christening it "kin selection."[33] This caused a lifetime of bad feelings between the two men. How ironic and sad that selfish competition for priority caused a moral lapse at the origins of scientific studies of altruism. Maynard Smith was an inspiring conversation partner, generous with his patience, as I asked him ignorant question after question about group selection. Hamilton was a distracted genius who was curious about everything, and conversations with him about mental disorders inspired me. The two were eventually able to talk, but the relationship was forever strained. Their hard feelings foreshadowed continuing intense and sometimes mean-spirited conflicts about cooperation that still continue.[34,35,36]

Mutual helping is another potent explanation of social behavior. If two animals groom each other simultaneously, both benefit and there is no opportunity for cheating. If two people turn over a heavy rock, both benefit from anything underneath. Birds that eat ticks off the backs of livestock get a meal and the animals get reduced parasites. Such mutualism is everywhere once you recognize it.[37,38,39,40]

Trading favors explains most helping between nonrelatives. If helping episodes are separated by time or place, cheating is possible. If two people are turning over rocks separately to look for gold, one could secretly pocket the treasure. A person who helps someone else build a shed may or may not get help later when he builds his own shed. If you drive someone to the airport, you may or may not get a lift when you need it. Reciprocal favor trading benefits both parties if cheating can be controlled.

The idea has a long history, but its importance for the biology of social behavior came to attention in a 1971 article by the biologist Robert Trivers.[41] A game called "the prisoner's dilemma" provides a great way to study how people do and don't reciprocate help. It gets its name from the situation in which the police are interviewing two criminal collaborators separately. Each is told that if they confess first (defecting), they will get off easy, but if the other person confesses first, they will get a severe punishment. If neither confesses despite the risk that the other one will defect (both cooperate), both benefit by getting only a moderate punishment. This game lends itself to computer modeling and games you can play with real people. Hundreds of studies have investigated how people trade favors. My friend and colleague the political scientist Robert Axelrod analyzed much of this work in his landmark book *The Evolution of Cooperation*.[42,43]

If the prisoner's dilemma game is played over and over, the best strategy is called tit for tat, that is, doing what the other person did on the previous move. This maximizes benefits when paired with a cooperator (who won't confess) but avoids exploitation if the other person defects. The game usually plays out in long sequences of cooperation, followed by stubbornly persistent bouts of mutual defection, exactly what one sees in many relationships.[44,45,46] Steady cooperation maximizes the combined benefit (3 to each partner in the table below), but one player can get a payoff of 5 by defecting on a turn when the other cooperates.

If the situations that recur in the process of trading favors have fitness consequences, they should have shaped emotions to cope with those situations. They have.[47,48,49,50] After repeated experiences of cooperation, trust and friendship grow. Especially generous behavior arouses gratitude. Anticipated defection arouses suspicion; experiencing a defection arouses anger. Temptation to defect arouses anxiety and defection arouses guilt, both aversive emotions that inhibit hasty selfishness.

If you are tempted to do something that will betray a commitment, anxiety inhibits hasty self-interested behavior. You will be late for work if you give your friend a ride to the airport, but if you owe the person a ride, you need to do it. If you don't, guilt will motivate apologies, and reparations will be needed to reestablish trust. Alternatively, you could try to devalue what the other person provided for you. Most arguments are about who violated what expectations.

EMOTIONS SHAPED TO COPE WITH THE SITUATIONS THAT ARISE IN EXCHANGE RELATIONSHIPS[51]

EMOTIONS AROUSED BY SITUATIONS IN RELATIONSHIPS	OTHER COOPERATES	OTHER DEFECTS
YOU COOPERATE	(3 for each) Friendship Trust	(0 for you, 5 for other) Suspicion (before) Anger (after)
YOU DEFECT	(5 for you, 0 for other) Anxiety (before) Guilt (after)	(1 for each) Disgust Avoidance

Although the reality of social life is far more complex, this simple table provides a useful guide to the origins and utility of social emotions.[52] Anger signals that a betrayal has been recognized and apologies and reparations will be required to keep the relationship going and to avoid spiteful revenge.[53] People who feel they can't leave a relationship are reluctant to express anger, leading to passive-aggressive behavior or sullen withdrawal that limits cooperation and fuels chronic conflict. Such situations are at the core of much neurosis and many marital problems. The psychologists Timothy Ketelaar and Martie Haselton have advanced this construct much further,[54,55,56] but clinical applications remain to be developed.

Something Is Missing

The explanation of social behavior by kin selection, mutual benefits, and trading favors is one of the great scientific advances of our time. Together, they explain almost all cooperation.[57,58,59,60,61,62,63] But not quite all. They have trouble accounting for people who lie awake nights feeling guilty because of a minor misstep no one else knows about. They don't provide a full explanation for the huge sacrifices made in committed relationships. They don't explain fighting to defend the group despite knowing that death is inevitable. And they can't explain why, for every sociopath, there are ten people who worry constantly about how to avoid offending others. Humans have extreme prosocial tendencies that need additional explanations. Providing them is a major academic endeavor that is making progress.[64,65,66,67,68,69,70,71,72,73,74,75,76,77,78,79,80] The key to a general solution comes from recognizing that altruists who associate selectively with other altruists reap advantages compared to others who merely trade favors with random others.

Simple geographical proximity is the simplest mechanism; the offspring of altruists will likely live close to other altruists. This is relevant even for bacteria. Because they divide fast, bacteria are usually surrounded by close relatives, so bacteria that contribute to the common good, for instance by allocating resources to manufacture a substance that digests host cells, derive advantages for their own genes.[81,82]

Humans have many ways to find and stay close to good partners.

Avoiding jerks results in more time spent with generous types. Leaving suboptimal partnerships results in selective association with altruists.[83] Gossip provides invaluable information about whom you can trust.[84] Hiring committees spend hours checking references for good reason. Such models of selective association among altruists are sometimes called group selection, but this creates confusion. As the biologist Stuart West said incisively, "An alternative is to state as simply as possible what they are—models of nonrandom assortment of altruistic genes."[85]

Descriptions of cultural group selection developed by anthropologists Robert Boyd and Peter Richerson provide a major explanation for deep cooperation and intense altruism.[86] Groups with cultural norms to sacrifice for the group grow faster than other groups. Groups can give advantages to individuals who obey the norms, creating selection for the tendency to do what is good for the group. Individuals can benefit the group by punishing cheaters, but rewarding cooperators is usually more effective and less dangerous. A recent article by Richerson and colleagues reviewed extensive evidence for the power of cultural group selection.[87] The article is convincing, but it argues that altruistic behaviors that cannot be explained by group selection, mutualism, kin selection, or reciprocity must be therefore explained by cultural group selection. However, there are at least two other ways that selection can shape capacities for cooperation: commitment and social selection.[88]

Commitment

Commitment is not just keeping promises to a spouse. In game theory, commitment can explain altruistic acts that have no guaranteed or even expected return benefits.[89,90,91,92] The core idea is paradoxical: convincing others that you are committed to some future actions that won't be in your interest can influence their behavior powerfully. Promising to stay with someone in sickness or in health can cement a relationship with a better partner than would otherwise be possible and, hopefully, also get you help when you are sick. Threatening a nuclear response to an attack is far more irrational, but it is a powerful influence if others believe you would do it.

Mutually assured destruction has prevented war so far, but commitment strategies are unstable, so civilization as we know it could end at any time.

Relationships based on commitment are more valuable than those based on reciprocity. Evolutionary psychologists John Tooby and Leda Cosmides have written profoundly about "the banker's paradox."[93] Banks operate on reciprocity only: they are glad to lend you money when you have collateral, but when you have nothing and really need financing, they won't even talk to you.

Relationships based on commitment provide help when people need it most: when they have little to offer in return. The challenge is to convince others that you will, in some future situation, do something that will not be in your own interest. The related challenge is to convince yourself that others will help you when there is no way to enforce the obligation. The solution is to go ahead with non-self-interested actions that demonstrate your commitment. Skip the big game to stay home and help her nurse her cold. Cancel the big presentation to go on the planned vacation. Before you know it, what may have started as a manipulation turns into an enduring commitment.

Such strategies are not all love and roses. Gangs that demand protection money are using a commitment strategy. They don't want to burn down restaurants, but to convince business owners that they will do such an irrational thing, they must occasionally do it. Commitment explains behaviors that other theories of cooperation can't.[94]

Closed groups that demand substantial sacrifices from members make commitment strategies safer and extraordinary altruistic behaviors possible. Many religious groups require extensive study and sacrifice before membership is granted. Such groups emphasize the importance of helping because of emotional and moral commitment, not self-interest. If you tell the leader of a church that you want to join because you would like to get help when you get sick, you will likely be told that you just don't get it; members are expected to help others willingly from their hearts, not because they want to get something. The paradox is that those whose helping is motivated by commitment often get more help when they need it than those who negotiate explicit contracts.

Social psychologists contrast "communal relationships," based on emotional commitments, with "instrumental relationships," based on exchange.[95] Sly researchers have set up experiments that call attention to how friends trade favors; the participants protest and object to having their actions portrayed as trying to get something. They want to view their friend's actions, and their own, as motivated by caring and commitment.

The perils of analyzing exchanges in communal relationships were brought home to me when I was being taught how to do marital therapy by analyzing resource exchanges between spouses. We helped spouses make lists of what each spouse contributed to the relationship and then helped them negotiate a new contract that specified who would contribute what. The therapy brought couples closer, but mainly, it seemed to me, because of their shared conviction that the would-be therapists knew nothing about how real marriages actually work.

Psychotherapy relationships are instrumental because a fee is paid in exchange for help. However, they generate feelings of commitment that are often crucial to their success. This is why negotiating the appropriate distance between therapist and patient is a constant source of tension. I wonder if the distinction between formal and informal forms of address in many languages signals whether a relationship is based on emotional commitment or instrumental exchange. I ask my patients to call me Dr. Nesse.

Social Selection

Commitment explains some things, but others still don't fit. Tendencies to genuinely moral behavior persist in our genomes. An exceptionally attractive young woman provided loyal care for her husband after he slipped off a roof and had permanent brain damage that left him severely disabled. Some people devote their lives to helping others selflessly. Many people take great satisfaction from volunteering to feed the hungry, build houses, or tutor students. Some avoid eating meat in moral protest against the way animals are treated. And many wash out containers carefully and pay extra to get them recycled. Moral behavior is everywhere.

Morality requires following rules instead of calculating what most benefits the self. It does not guarantee a benefit in return. It can give emotional satisfactions, such as pride in doing what is right, but where does pride come from? Moral actions are expensive. What else has natural selection shaped that is expensive? Peacocks' tails. That line of thinking took me back, again and again, to articles by the theoretical biologist Mary Jane West-Eberhard about "social selection."[96,97]

She found a solution that I think helps explain our moral capacities and extraordinary social sensitivity: because individuals pick the best available partners, those who do what it takes to be a preferred partner get big benefits. The benefits of being preferred as a sexual partner shape extremely expensive displays such as the peacock's tail. If, as evolutionary psychologist Geoffrey Miller has suggested, people prefer altruistic sexual partners, that would select for altruism directly.[98] West-Eberhard pointed out that sexual selection is a subcategory of social selection, and that individuals preferred as social partners also get big benefits because they get the best possible partners.

"Social selection" is not an ideal term because it has different meanings in different fields. "Partner choice" is closer to the core idea, but choosing partners is only part of the story; rejecting or punishing partners is also important.[99,100] "Partner selection and rejection" captures the essence of an evolutionary process that has made us capable of goodness. People with tendencies to help their friends generously are preferred as social partners, so they get the best partners and all the attendant fitness advantages.[101] This process may have been crucial for making humans extraordinarily cooperative and capable of creating culture.[102]

For most species, close social partners other than relatives are either nonexistent or nearly interchangeable. That was probably the case for our human ancestors until some tipping point in the past hundred thousand years, when selecting especially capable, generous partners began to give advantages. The benefits of having relationships with the best possible partners shaped tendencies to generosity and loyalty. West-Eberhard described how the process of social selection could enter a runaway phase in which a preference for partners with certain traits gives advantages to those who have those traits, giving even more advantages to those who choose carefully. The resulting prosocial traits are as expensive and dramatic as a peacock's tail.

Social psychologists have found evidence for "competitive altruism."[103,104] People spend extraordinary amounts of time and money to display selfless altruism. Cynics attribute this to sly manipulation strategies, noting the charitable donations made by swindlers such as Bernie Madoff. However, altruism is often real, sometimes even without any expectation of reward, except for the feeling of pride for being a good person—and perhaps the hope that it will lead to better partners. There is even recent evidence that less generous people try to protect their reputations by attacking others who are especially generous.[105]

The renowned anthropologist Sarah Hrdy has suggested that all of this may have gotten started when mothers began cooperating to care for children.[106] A human mother can have twice as many babies in a decade than a chimpanzee can, not because human mothers are more efficient foragers but because cooperation networks provide help and resources that allow a much shorter interval between offspring.

Related ideas have been developed in several fields using several designations. David Sloan Wilson uses trait-group models to describe a process that makes cooperation possible.[107] In economics and biology, the role of partner choice has been explored and developed by Peter Hammerstein and Ronald Noë, among others.[108] A related process can even explain the symbiosis of plant roots and associated bacterial nodules.[109,110] The nodules capture nitrogen from the air and make it available for the plant, and the plant provides nutrition the bacteria need to grow. A nodule that tries to take a plant's resources without providing fixed nitrogen is dropped. A plant that tries to take the fixed nitrogen without providing nutrition gets abandoned by the bacteria. Cooperation is enforced by partner selection and rejection.

Flowers illustrate the expense of competing to be chosen. Large, colorful, fragrant blooms with nectar and pollen use valuable calories that could otherwise be put into leaves, roots, and seeds. However, big spending is essential because blossoms compete to be chosen by pollinators.

Social selection models explain how selfish choices can create strong selection for generous individuals. Individuals with the most to offer choose the best available partners, thus automatically bestowing fitness benefits on the most generous individuals in a group. The process is a version of Adam Smith's invisible hand.[111] Self-interested choices made by merchandise creators and consumers create an economy that produces more goods for all at the lowest cost in the proportions needed. Self-interested partner choices shape biological capacities for moral passions and genuinely moral behavior that make deep cooperation possible for human social groups.

Like all good ideas, social selection is not completely new. Two hundred years before Darwin wrote, the Scottish philosopher Thomas Hobbes described the fate of fools who advocate breaking promises in his Third Law of Nature: "That men performe their Covenants made."

> The Foole hath sayd in his heart, there is no such thing as Justice; and . . . there could be no reason, why every man might not do [whatever he wanted to]: and therefore also to make, or not make; keep, or not keep Covenants. . . . From such reasoning as this, Successfull wickedenesse hath obtained the name of Vertue. . . . [However,] [h]e therefore that breaketh his Covenant . . . cannot be received into any Society, that unite themselves for Peace and Defence, but by the errour of them that receive him . . . if he be left, or cast out of Society, he perisheth.[112]

Such fools still abound, emboldened by thinking that selfish genes must make selfish people and enabled by mass societies that allow anonymity and movement between groups.

People prefer partners with plenty of resources. So to get the best possible partners, people show off their resources along with their generosity. Here, too, extreme traits are obvious. Anthropologists describe potlatch ceremonies in which wealthy individuals destroy prized possessions to prove they can afford the loss. Related conspicuous consumption drives much of the economy.[113] Fancy cars and sneakers aren't much better than cheaper ones, but they are expensive, and therefore honest, signals of wealth. Ten-thousand-square-foot homes are rarely fully used, but they create connections with others who also can consume equally conspicuously.

More in tune with everyday life, everyone wants to be someone, to be valued and appreciated for their special contributions and expertise. This makes every arena competitive. In sports this is overt; in music and drama only slightly less so. Bird-watching seems egalitarian, until you actually listen in as twitchers talk. Model train enthusiasts wield their specialized knowledge with the flair of Supreme Court lawyers. People can't help it; they turn every pastime into a competition. These competitions make life wonderful and interesting and provide meaning, occupation, and camaraderie for almost everyone.

I once spent a pleasant morning with Sarah Hrdy watching a flock of wild turkeys. The toms walked a few paces, then fanned out their huge tails, walked a bit more, and did it again. It seemed as silly as it was impressive. But we humans spend our days creating similar displays, not just to impress mates but to show that we are desirable social partners. Our constant efforts to impress and please others make life rich with interest and potentially full of meaning and love.

Social Anxiety and Self-Esteem

Social selection has big implications for mental disorders. When I began treating patients, many wanted help to make them less sensitive to what other people thought about them. It was the 1970s zeitgeist: I'm okay, you're okay, let's shed stifling social conventions and follow our bliss. Escaping conformity seemed like a laudable goal. I did my best to help patients achieve those aims, usually with only modest success.

As I came to understand how partner selection shapes relationships, I gradually recognized why social anxiety is overwhelmingly common. Natural selection shaped us to care enormously about what other people think about our resources, abilities, and character. This is what self-esteem is all about. We constantly monitor how much others value us. Low self-esteem is a signal to try harder to please others.[114,115] However, trying harder to please others often conflicts with competing for status, creating plenty of conflicts that you hear about in psychotherapy.

Big life decisions about whom to marry, whom to work for, whom to hire, or whom to admit to a social group all involve careful assessments. We try to select honest, cooperative, generous people with plenty of resources who will work hard to benefit us and our group. The benefits that go to those chosen help explain the extraordinary potential cooperativeness of humans compared with any other species. This is what makes life bearable, and even good and wonderful, for many people.

However, some people make apparently heartfelt promises that are revealed to be mere manipulation the moment they get what they want. Some people hear about guilt or social anxiety and don't know what people are talking about, any more than a color-blind person can grasp the experience of "green." Such sociopaths aren't bothered by such aversive emotions, and they have no compunctions about manipulating, cheating, lying, and taking advantage of others. Those who are crude about it tend to be excluded from social groups, sometimes by being locked away in prison. Subtler sociopaths use their skills to exploit victim after victim.

Such tendencies are highly heritable, but they persist. An article by the evolutionary psychologist Linda Mealey suggested that the genetic tendency to cheat would become more common in groups where most people were exploitable cooperators but would decrease in groups where cheaters are prevalent. The two forces would stabilize to maintain a certain ratio of cheaters to cooperators.[116] I've never found this argument persuasive; full-fledged sociopaths are extruded from small societies or killed,[117] and many have signs of minor brain damage.[118] Mealey's theory certainly is provocative, however. It becomes more compelling in mass society, where people can move between groups, leaving bad reputations behind.

Sociopaths are a danger not only because they exploit people but because they undermine trust. The experience of betrayal changes people. Betrayal by a parent can create distrust of everyone for a lifetime, distrust that makes deep relationships impossible. Several patients over the course of my career have told me spontaneously, at the end of many months of therapy, that they had never really trusted anyone before. Such comments are not just gratifying, they reflect a crucial core ingredient of therapeutic success. Experiencing a trusting relationship and acceptance despite their flaws gives people a vision of what they and their relationships can become. It can give them the courage to change their self-protective, self-defeating ways. It can open them to new relationships that offer new life paths and opportunities. Short-term treatments can't provide anything similar. Changing beliefs about the self and other people requires developing long-term authentic personal relationships.

For most people, genuine caring is intrinsic to relationships with parents, siblings, and spouses. It also extends to friends and sometimes especially intensely to dogs and cats.[119] We care about our pets because they care about us—as well they should after thousands of years of domestication by social selection. Even before systematic breeding, people preferred some dogs and cats to others. Preferred pets got more food, shelter, and opportunities to breed. A few hundred generations later, our pets exemplify exactly what we most value: they are loving, loyal, affectionate, adorable, and eager to obey—well, dogs at least. On occasion patients have told me that a parent loved the family dog more than them. I used to assume that meant the parent was truly terrible, but gradually I have come to realize that sometimes it reflects the depth of a relationship with a very special partner from a domesticated species bred to be the exact kind of partner we most prefer.

We humans have also been domesticated thanks to choices made by other humans.[120,121,122,123] We choose partners and friends who are honest, trustworthy, kind, generous, and, when possible, wealthy and powerful. People with extremes of those qualities get partners with similar qualities, to their mutual advantage. This process creates "the nonrandom assortment of altruistic genes" that Stuart West recognized as the core ingredient for natural selection to shape the capacity for altruism.[124] We are the beneficiaries, but we also bear the costs. Social anxiety and constant concern about what others think about us are the price we pay for deep relationships. Our capacity to feel grief is another.

Grief

It always seemed to me that grief could be useful, but I did not think deeply about the question until I took on a large research project. When I started a new position at the University of Michigan Institute for Social Research, I met with the director. He asked me what project would most advance my research—blue sky, anything. I told him I wanted to understand what low mood is for and that the best way to study that would be to find people who had little capacity for experiencing grief and see what goes wrong in their lives. The study would obviously be impossible, I explained, because it would have to assess people before the loss of a loved one and again after.

The director paused, gave me a quizzical look, and said, "What if I told you that the world's largest prospective study of bereavement has already been completed, that the data are in a computer awaiting analysis, and that the original researchers have all moved on to other places and projects?" I instantly realized the incredible privilege and opportunity—and my obligation to engage in years of effort to analyze the data.

He sent me to James House, the noted sociologist who had helped design the original project. He said the study had included a random sample of thousands of couples of retirement age who were interviewed for hours to measure thousands of variables. The researchers had then checked the obituaries every month. When a study subject passed away, they contacted the surviving spouse to request an interview that covered every aspect of bereavement, depression, health, and social and physical functioning. These follow-up interviews were conducted at six months, eighteen months, and forty-eight months after the loss.

The data set was a gold mine. Most research projects on grief ask people to recollect what health and relationships were like before the loss, but such data are untrustworthy because memories are unreliable and influenced by the loss. The Changing Lives of Older Couples (CLOC) project studied people in extraordinary depth before any loss occurred.[125]

I spent the next three years organizing a research team and getting funding to analyze the data. Others had devoted whole careers to understanding grief. Some of the best, especially psychologists Camille Wortman and George Bonanno, were generous enough to join the project and provide essential guidance. A young sociologist, Deborah Carr, became my research partner; her effort and expertise were essential to the project's success.

We were surprised by many of the findings. For instance, many clinicians think that "delayed grief" is common and a precursor of future problems. But hardly any of our subjects experienced intense grief after an initial period without much grief. Another idea, one still common among psychiatrists, was that recovery required getting in touch with grief and that avoiding "grief work" caused problems later. We didn't find that, either. We also thought that sudden losses caused more grief. Also not true.[126]

One of the most profound findings contradicted my psychiatric training. I had learned that severe or prolonged grief was usually caused by an ambivalent relationship with the deceased. That was based on Sigmund Freud's idea that unconscious anger toward the lost loved one would be turned against the self and show up as depression. I spent many hours trying to help bereaved depressed patients get in touch with such unconscious anger. It was shocking to discover that our data provided no support whatsoever for the idea. People with ambivalent relationships before the loss tended to have less grief than other people. As Homer Simpson would say, "D'oh!" The best predictor of depression after a loss was also no surprise at all: having depression before the loss.

What about my target group, those who reported little grief? There were plenty of them, but they tended to be just about the same as other people in terms of their other relationships, their health, and their ability to cope with life. My hypothesis that such people would show dire problems was wrong. However, when I delved more deeply into their individual records, I rediscovered something that I had learned many times before: people are enormously subjective. A few people who reported no grief symptoms when interviewed six months after the loss said in the interview eighteen months after the loss that they had experienced intense grief right after the loss. For others, it was reversed. At eighteen months after the loss, they recalled no grief previously, but the data at six months revealed substantial symptoms. People are subjective beings.

Grief is so tragic and so awful that you have to wonder why it exists. There are two main possibilities: it could be a useless side effect of mechanisms that make deep relationships possible, or it could be a special form of sadness that offers benefits like those sadness provides after other losses.

Few researchers have taken on this question. The British psychologist John Archer wrote a lovely book arguing that grief is the price of love.[127] He argued that grief itself is useless but pain after loss is necessary for close bonds to be meaningful. In his view, grief is an unfortunate side effect of natural selection being unable to create the benefits of loving relationships without also giving rise to incredible pain.

This doesn't seem plausible to me. A grieving person's suffering, disability, and lack of energy can be so desperate that you would assume selection would find some way to allow relationships to be warm, deep, and secure without so much suffering at their loss. Months and years of poor sleep, poor appetite, hopelessness, and lack of motivation take a huge toll. Seven percent of people develop complicated grief that impairs their functioning for years.[128,129,130] If it is just a side effect that natural selection could not fix, it is a particularly stupid, awful one. If a drug were found that would eliminate grief, should we use it? An answer requires finding out if and how grief is useful. And that requires understanding why sadness exists.

Sadness in general seems to come too late to do any good. The loss has already happened. But loss is a situation that has recurred over and over in every life since the beginning of time. Sadness was shaped to cope with the situation of loss.[131] But how can it help?

Pretend for a moment that you are in the horrifying situation of watching one of your children being pulled out to sea in a riptide. Would you just go on eating your lunch? No way. The first thing you would do is to scream to get help rescuing your child. You would simultaneously get all other children out of the water as you dive in and try to rescue the missing child, even knowing the danger and that it is probably too late. If you were sensible enough not to swim out or fortunate enough to get back to shore safely, grief would promote endless rumination about what you could have done to prevent the loss. This would help prevent a repetition with other children. Your sobbing would signal your need for help and warn others about the danger.

When a child dies of cancer or pneumonia, speculating about what you might have done to prevent it is mostly useless. However, the tendency to blame is built in, so people do it anyway, blaming themselves, doctors, anyone who was involved. Those motives can create marvelous initiatives, Mothers Against Drunk Driving being a spectacular example. Every community has organizations dedicated to preventing the kind of sickness or accident that carried off a loved member of the community.

In our ancestral environment, loved ones must often have simply not returned to camp. Searching for them would have been essential. A loss creates mental preoccupation and a search image tuned to detect relevant cues. In the weeks after a loss, bereaved individuals often think that they see or hear the lost loved one. Tiny random sounds or sights are misinterpreted as the person's voice or form. Visual and auditory hallucinations arise. Such experiences are sometimes interpreted as wish fulfillment, but a more plausible explanation is that they are products of a search image that makes it easier to find the missing person. False alarms in such a system would be normal, useful, and experienced as ghosts.

Anniversary reactions are also common and fascinating. Many people occasionally experience sadness that seems unaccountable, until they realize it is the anniversary of a loss. I doubt that anniversary reactions are adaptive in general; however, in ancestral environments many opportunities and dangers recur with seasonal regularity. So smelling overly ripe apples in an orchard may bring back vivid memories of a fall long ago.

CHAPTER 10

KNOW THYSELF—*NOT!*

If . . . deceit is fundamental to animal communication, then there must be strong selection to spot deception and this ought, in turn, to select for a degree of self-deception.

—Robert Trivers,
foreword to *The Selfish Gene*, 1976

Too much sanity may be madness. And maddest of all, to see life as it is, and not as it should be!

—Miguel de Cervantes Saavedra,
Don Quixote

The Animal Behavior Society is an organization of scientists who investigate why animals do what they do. They study how natural selection shapes brains that give rise to behavior that maximizes fitness. This seemed like crucial knowledge for a psychiatrist, so I went to the society's annual meeting. I expected to come away with new ideas, but I was completely unprepared for what happened: in the middle of the annual banquet I realized that I would have to spend years trying to understand psychodynamics in evolutionary terms.

The first morning of the meeting included a symposium on whether animals have consciousness. Another symposium was about why individual animals that experience early harsh environments become risk takers that start reproducing sooner. If life is likely to be short, doing whatever it takes to reproduce early will be worthwhile. This simple notion immediately triggered thoughts about patients who were abused as children and grew up to be reckless adults. Studies of what is called "fast versus slow life history theory" have developed into a major line of research in evolutionary studies of behavior.[1,2,3]

At lunch the scientists at my table thought it was great that a psychiatrist had a serious interest in animal behavior, but they made plenty of jokes about Prozac. Then one said something that surprised me: "If you are a psychiatrist, then you must know that the purpose of the unconscious is to stay unaware of our motives so we can better deceive people." I said that I knew about the idea from conversations with the biologists Dick Alexander and Bob Trivers, who first came up with it, but that it was by no means widely accepted. Several at the table disagreed, citing the ubiquity of deception in the animal world: camouflaged butterflies, birds that pretend to be injured to lure predators away from the nest, cannibalistic fireflies that lure male victims by imitating the female's flash.[4,5] They explained that all communication systems get exploited, creating ever escalating arms races between strategies for more subtle deception and more powerful ways to detect deception, that create ever more complex signals. Their fascinating comments were certainly relevant to human relationships.

At the banquet the next day, I sat with a different group. The conversation turned to how understanding the evolutionary origins of cooperation could help people get along better. After a few minutes of discussion one person said, "But we all are basically selfish, aren't we? It is just that the unconscious hides our motives from us and others." The same idea again! Something in my mind flipped. If animal behavior researchers were confident that natural selection shaped our capacity for keeping things unconscious to allow us to better deceive others, I had to investigate. If the idea was true, it had the potential for grounding psychodynamics in biology. If it was false, it was a clever meme that could harm relationships.

University of Michigan biologist Richard Alexander wrote, in a 1975 article, "Selection has probably worked against the understanding of such selfish motivations becoming a part of human consciousness, or perhaps even being easily acceptable."[6] The idea got more attention in the foreword Robert Trivers wrote in 1976 for *The Selfish Gene*. He said, "There must be strong selection to spot deception and this ought, in turn, to select for a degree of self-deception, rendering some facts and motives unconscious so as not to betray—by the subtle signs of self-knowledge—the deception being practised."[7]

Trivers went on to write several papers and a book arguing that self-deception evolved to make it easier to deceive others.[8]

Trivers and Alexander didn't know much about psychoanalysis, however. It is based on the observation that our behavior is influenced by unconscious ideas, emotions, and motives, and that powerful ego defenses keep some things out of our consciousness. Psychoanalysis is a strategy for getting around these defenses, thus revealing things previously hidden by repression and thereby reducing self-deception. As the psychoanalyst Heinz Hartmann put it, "Indeed, a great part of psychoanalysis can be described as a theory of self-deception."[9]

The evidence for repression that inspired Freud came from otherwise unaccountable symptoms. My own work provided plenty of examples. The neurologists asked me to evaluate a middle-aged woman whose right arm had been paralyzed for three months. With a sudden onset, no precipitant, and no viable neurological explanation, they thought the cause was psychological. When I met the patient, she held her right arm limp in her lap. On neurological examination, she was able to shrug her right shoulder slightly but otherwise could not move her arm or fingers. Reflexes were normal. Sensation to touch and pinprick was intact. Arm musculature was reduced only a little. There were no twitches or contractures.

When I asked if she had been under any stress, she said, "No, not really, except for my arm is paralyzed, so I can't do anything." She mostly took care of her house and her two children, who had recently started high school. When asked about her husband, she said, "It's the usual, he's a man, you know." She refused to provide details but suggested indirectly that her husband was a philanderer who had little sympathy for her arm problem. She then immediately said, "But I am here just to get help with this paralyzed arm, not to talk about my husband." As we were concluding the mostly unproductive interview, I asked her, "So if your arm could be miraculously cured, what would you do with it?" She became visibly emotional, and, to my incredulous eyes, she raised her right fist to her shoulder and then brought it down sharply as she said, "I guess I'd just put a knife through his back!" I said, "You raised your arm!" She said, "I did not, it's paralyzed."

Doctors at the medical clinic where I worked often asked me to see patients who were having hard-to-explain spells. They invited me to see a teacher who had fainted several times at work, resulting in three ambulance trips to the emergency room. She was a single, otherwise healthy middle-aged woman who denied having depression and anxiety. After half an hour, I still had no clue as to what was wrong, so I asked her the exact moment and place of her first fainting episode.

She said it had been after lunch, just as she was leaving the teachers' lounge. I asked her what happened next. There was a significant pause, and her voice changed slightly as she said, "I guess they called the ambulance and helped me in." When I asked if she could remember who helped her, she got an odd look on her face, and then said, "I think it was Bob." I asked about the other fainting episodes, and she emphasized that it was just a coincidence, but Bob had caught her each time. I asked her to tell me more about Bob. She said that he was popular, attractive, and helpful, "just a very nice man."

She returned for another session later that week and said our conversation had made her realize that she should tell me that she had had a crush on Bob for a year. She stressed that she was sure it had nothing to do with her fainting episodes, even as she described him carrying her in his arms to the ambulance three times. She insisted strongly that she had no interest in having a man in her life.

A man was referred to our anxiety clinic because he had experienced several months of tension, nervousness, and sleeplessness. There was a moderate family history of similar anxiety, but he'd never had symptoms until recently. I asked about stressors and life changes. He said that nothing was different, that everything was going fine at work, and that he was looking forward to his wife having a second baby in a few months. I asked if the pregnancy was causing stress. He said no. He then quickly went on to describe his deep commitment to his church and the importance of his religious beliefs and church projects. When asked about the projects, he described an antipornography group he had started. He and a few other church members met with local storeowners to try to convince them not to carry pornographic magazines. He had started the group about a month after his anxiety had started.

I asked if anything else had happened around that time, and he said, "No. There have been some changes in the neighborhood, but nothing bad." I asked him to say more, and he described a woman moving in next door after a divorce. He had helped her move boxes into the house. After a pause he said, "I'm not really sure what kind of woman she is." "How so?" I asked. "Well," he said, "she invited me in for a drink, but I don't drink. Then she suggested that I should come back later in the evening. That just didn't seem right." As you may have suspected, the date of her move coincided with the onset of his anxiety.

Repression Is Real

Many people think that repression mainly keeps traumatic memories from consciousness. That was Freud's original idea, but it is contentious and not that relevant to a modern perspective.[10] Freud shifted his view as he observed what kinds of things are repressed. Overwhelmingly, they are socially unacceptable wishes, memories, desires, emotions, and impulses. Being in love with another teacher who is married. Wanting to murder your husband. Getting turned on by an invitation from the attractive divorcée next door.

Although the reality of repression is well supported, many deny it. Some even repress it. When I began my career, psychoanalytic ideas were dominant. The chair of nearly every major psychiatry department was a psychoanalyst. They have all been replaced by neuroscientists. Purged is more accurate. Psychoanalysis is ridiculed, and those who practice it are held in contempt by many academic psychiatrists. It's a bit dangerous even to acknowledge, as I am doing here, that some psychoanalytic ideas are valuable.

It is easy enough to find psychoanalytic ideas ripe for ridicule. The credulous tendencies of some psychoanalysts were brought home to me by an article in a psychoanalytic journal, intended as a friendly spoof, about the symbolic meaning of ingrown toenails. Alas, many took it seriously, making the author's point more strongly than he had intended.

It is unfair, however, to use such examples to dismiss all of psycho-dynamics. Preposterous extremes are easy to find in every field. Some learning theorists try to explain and treat every psychiatric disorder, even psychosis. Some neuroscientists make grand claims that all mental problems are caused by something broken in the brain. Some family therapists think most disorders are caused by family dynamics. Some evolutionary psychologists propose wild sexy ideas that get lots of attention. And some evolutionary psychiatrists make preposterous claims about the adaptive significance of mental disorders. Every perspective gets pushed to extremes that dirty the water. But there is a baby in every bathtub. The baby, for psychoanalysis, is the fact of repression.

Repression poses a first-rate evolutionary mystery. "Know thyself" always seemed to me to be a practically useful maxim as well as a virtue. Like most people, I assumed that objective perceptions of inner and outer reality would maximize fitness. But at that banquet, I realized my naiveté. Could objectivity harm fitness? How could I assess the hypothesis?

The things repression keeps from consciousness are not mundane events, such as our gallbladders contracting while we eat; they are powerful feelings and desires. Lust, hatred, and envy lurk in the depths. Our minds employ several strategies—psychoanalysts call them ego defense mechanisms—to keep such things out of conscious awareness, no matter how hard we try to get in touch with them.

While I was a college student working in a summer program at a mental hospital, I had a conversation with a psychologist and two other students while driving late one night. We were talking about people who are hard to get along with. I took the opportunity to complain about a nurse who didn't like me. They asked me for details, and I explained that the nurse was a bully who had strong opinions about everything and was unsympathetic to young people. They asked me for specific examples, but I had trouble coming up with any. After I complained about her for another ten minutes, the psychologist said quietly, "I think you're probably projecting." I had no idea what she was talking about. She went on to say, "There isn't much evidence that she is criticizing you, but you clearly dislike her intensely, so you may be denying that and instead thinking that she dislikes you." "That's ridiculous," I said. Then one of the other students said, "Or else you are turned on by her." It wasn't until I was well into my training as a psychiatrist that I realized that they were probably right, at least with the first hypothesis, and that we all have false beliefs about other people and ourselves.

I returned home from the Animal Behavior Society meeting determined to figure out why we have repression and psychodynamic defenses. They distort reality. They create symptoms. They cause interpersonal conflicts. Psychotherapy that helps people get in touch with previously unconscious material can be very helpful. You would think that our minds would provide us with accurate self-knowledge without all the time and trouble of psychotherapy. But actively maintained obstacles block access to much that could otherwise be conscious. Something very interesting is going on.

That mechanisms outside of consciousness guide behavior isn't surprising. Bacteria and butterflies get along just fine without anything like human consciousness. The origins and functions of consciousness of the human sort have been debated for centuries. This is not the place to review them, but there is some agreement that the capacity to create internal models of the external world can be useful.[11,12,13,14] Mental manipulation of such models allows comparing the likely outcomes of alternative strategies without the risks of actually doing things. Which is why, as you consider pressing "send" on your carefully crafted angry resignation email, your ability to predict the future makes you pause.

Coping with the inordinate complexity of social life has selected for larger, more capable human brains. The anthropologist Robin Dunbar has shown that the brain size of a given species of primates is strongly correlated with group size and social complexity.[15] He and others argue convincingly that for humans, most resources are social resources, and getting and keeping them requires constant mental processing of possible outcomes of alternative courses of action.[16]

Modern media boost the stakes exponentially. Perhaps you heard about the woman who thought she was sending a cute tweet to a few friends, just as she got on a flight to Africa, about being unlikely to contract a sexual disease because she is white.[17] When she arrived, she turned on her smartphone to discover that her tweet had gone viral and she was now unemployed and the object of worldwide scorn. The mechanisms our minds use to anticipate the results of our actions are inadequate for coping with modern media.

The question is not why there is an unconscious; it is why some events, emotions, ideas, and drives are actively suppressed and kept from consciousness: in a word, repression and ego defenses to enforce it. There are two global alternatives. Repression could simply be an unavoidable limitation of the cognitive system. Perhaps selection could not shape a system with access to everything, or the obstacles are useless by-products of some other system. Those explanations are just barely plausible. Much unconscious content is not just unavailable; it is actively blocked from consciousness by specialized mechanisms called ego defenses.

A brief pause here, as I return after procrastinating for a day. I tried to force myself to write; a deadline is looming. But I just couldn't. I asked myself why and decided I was just tired. Then I let my mind wander. It went quickly to imagine critics who might dismiss this entire book just because it says that some aspects of psychoanalytic theory are correct and useful. Worse, I realized that I have been writing as if only fools don't recognize the reality of repression. This led to the memory of my first meeting with Robert Hatcher, the psychologist who supervised my first psychodynamic therapy case. I began by telling him that I really didn't believe all that stuff about the unconscious. He didn't argue with me. He simply said, "You will make your own decision about that. But to see for yourself, you need to listen carefully for many sessions, say very little, and write down everything the patient says, so we can review the transcript together."

Listening carefully as someone says whatever comes to mind reveals connections between apparently meaningless jumps from topic to topic. One minute a patient is talking about having coffee in an outdoor café, the next about a Japanese colleague. The sun reflecting on the glass tabletop created an association with the rising sun, and thoughts veered off to Japan. One minute a young woman is talking about her resentment that her father is more interested in her brother's football games than her soccer matches, and then she goes on immediately to criticize her father for having so many tools. My conviction about the reality of unconscious influences comes from hours of listening to free associations.

Psychological Studies of the Adaptive Unconscious

These are, however, only anecdotes. They have convinced me that the mind has mechanisms that actively block access to certain kinds of mental content. Appropriate skepticism is countered by the dozens of studies conducted by social psychologists to document the reality of the adaptive unconscious. Social psychologists hardly see eye to eye with most psychoanalysts. The University of Michigan psychiatrist/psychoanalyst/philosopher Linda A. W. Brakel is one of the rare psychoanalysts whose work bridges the gap. She has reviewed the evidence that most of our actions are influenced by primary process thinking, that is, the a-rational machinations of the unconscious mind, and concludes that primary process thinking can enhance Darwinian fitness.[18] Another is Timothy Wilson, who describes many experiments that demonstrate unconscious processing in his lovely book *Strangers to Ourselves: Discovering the Adaptive Unconscious.*[19]

Wilson conducted a particularly influential project with the University of Michigan psychologist Richard Nisbett.[20] They showed the same movie to two groups. One group watched the movie over loud noises from a jackhammer, the other in a quiet room. Afterward, the subjects were asked if the noise influenced their ratings of the movie. The ones who had heard the jackhammer were confident that it lowered their ratings. However, the data showed that it had had no effect. In another study, two groups of students watched different versions of an interview. In one version, the actor was warm; in the other, the same actor was cold. They rated the warm actor as attractive and his foreign accent as appealing. When the actor was cold, he was viewed as unattractive and his accent seemed irritating. However, the subjects attributed their dislike of the cold version of the actor to his appearance and his accent.

John Bargh and colleagues provide many more examples of unconscious thinking.[21,22,23] We imagine that our decisions about who to vote for are products of thoughtful deliberation, but studies show that most decisions are evident in the first second of exposure to a photo of the candidate. You can tell if a sentence is grammatical even though you may have no idea about the rules of grammar. You awaken in the night with the answer to a complex mathematical problem—or the realization that you forgot to include a big item on your income tax form.

Split-brain research provides more dramatic examples. The pioneering neuroscientist Michael Gazzaniga studied P.S., a patient who had had surgery to divide the right and left halves of the brain to relieve intractable epilepsy.[24] Gazzaniga arranged an apparatus that projected an image of a winter scene to the right half of the brain and a chicken claw to the left half of the brain. The patient was able to describe the chicken claw, thanks to language processing happening in the left half of the brain. P.S. had no conscious awareness of the winter scene. However, when he was asked to choose one of several pictures using his left hand (which is connected to the right half of the brain), he pointed to a snow shovel. When asked to explain the choice, the patient said, "You need a shovel to clean out the chicken coop." He made up the story to explain a choice that was influenced by the unconscious influence of the winter scene. As Gazzaniga put it, "The interpreter tells the story line of a person. It's collecting all the information that is in all these separate systems that are distributed through the brain." An article by Carl Zimmer summarizes Gazzaniga's discovery by saying, "While the story feels like an unfiltered picture of reality, it's just a quickly-thrown-together narrative."[25] We make choices outside of consciousness, then make up stories to explain our behaviors.[26] As Wilson put it in his book, we are sometimes like children at an arcade race car–driving game who imagine that they are steering the car, when they are only watching a video preview.

Hundreds of research studies show that prejudice is influenced by unconscious biases. One method flashes pictures of people of different races paired with neutral or positive images. Implicit bias is confirmed by the faster reaction times to negative images paired with faces from a racial outgroup.[27,28] Subjects in such experiments protest that they are not biased, but powerful mechanisms keep unconscious processes out of consciousness.

Why Can't We Access Our Motives and Emotions?

Unconscious cognition is ubiquitous. Psychodynamic defenses such as denial and projection are real and powerful. The question is if and how they could have provided selective advantages. Like most everyone else, I began by assuming that we should look for one explanation. Soon I found two. Now I realize that there are many.

The idea proposed by Alexander and Trivers, that selection shaped the unconscious to make people better at deceiving and manipulating others, spread fast because it is paradoxical and disturbing. It amplifies the selfish-gene meme by making even the most moral acts appear to be disguised selfishness. Cynics take delight in the idea because it confirms their beliefs that everyone is selfish and that moral pretensions are mostly hypocritical. As the evolutionary biologist Michael Ghiselin put it, "Scratch an 'altruist' and watch a 'hypocrite' bleed."[29] Others are appalled by an idea that undermines the possibility of genuine moral commitments. I certainly was.

A year spent learning more about psychoanalysis and the evolution of altruism breached my defenses. I finally acknowledged that Trivers and Alexander were at least partially right. Sometimes, even often, people pursue selfish aims even as they strenuously and sincerely deny that they have any such motive. Women sometimes act seductively and then, when a man responds, express outrage at the idea that they had any such intention. Men sometimes make convincing and sometimes sincere midnight expressions of undying love that evaporate like a mist in the morning sun. Especially when sex is involved, people sometimes deceive themselves in the service of better deceiving others.

Although benefits can come from deceiving others, this provides only a partial explanation. Self-deception can also help preserve relationships by keeping us unaware of the inevitable minor betrayals in everyday life.[30] If someone stands you up for a lunch date, it is often best to just carry on with an otherwise good relationship; otherwise it is easy to slip into a critical mind-set that calls attention to previously invisible minor violations. Relaxed relationships are hard for people who are acutely aware of every tiny defection.

Another possible explanation for repression is that it minimizes cognitive disruption by keeping upsetting thoughts out of consciousness. If you are about to give a lecture, it is better to forget temporarily that your spouse said at breakfast that a serious conversation is needed soon. Avoiding distraction fits many examples. However, something more intense seems to be involved in cases like that of the woman with the paralyzed arm.

Also, repression is rarely perfect. The mind returns to current life problems the same way the tongue returns to a canker sore. And sometimes the unconscious insinuates itself in surprising ways: putting the keys in the garbage, forgetting the way to the wedding.

The benefits of focusing the mind's limited processing power on a few important things can explain suppressing certain thoughts or motives, but it does not necessarily explain the active way that repression prevents all awareness of some things. I suspect that keeping some desires out of consciousness is a major function of repression. We can get only a fraction of what we want. Gaps between what we have and what we want generate envy, anxiety, anger, and dissatisfaction. Keeping unsatisfiable desires out of consciousness not only avoids mental suffering, it also allows us to focus on projects that are possible, instead of ruminating about those that are not. More important, it allows us not only to appear to be, but also to actually be more moral than would be otherwise possible. Thanks to social selection, being good increases fitness. Repression makes it easier to appear good and to be good.

Too Aware of What Is in There

The utility of repression is revealed by cases where it is missing. During a psychotic episode, people experience unconscious content that the rest of us are never aware of. Their sexual and violent visions can be frightening. It is chilling to listen to cannibalistic fantasies. However, such patients are experiencing a global collapse of cognition, so their experiences are not that helpful for understanding ordinary repression.

Patients with obsessive-compulsive disorder (OCD) have a more focused repression deficit. People with OCD do things over and over again, such as washing their hands or checking to see if they locked the door. This isn't simply because they are careful; it is because they fear that some tiny misstep or momentary memory lapse might lead to a catastrophe that will harm others.[31,32,33,34] A graduate student could never be sure she had turned off all the gas jets when she was the last to leave the laboratory for the night. Visions of the building blowing up made her go back to check, not once but five times or more. Another woman couldn't get to work because she kept returning home to check to see if her curling iron had been turned off. She unplugged it and put it in a drawer. But when she left the house, she wondered if it might still have been hot, so she drove home to check yet again.

Another patient had trouble in large grocery stores whenever he saw elderly women with thin necks. He feared that he might suddenly put his hands around one of those necks and twist it. While driving, patients with obsessive-compulsive disorder often fear that they might suddenly swerve into oncoming traffic. Others fear that they have inadvertently hit someone and didn't notice. Some drive around the same block again and again, sometimes calling the police to ask if anyone has reported an accident. Then there was the physician who had to wash his hands for hours before going home for fear that he might give a dire infection to his wife and children.

People with OCD don't carry out the horrendous actions they fantasize, and the terrible outcomes they fear don't happen, but they are never sure, so they engage in repetitive protective rituals. The symptoms give the strong impression that OCD patients are aware of hostile wishes in a way that normal people are not.

OCD can be caused by brain damage. A part of the brain called the caudate nucleus is smaller than usual and contains excesses of inflammation markers in people with OCD.[35,36,37] The caudate is abnormal even in children with mild OCD symptoms.[38] The changes are too small to be diagnostic, but they are real. Further intriguing evidence suggests that autoimmune responses to streptococcal infections can damage the caudate the same way rheumatic fever damages joints and heart valves.[39,40]

OCD is, in some ways, the flip side of paranoia. People with paranoia have an unreasonable fear that someone else might harm them. Many people with OCD have an unreasonable fear that they might harm someone else.

Patients with obsessive-compulsive personality disorder are very different from those with OCD.[41] Obsessive-compulsive personality illustrates the perils of excess objectivity and conscientiousness. Such patients tend to follow rules, fulfill their obligations, and expect others to do the same. Their expectation that everyone should comply with their high standards puts other people off. A light left on in an unoccupied room becomes a moral transgression of the highest order. Confronting energy-wasting miscreants becomes an exercise in frustration that wrecks relationships.

Extreme objectivity and conscientiousness have a high price. Less awareness of obligations and minor mistakes makes life better.

Some patients are incapable of making decisions. This is a big problem in the ER in the middle of the night when a patient vacillates for hours about whether or not to accept an offer of hospitalization. But it is also a problem for many people whose decisions don't stick. One woman spent months deciding that a BMW was the perfect car for her, then, hours after the purchase, became convinced that it was a mistake. Most of us are protected against such ambivalence by what social psychologists call dissonance.[42,43] Once a decision is made, people see all the reasons why their decision was smart and why the other choices were not as good. In a typical psychological experiment, people are asked to examine several coffee mugs and say how much they value each one. Then they are given one of the mugs. The people who are given their second-choice mug soon find reasons why it is superior to their first choice. This is irrational. However, such subjectivity puts decisions in the past so people can move on to other concerns.

Inhibiting Selfish Motives

People repress selfish motives and those that violate local mores. Freud's original model of mental conflict fits this well. He viewed the unconscious as a swirling cauldron of socially unacceptable impulses that are inhibited by the superego. The ego mediates, allowing acceptable impulses and repressing the rest. Our fantasies wander across wide realms of possible actions. Anxiety blocks some routes completely without us even being aware of it. Other fantasies go a long way down a pleasurable but unrealistic path. A few paths are open all the way. However, there is always a tension between desires and inhibitions.

The conflicts Freud saw at the root of many problems have a straightforward evolutionary interpretation: the central trade-off in social life is between actions that give short-term personal pleasure at long-term social costs versus those that inhibit immediate selfish motives to get social benefits later. Illicit sex now that will have long-term costs to reputation and relationships is a fine example. Other species are much less able to inhibit their behavior. We can control our impulses, at least most of us most of the time, thanks to a capacity for repression that helps us inhibit as well as conceal selfish impulses whose expression would make cooperation and commitment impossible. This is close to the opposite of what Alexander and Trivers proposed. Instead of making sly unconscious pursuit of anti-social motives possible, repression keeps us from even being aware of them, making us more desirable social partners who are capable of moral behavior.

The two sides of this trade-off at the root of mental conflict are supported by genetic studies that have found two global pathways to mental disorders.[44,45] One pathway is via internalizing, that is, inhibition, anxiety, self-blame, neurosis, and depression. The other pathway is via externalizing, that is, by pursuing self-interest with little inhibition in ways that often lead to social conflicts and addiction. For the first group of patients, social selection has worked all too well; they are acutely attuned to what others want, and they work hard to please others. For the second group, the tendency to pursue self-interest leaves them with limited moral moorings or committed social support. Most of us muddle along somewhere in between.

These two global strategies are closely related to fast and slow life history strategies and their possible relationship to mental disorders.[46] Early adversity has been proposed to discount the perceived value of long-term benefits and set behavior to take advantage of opportunities now, even at the expense of long-term relationships.[47,48,49] This may help explain the association of early adversity with borderline personality.[50]

The Enlightenment

The idea that repression and lack of self-knowledge can be beneficial is disturbing. Ever since the Enlightenment, hope for progress has been pinned on reason, respect for facts, and critical independent judgment.[51] This is threatened by the idea that our tendencies to deny facts and distort reality may be useful adaptations shaped by natural selection. However, I think a case can be made for the crucial role of repression in fostering high-level cooperation and actions for the good of the planet. On the other side, unconscious distortions also foster the tendency to tribal thinking that is now in such unfortunate ascendance.

I would like to think that objectivity maximizes fitness, but life in human groups demands patriotic loyalty to the in-group. Objective individuals are devalued and rejected. For sport fan groups this is not much of a problem, except for the unwary individual who suggests that the home team just isn't any good. However, groups advancing neuroscience, psychoanalysis, behavior therapy, family therapy, and, yes, evolutionary psychiatry also tend to insist on loyalty to the core schema. Ideas and facts that don't fit are ignored, opposed, and even repressed. Individuals who are excessively objective or sympathetic to other views are excluded. The tendency is deep and probably useful for our genes, but it can be poison for those searching for truth in the connections among different fields.

PART FOUR

Out-of-Control Actions and Dire Disorders

CHAPTER 11

BAD SEX CAN BE GOOD—FOR OUR GENES

Of all the obstacles that God designed for our learning, I think the one that He or She most fiendishly designed is sex. God built into us a feeling that we can solve the problem of sex and be forever sexually fulfilled . . . when actually we never can.

—M. Scott Peck,
Further Along the Road Less Travelled, 1993[1]

The only unnatural sex act is that which you cannot perform.

—Attributed to Alfred Kinsey[2]

Here is a sex fantasy on an epic scale. Not the usual kind about a few extraordinary bodies with exaggerated sex organs engaged in erotic gymnastics. This fantasy, instead, imagines all members of our species having reliably great sex. They all find partners whom they desire and who desire them. Partners have coordinated levels of libido, and they always want sex at the same time. Sexual quirks and fetishes are coordinated for mutual satisfaction. The plumbing and wiring of the sex organs are so reliable that problems never interfere. Orgasms are glorious body- and soul-shaking simultaneous experiences that leave both partners completely satisfied. And people desire sex only with their partners—or else they are fine with their partners having sex with other people.

Alas, it is just a fantasy. People long for partners they can never have, and many have little desire for the partner they do have. They want more sex than their partners, or less, or different. They are preoccupied by fantasies that can never be fulfilled in real life. They worry about impotence or lack of arousal. They have orgasms too soon, too late, or not at all. And jealousy creates frustration and sadness beyond measure.

You would think that natural selection would've done a better job. Sex is the key to reproduction, so of all functions, it should be the object of strong selection. It is. That's the problem. Selection shaped our brains and bodies to maximize reproduction at enormous costs to human happiness.

Sexual problems and frustrations are ubiquitous, but honest talk about them is rare, even in this age of unparalleled openness. Listening to your friends, you might think that most everyone has great sex several times a week. However, you probably know as little about their actual experiences as they know about yours. Psychiatrists hear things others don't. Here are snippets from stories I have heard in the clinic and the psychiatric emergency room.

"My life is over, I have to kill myself. I came home early from a trip and found my husband in bed with my best girlfriend. I can't sleep, I can't eat, there's not even anyone I can talk to about it, because she was my very best friend. And he is my boss, so I am going to be a bag lady. I have been thinking about killing him or both of them. I will never trust any man again."

"I'm so frustrated I don't know what to do. My wife is addicted to candy, and she has kept gaining weight, so she now is three hundred pounds, but she still demands to have sex and I just can't do it anymore. I don't want to leave her, and I don't want to go around with other women, but she keeps demanding sex. What should I do?"

"Nobody wants me. All I want is a reasonably nice guy who wants to share a life and raise a family. But I am thirty-five and sagging and I never was a great looker, and the only guys who want to go out with me just want to have sex. Maybe I should try finding a woman, but I am not really into that. My whole life I have had this fantasy of raising kids in a little house with a white picket fence, but I guess I am already an old maid. There is no point to anything."

"I can't come, except sometimes with the vibrator. There has to be something wrong, but I have always been this way. The books say that you have to relax and keep trying, but that isn't working, and I think my boyfriend knows I am faking orgasms. Is there some kind of Viagra for women?"

"I work on a farm, and no one knows about this, but I keep doing it with the sheep, if you know what I mean. I try not to, but something comes over me, especially at night, and I just can't stop myself. If anyone finds out, my life will be ruined. Is there some kind of drug you can give me that will make me stop?"

"My husband, I married him because he was the first nice guy who ever said he loved me. But, to be honest, I was never interested in him sexually. What has happened is, I am sneaking off to meet this guy from work. I tell my husband I have to work late, but he is getting suspicious, especially since I am even less interested in sex with him. But the guy from work, he isn't nice at all; in fact, he's married and a real jerk a lot of the time. You've got to help me. I don't know what to do."

"We have two problems. He usually comes even before getting inside, and for me it just hurts anyhow."

"Can diabetes make it so things, you know, don't work? Most of the time with my wife it's just limp. But other times it stands up and salutes, so maybe it isn't the diabetes."

"I've got two girlfriends, and it's tearing me up. They don't know about each other, but they suspect something. I want them both, but I can't keep this up much longer. I can't afford them both, for one thing. I need help, or my whole life will be down the tubes."

"I love my husband, but he always wants blow jobs and other stuff and says if I don't do it he will find somebody else who will. He's okay otherwise, and I guess I want to stay with him . . . well, I got nobody else."

"I did something I shouldn't have and caught herpes. My husband will kill me if he finds out. You have got to put me in the hospital and cure me or something or at least keep me from going home, 'cause if I go home he will jump me, and then he will get it, and that will be the end of everything."

And finally there was the patient who walked up to our clinic check-in window for his first appointment and began by blurting out, "I'm a premature ejaculator."

Sex talk is everywhere, but serious talk about sex is risky because people have such different ways of coping with its problems. Some revel in their sexuality, not wanting to hear anything about problems. Some fear it and avoid it. Others try not to think about it. Most muddle through, finding satisfaction as best they can and enjoying a laugh about the rest. All four groups get uncomfortable when confronted with the reality that sexual desire can be neither completely suppressed nor fully satisfied. Sex problems match its pleasures, for good evolutionary reasons.

Our question is, as usual, not why some people have problems; it is why sexual problems exist at all. Why are they so amazingly and unfortunately common? The most important answer is simple: natural selection shaped us not for happiness or pleasure but to maximize reproduction.

Finding—and Being—a Desirable Partner

Most humans are choosy about who they mate with. Very. As you know from cruel experience if you are over thirteen years old and not stunningly attractive. If you are very attractive, you experience the problem from the other side: constant approaches, manipulation, and deception, compounded by the envy of those who can't imagine, much less sympathize with, your problems.

The preference for healthy, young, attractive mates has an easy evolutionary explanation: it results in children who are likely to be healthy and attractive, who are likely to have more children of their own.[3] The preference for partners who are kind, strong, helpful, rich, high-status, hardworking, and devoted is at least as useful.[4] It results in more resources and more help, which result in more children, who are likely to be more successful and will have more grandchildren. That, for natural selection, is all that matters.

Choosiness is great for our genes but not for us. Few people can have the partners they most want. Most people are dissatisfied with themselves, because they are not the partner everyone else wants. Their dissatisfaction motivates vast expenditures of time, money, and effort on diets, cosmetics, grooming, fashion, lessons, plastic surgery, and preparing for diverse social competitions. A vast swath of life is taken up by judging, being judged, and getting prepared for being judged in the mating competition. It is brutal. One friend who complained about not finding a suitable partner was told by another friend, "You are an eight chasing tens but being chased by sixes."

Modern media make it worse. In a hunter-gatherer society with only half a dozen possible mates within walking distance, hopes for a spectacular partner could be kept within bounds. Today, most of us see billboards several times daily with nearly naked svelte models offering a direct wide-eyed gaze of sexual invitation. We browse magazines with airbrushed images of fantasy figures lounging invitingly. On television, fabulously sexy, talented, energetic, rich people seem eager to please their partners in every way. Even on Facebook, seeing the positive side of our friends' relationships arouses envy, even when we know better.[5] Then there is pornography, transforming every conceivable fantasy into apparent reality, stimulating desires that are impossible to satisfy. Our real-life partners can't compete. Neither can we.

Awash in stimulation, our imaginations transformed by the virtual reality of modern media, we are rarely satisfied with ourselves, our partners, or our sex lives. A lovely little study conducted by the evolutionary psychologist Douglas Kenrick asked men to rate their satisfaction with their partners. Before filling out the questionnaire, half waited in a room with books about abstract art, the others in a room with copies of *Playboy*. Just browsing centerfolds made the second group's satisfaction with real partners plummet.[6]

Natural selection has created psychological mechanisms that help keep these problems from getting out of control. The capacity for repression is one. But even more important, our mating pattern is peculiar for a primate. Fathers invest inordinately in their children. We get attached to our partners.[7,8] Better yet, most people fall in love, idealize one partner, and lose interest in others.[9] Pause a moment to marvel at romantic infatuation. It superbly demonstrates the value of subjectivity. As George Bernard Shaw put it, "Love is a gross exaggeration of the difference between one person and everybody else." Infatuation focuses desires so sharply that all others fade from sight. Such subjectivity can make life wonderful.

Alas, it is usually only partial and temporary. In *The Devil's Dictionary*, Ambrose Bierce defined love as "A temporary insanity curable by marriage."[10] The article in the *New York Times* viewed the most times in one month in 2017 was entitled "Why You Will Marry the Wrong Person."[11] Many people have enduring satisfying intimate relationships, but problems are rife.

Sometimes the problem is not the availability of partners but their social acceptability. While still condemned in some cultures, homosexuality is increasingly recognized as a deep template that individuals cannot control or change. The most common question I get from the audience after a lecture is how evolution explains homosexuality. I usually try to duck the question because it is so fraught and no answer is widely accepted, but several possibilities have been suggested.

One is that male homosexuals may nonetheless have many children. Perhaps, like in the movie *Shampoo*, apparently gay men can get away with liaisons with women that other men can't. That is unlikely; homosexual men have only about half as many children as heterosexuals, which is not surprising, since most have little sexual interest in women.[12]

In his book *Sociobiology*, Edward O. Wilson suggested that homosexuality is an adaptive strategy when resources and mates are scarce.[13] Some birds use this strategy routinely.[14,15] If no nesting sites are available, young birds stay at the parental nest helping to rear younger siblings who share half of their genes instead of wasting effort on a nest that is likely to fail. This is not like most human homosexuality, however; birds that help at the nest are happy to mate the moment a viable nest site is available. Also, homosexual humans are not necessarily lacking in resources, nor do they reliably dedicate their lives to helping their siblings. Wilson's hypothesis fails.[16]

Plenty of other possible adaptive benefits have been proposed for homosexuality.[17,18] Same-sex intercourse is not a mystery; it is widespread in many species and can have many explanations, both functional and nonfunctional.[19,20,21,22] The mystery is why individuals would turn down opportunities for sex that could result in offspring.

One of the few well-established relevant facts is that the likelihood of a man being homosexual is directly proportional to how many older brothers he has.[23] This suggests that a pregnancy with a son changes the mother's physiology in some way that can influence future sons. This was only informed speculation until a 2018 report by Ray Blanchard and colleagues that mothers of gay sons have especially high levels of antibodies to a protein, NLGN4Y, that influences sexual differentiation of the brain.[24] This has not been confirmed, and it is by no means the full story. The number of older brothers can explain only a fraction of men who are homosexual;[25] genetic factors are relevant,[26] and cultural factors are strong. Also, none of this research bears on female homosexuality. For now there are far more questions than answers. The contribution of an evolutionary perspective is to recognize that tendencies that lead to intercourse between members of the same sex have many explanations, but a lack of interest in sex that might lead to offspring needs explanation.

Uncoordinated Desires

Most young couples want to have sex every few days. That is just about how long an egg remains fertile, so that frequency maximizes pregnancies. It is also about how long couples in ancestral environments are likely to be separated because of hunting and gathering expeditions. Partners separated for a few days are usually eager to get back together; that is very good for them, their fertility, and their reproduction.

For many couples, however, one person wants to have sex more often. If the other acquiesces out of duty or fear, romance is liable to fade. Even if the partners have generally matched levels of libido, temporary periods of mismatch result from sickness, pregnancy, worry, and fatigue. Or one partner may be taking an antidepressant that torpedoes sex drive. In the Woody Allen movie, Annie Hall's therapist asks her, "How often do you have sex with your husband?" She replies, "Constantly. I'd say three times a week." Her husband's therapist asks him, "How often do you have sex with your wife?" He replies, "Hardly ever. Maybe three times a week." Sometimes it is the other way around; many women would like to have sex more often than their partners.

Most couples muddle through their differing desires with some combination of acceptance, denial, satisfying the partner despite a lack of desire, masturbation, and humor. However, the classic line from the comedian George Burns applies all too often: "About marriage and sex . . . After marriage you can go longer . . . and longer . . . and longer . . . without sex." Natural selection did not shape a mechanism to coordinate levels of sexual desire. That is not just too bad, it is a tragedy.

The situation a patient described in the ER one night is common: "My wife doesn't want to have sex, and I don't know what to do. I want to stay with her, but I also want to have a sex life." I recall vividly the succinct advice the patient received from the senior doctor: "Well, you have four choices: you can go to sex therapy; you can get a divorce; you can have an affair; or you can stay in the marriage and masturbate. You just have to choose." Providing such terse advice after only a brief conversation seemed brusque to me, but it nailed the quandary experienced by millions.

You would think that some culture would have found a solution that could maintain long-term, mutually satisfying relationships and full sexual satisfaction, but all solutions involve trade-offs. Enforcing monogamy causes dissatisfaction. Allowing sex with others arouses jealousy, conflicts, and breakups. Most cultures have emphasized controlling sexuality to preserve relationships. Now, however, some people are trying to control attachments to preserve sexual opportunities. Some whose sex life consists of casual hookups avoid having sex repeatedly with the same person to avoid attachment and subsequent grief when the relationship ends.

It is so easy to talk about having sex, as if most couples just have plain intercourse, and that is that. However, desires for special kinds of sex cause plenty of problems. Wanting oral sex or not is a common source of conflict. The deep connections among sex, submission, and domination take us to a different realm, one that has been explored in depth by early evolutionary psychiatrists.[27] Some couples enjoy bondage and discipline games, but for many more, trying to get a partner to play that special role is an exercise in manipulation and frustration. In a very old joke the masochist says, "Whip me"; the sadist replies, "No."

Fetishes are fascinating. Why do some people require four-inch heels or shiny black leather for sexual arousal? "People" is not the right word— big-time kinks are overwhelmingly a guy thing. A woman wrote to a sex advice columnist to ask, "Where can I find a man who doesn't have such perversions?" The columnist's reply: "In the grave."

You would think that natural selection would ensure that men consistently prefer intercourse with women because that would maximize the likelihood of pregnancy. However, some men would rather get a hand job while in handcuffs. Getting aroused by cues that are not quite spot-on harms fitness for females much more than for males.[28,29,30] For females, choosing a good mate is essential because the number of children women can have is strictly limited by the enormous investment required.[31,32,33] For males, anything that somewhat resembles a mate, or has been associated with a mate, might be worth pursuing; the costs are low, and the reproductive benefits could be big. That is why men have a tendency to imagine that small friendly gestures are sexual invitations, a phenomenon UCLA evolutionary psychologist Martie Haselton explains using an expanded version of the Smoke Detector Principle, error management theory.[34]

This doesn't explain fetishes, however; it only explains why they are less costly for men. Many fetish objects are things that are especially salient to a toddler, such as feet, shoes, and being spanked, suggesting that early imprinting may connect such cues to desire.[35] One patient reported he could only get aroused by getting someone to put him in diapers. Such fetishes seem like pathological side effects of a system that connects certain stimuli to libido early in life, to no purpose I can imagine.

Arousal and Its Absence

Lack of sexual arousal is not only more obvious for men than women, it is more harmful to fitness. The causes are many, including drinking, fatigue, medications, atherosclerosis, neurological damage, hormonal problems, and anxiety. All except the last are simple failures of the mechanism, for one or another reason. Anxiety, however, is a different matter. Having an erection subside in the face of danger is unwelcome but, as suggested in the book *Zoobiquity: The Astonishing Connection Between Human and Animal Health*,[36] possibly lifesaving if someone nearby is likely to attack or, possibly worse, gossip. This can initiate a vicious cycle. Fear about performance adequacy causes anxiety that decreases performance, causing more anxiety and worse performance, in a feedback cycle that a frustrated partner can aggravate dramatically by a humiliating comment.

Biotechnology has solved most such problems. Who would have predicted, twenty years ago, that a drug could make erections reliable? Viagra has been a miracle for millions. The market for erectile dysfunction drugs is now about $4 billion a year.[37] Pharmacology has changed the sexual world, to the pleasure of many men and women—and the dismay of some women, who had thought they were done with all that.

Arousal difficulties for women are less obvious but more common. Lack of physiological arousal for women usually goes together with lack of psychological arousal, but sometimes the mind is eager but the flesh balks. No drug has yet been found, however, that reliably increases female arousal. Sometime soon such drugs probably will be discovered, and the sexual world will change again. How? Now is the time to predict the unexpected consequences. You first.

Climaxes Out of Sync

Books about sexual disorders all have whole chapters about premature ejaculation in men but nothing about premature orgasm in women. They all have chapters about women who experience delayed or absent orgasms but give only a nod to men with the same problem. No book explains why it is men who climax too quickly and women who climax too late or not at all. This lack of synchrony may be an especially unfortunate example of natural selection maximizing reproduction at a cost to happiness.

Why female orgasm exists at all has inspired a contentious debate that continues despite the arguments in more than fifty published papers. Those on one side argue that female orgasm gives specific fitness advantages, perhaps by selectively taking up sperm from preferred partners or increasing bonding.[38,39,40] Spirited opponents, whose position is well summarized by Elisabeth Lloyd's comprehensive review, say that female orgasm is a by-product with as little adaptive significance for women as nipples have for men.[41]

A recent evolutionary sophisticated perspective by Günter Wagner and Mihaela Pavlicev suggests that orgasm had its origins in the mechanism in many species that induces ovulation after mating, and that female orgasm in humans is a vestige of that system.[42,43,44] They also note that the clitoral equivalent in other species is inside the vagina and its displacement outside is a product of natural selection. Their conclusions seem sensible. However, even if female orgasm is a vestige, the tendency for men to climax before women needs explanation. One possibility is that orgasm is slower in women simply because the mechanisms that regulate it are not subject to selection. However, studies show that the speed of reaching orgasm is influenced by genes but not by other things such as social or marital status.[45,46]

An alternative explanation is that pregnancy is more likely for women who have slower orgasms than their partners and men whose are faster. Ejaculation that is genuinely premature, that is, before entry, poses huge costs to fitness. But that is rare compared to climaxing "before the person wishes it," as premature ejaculation is sometimes defined. On confidential surveys, a third of men report premature climax.[47] The definition William Masters and Virginia Johnson used—unable to continue until the partner is satisfied 50 percent of the time—would boost the percentage higher yet. A study of 500 couples found that the duration of intercourse ranged from under half a minute to more than forty minutes, with an average of about five minutes.[48] Following the usual definition of pathology as the most extreme 1 or 2 percent, climax in less than one minute is considered abnormal.[49] However, some primates ejaculate in seconds. Five minutes is a relatively long time. Is the long duration of human intercourse, as some have suggested, to scoop out sperm that may already be there from another man?[50,51,52] To cement the emotional bond? Or is it just an accident of physiology? Despite available data on sex in many primates, no answer is confirmed.[53]

Maximizing reproduction requires that a man's climax occurs when the penis is in the right place to get sperm to the egg, then stopping.[54] Continuing intercourse can pull sperm away from their path.[55,56] So after orgasm men experience extreme sensitivity that benefits their genes; too bad about what is good for their partner's pleasure. A refractory period that makes repeated intercourse impossible for an interval of minutes to hours further ensures that there is time for the sperm to get on their way.

For a woman, any genetic tendency to sometimes stop intercourse before her partner ejaculates will be selected against. Imagine, for a moment, if women had the same sexual response cycles as men. They would often have orgasms before their partners, then become sensitive and stop, making conception exceedingly unlikely. Such a system would have dire fitness costs, but early orgasm is not a problem for women. They take much longer than men to reach orgasm, 75 percent never reaching orgasm from intercourse alone in one study.[57] After a climax, instead of stopping, most women are happy to continue for a time, and some go on to have multiple orgasms. A few, however, become sensitive or sore and want to stop. You would think it would be easy to find out how often women want to stop intercourse after orgasm but before their partners ejaculate, but I can't find a published scientific study. On the internet, however, many women report becoming extremely sensitive and stopping intercourse after having a climax. If that happens to more than a very few women, it would select for delayed orgasm.

Given these complications, it is not surprising that lack of synchrony is common and that climax is consistently faster for men. The results from one large national survey showed that 25 percent of women but only 7 percent of men could not reach orgasm. Climaxing too early was reported by about 30 percent of men but was not even measured for women.[58] In another study, only 10 percent of women reported consistently reaching orgasm by intercourse alone.[59] According to a 2013 survey by Elizabeth Armstrong, men reported orgasms three times more often than women in short-term relationships, but the rate of orgasms went up dramatically for women in long-term relationships.[60] It is unclear if that is explained by stable relationships or by men not rushing and learning what to do.

The global conclusion is simple: men have no trouble reaching orgasm, while many, or even most, women do. According to a 1999 study published in *The Journal of the American Medical Association*, 43 percent of women suffer from "female sexual dysfunction."[61] That figure spurred debate and better research that challenged the idea of using the male pattern of sexual response to define what should be normal for women.[62]

A proximate reason for lack of synchrony is the location of the clitoris. If it were located a bit closer to the vagina, it would receive more stimulation during intercourse, resulting in faster orgasms—even if perhaps fewer pregnancies. The logic is compelling, but the hypothesis needs to be tested. Here is the study: find 1,000 women who are not using birth control, measure the location of the clitoris, and see if women whose clitoris is further away from the vagina have fewer orgasms but more babies over the course of a decade. Some studies are as impractical as they are unethical.

A more feasible study would measure the distance between the clitoris and the urethra to see if orgasms are more common if the clitoris is located where it gets more stimulation. Princess Marie Bonaparte did the study and published the results in 1924 under the pseudonym A. E. Narjani.[63] The princess, a great-grandniece of Emperor Napoleon I of France, had difficulty reaching orgasm. She also had obsessions, anxiety, and other symptoms, perhaps because her mother died within a month of her birth and her father was far more interested in his studies of glaciers than in her.[64]

In 1925, she turned for help to Sigmund Freud, who was soon seeing her for two hours each day, while tapering off his relationship with Lou Andreas-Salomé, another woman admirer.[65] When the princess declared her love for him, Freud was reportedly delighted. Bonaparte was not only beautiful and royal, she was rich—really rich. Her mother's father owned property in Monaco, including the casino. When the Nazis threatened Freud, she paid the ransom to get him to England.

It was to Bonaparte that Freud said, famously, that there was one question he had never been able to answer: "What do women want?"[66] We don't know if she replied, "Reliable orgasms," but it seems likely. Bonaparte was not only searching for help for herself, she was a scientist trying to explain the problem. The study she conducted measured the distance between the clitoris and the urethral opening in 200 women and asked 43 of them how often they had orgasms. She concluded that orgasms were more frequent in women whose clitoris was positioned to get more penile stimulation. She took her theory seriously, arranging to get experimental surgery in 1927 to relocate her own clitoris, even publishing a description of the surgical technique.[67,68] The procedure did not work. Her love life was nonetheless active, including a long affair with French premier Aristide Briand, among other men. She later cofounded the Paris Psychoanalytic Society and practiced psychoanalysis until 1962.

A 2011 article by sex researchers Elisabeth Lloyd and Kim Wallen reanalyzed her data, along with data published in 1940 by the psychologist Carney Landis.[69] They confirmed Bonaparte's basic hypothesis that the location of the clitoris influences the frequency of orgasms. This whole approach is, of course, penis-centric, neglecting fingers, tongues, and vibrators, which are more effective ways to reach orgasm. It also illustrates the human tendency to try to figure out what is "normal" and to neglect the huge variation among individuals, couples, and cultures that influences how couples have sex. However, Bonaparte gets credit for doing remarkably bold science on a delicate good question nearly a century before her successors.

Relationship Problems

For humans, sex involves much more than choosing partners, arousal, and climaxes. For most of us, intimate relationships are the most meaningful in our lives. They are also fraught with conflict, for good evolutionary reasons. Some of those reasons were summarized in chapter 9, but some are specific to sex.

For most primates, fathers contribute little to reproduction other than sperm and perhaps some protection of offspring.[70] The intense collaboration of male and female primates during the years of arduous child-rearing is, with few exceptions, distinctive to humans.[71,72,73] What selective advantages could possibly have shaped mechanisms that bind couples into commitments that involve years of child care and fewer mates? The key is that our mating patterns are like those of birds and for the same reasons.[74,75,76,77,78,79] Birds form partnerships to build a nest and rear offspring because they must. A single bird can't gather enough food. Even if it could, being away from the nest would leave the eggs to cool and the chicks to predators.

Human babies are born profoundly helpless, months premature compared to the babies of other primates. One parent cannot provide the care needed. What benefits can compensate for the enormous costs of providing twenty-four-hour care for months and extended care for years? The benefits of having a big brain and culture.[80] The heads of babies who matured several months longer in the uterus would not fit through the pelvic opening, endangering the life of both baby and mother.[81] Also, big brains become maximally useful if they are exposed to years of learning and opportunities to absorb cultural knowledge.[82,83]

Other clues confirm the peculiarities of the human reproductive strategy.[84,85] Most female primates have short periods of fertility each year that are advertised by red buttocks, pheromones, and provocative behavior. Female humans not only do not advertise their fertile periods, they are often completely unaware of them, to the consternation of women using the rhythm method to prevent pregnancy. Although some scientists disagree, several see concealed ovulation as useful because it can make a partner more confident of paternity.[86,87,88] Fighting a woman's established partner to mate only once is rarely worth it because on any random day, pregnancy is unlikely. So concealed ovulation gives men in sustained relationships greater confidence that they really are the fathers of their long-term partner's babies. This, in turn, shapes the motivation to provide long-term care to a child, half of whose genes are almost certainly the same as his. Comparative studies make it clear that the full picture is more complex, but the core idea remains important.[89]

The selective advantages of mutually supportive pair bonds shaped the mechanisms for maintaining them. One is the deep emotional attachment that develops between members of a couple.[90] Another is regular sexual intercourse, with its arousal of oxytocin and its tendency to facilitate emotional bonding.[91,92] Couples have sex during pregnancy and lactation, when no babies will result. But sex at those times nonetheless increases reproductive success by maintaining the pair bonds that are crucial to raising successful offspring.[93]

Those mechanisms help to maintain relationships, but they are unreliable in the long term. The anthropologist Helen Fisher has summarized cross-cultural studies to argue that the average human mating relationship lasts about seven years.[94] Men who have a tendency to want sex with women other than their primary partners tend to have more offspring than other men.[95,96] So it's not surprising that most men have a roving eye, at the least. In most of the hundreds of different human cultures, men are not prohibited from having more than one partner if they can afford it.[97] That doesn't mean women like it. A man's relationship with another woman can transmit disease and can reduce the time and resources available to the first partner and her children, so the tendency for women to object to such relationships is easy to understand.

Women also seek other partners. Sometimes this results in additional pregnancies, but it more often provides other benefits, including resources, status, protection, and possibly better genes for offspring, in addition to pleasure.[98,99,100] Men who try to prevent their partners from having such relationships will tend to have more children than men who are unconcerned about their partner's sometimes being pregnant with another man's baby. Male sexual jealousy reduces this risk, but at the cost of vast unhappiness, nasty fights, and much violence.[101]

Men and the power structures they erect use all kinds of strategies to try to control female sexuality. These strategies define, to a considerable extent, what a culture is like. The evolutionary historian Laura Betzig has devoted her career to studying the often sordid history of how men have controlled and used women's sexuality.[102] The rise of settled agriculture changed everything by making food storage and wealth accumulation possible.[103,104] Men soon used their wealth to control other men, and especially women, in harems. Genghis Khan apparently had more than seven hundred, explaining why about 8 percent of Asian men carry descendants of his Y chromosome.[105]

The general pattern is skewed reproduction, with some men having considerably more offspring than others. This has always been the case to some degree, but new genetic analyses show drastically decreased diversity on the Y chromosome, starting about 10,000 years ago, reflecting a sharp increase in reproductive skew.[106] That is about when the rise of agriculture made settled communities and wealth accumulation possible. The rise of market economies and complex societies that allow mobility changed things yet again so that groups of men now make and enforce rules that limit the ability of powerful men to hoard women.[107] Finally, in a transition that is just now under way, birth control and financial independence have given women political power that they are using to free themselves from male domination.

These are, however, mere nomothetic generalizations. They provide a useful foundation for understanding why marriage and other sexual relationships are often so difficult and why sexual disorders are so common. However, they say little about the diversity of cultures, to say nothing of those among individuals and couples within cultures. They don't begin to explain the complexities that swirl in most relationships. They do help to explain how a satisfying sex life with few difficulties is possible for many couples. Selection shaped mechanisms that make possible enduring committed relationships in which sex is one part of a rich tapestry woven over many years. An evolutionary perspective explains not only the prevalence of sexual problems but also the miracle of human love.

New Sex

New technologies are changing behavior, mores, and laws so fast that natural selection can't begin to keep up. The biggest change is the advent of reliable birth control. No longer intrinsically tied to reproduction, sex has become a recreation for many. Prohibitions against sex before marriage and with multiple partners are no longer necessary to avoid pregnancy. Attitudes are changing fast. The percentage of Americans who think premarital sex is "not wrong at all" went from 29 percent in the 1970s to 58 percent in 2012.[108] The fun is not risk-free. Control of sexually transmitted diseases looked, for a time, as if it would be reliably successful, but antibiotic resistance and epidemics of HIV and other diseases require condoms and caution more than ever before.

Another dramatic change is the earlier age at menarche, declining from an average age of sixteen to twelve.[109,110,111] The brain, however, doesn't mature any faster, so many people are wanting and having sex years before brains are ready to provide guidance.

Jealousy has decreased in the United States in recent decades, or at least its expression has become less acceptable,[112] but it is still very much a part of our nature.[113] Explaining its origins does not influence its power. I once heard a psychotherapist describe how he used his new evolutionary knowledge in couple's therapy. "I just explain to them," he said, "that men have built-in desires for sex with other women, so there is no need for a woman to get upset about occasional affairs." He did not say how this worked, but it is easy to imagine it helped couples unite in agreement that they needed to find a different therapist.

New media make sexually arousing images unavoidable in public and pornography available in private. A remarkable number, well over 100,000 professionals and untold more amateurs, are doing it in front of cameras so millions can watch.[114] The market for internet porn, estimated at about $40 billion per year a decade ago, has now shrunk dramatically, not for lack of interest but because so much is now free.[115] The market for vibrators and other sex toys has exploded, with big implications for relationships, as they are marketed to women as routes to equal opportunities for independent sexual pleasure.[116] Systems that allow remote control of vibrators via the internet make sexual interactions possible with partners thousands of miles away, although privacy may be an illusion; one manufacturer of such devices was recently found to be keeping records of episodes. Paying for sex remains against the law in many places, but fewer than before. Sex robots are just around the virtual corner.[117]

Where is sex headed? The only certainty is that new technologies are changing sexual options faster than cultures can change their traditions and far faster than natural selection can change our brains. I predict more pleasure, new problems, and better solutions informed by evolutionary explanations of why sex is both such a pleasure and such a problem.

CHAPTER 12

PRIMAL APPETITES

They are as sick that surfeit with too much as they that starve with nothing.

—William Shakespeare,
The Merchant of Venice, 1596 (1.2.5–6)

Positive feedback is sometimes fun, sometimes disastrous. It is thrilling to watch a small snowball get enormous as it rolls downhill or grand fireworks set off by a single match. But runaway trucks and heart attacks are disasters. A tiny rupture in a bit of plaque induces turbulence in a coronary artery that causes clot formation, narrowing the artery, causing more turbulence and more clotting, until a completely blocked artery causes a heart attack. Positive feedback in anxiety and mood disorders causes similar spirals that can be almost as dire.

Vicious circles are central to explaining eating disorders. Excess weight causes joint pain, fatigue, and embarrassment that make exercise difficult, leading to more obesity and still less exercise, in a spiral to sickness. Eating sweets creates a desire for more sweets, in what has been called sugar addiction.[1] Strains of bacteria in our guts that are fed straight sugar may manipulate us to eat the kinds of food that allow them to grow faster than other bacteria.[2]

Extremes and vicious cycles are prevented by systems that stabilize every aspect of the body. When body temperature drops, shivering turns on until the temperature is back to normal. When body temperature increases, sweating cools it down. Low blood sugar motivates eating and transforms starch stored in the liver into glucose. High blood sugar releases insulin, which moves glucose out of the blood and into cells. These systems work like thermostats to maintain homeostasis, the body's stable state.

When something gets too high or too low, they turn on. When things are back in the normal range, they turn off. How many such systems are there? Thousands. They control large-scale functions such as blood pressure, heart rate, breathing, and eating. They also keep the levels of thousands of different chemicals and hormones and rates of cell division within narrow ranges. They even regulate when genes are turned on and off. Complex self-stabilizing systems are the essence of life.

Failures of homeostatic control systems are the essence of disease. The systems that regulate body weight now fail more often than not. The percentage of adults in the United States with normal body weight has plummeted from 55 percent in 1962 to 44 percent in 1990, 36 percent in 2000, and 32 percent in 2008. The percentage who are obese—over 210 pounds for a five-foot, ten-inch person—has more than doubled since 1962, from 13.4 percent to over 34 percent.[3] In the United States, two-thirds of adults are overweight or obese.[4]

We don't need numbers to know we are overweight; we need only a mirror. So we decide to lose weight. Willpower should be able to control eating. After all, we make a conscious decision to open the refrigerator. We voluntarily open the ice cream and put it in a bowl. It can't go down the hatch unless we lift a spoon and open our mouths. Even swallowing is voluntary. So millions of people decide to crank up their willpower and go on a diet.

Usually, weight declines for a few weeks or even months. However, 90 percent of the time weight goes back up, often above the starting point.[5] Talk about pursuing an unreachable goal! Trying to control their weight makes millions of people feel terrible, not only about their bodies but also about their lack of self-control. Every day they (we) tell ourselves we will not overeat. Most days we fail, and we blame ourselves.

Failure to lose weight not only makes us less attractive, it also causes frustration, demoralization, low self-esteem, and justified fear of diseases and death. Compared to normal-weight people, obese people are

50 percent more likely to suffer from a chronic health problem.[6] That is the same increased risk as aging from thirty to fifty and more than twice as much as being a smoker.[7] It accounts for about 300,000 deaths in the United States each year.[8]

The solution seems obvious: try harder. We should be able to control ourselves. Eat less. Exercise more. Well-meaning professionals keep explaining this. Again and again. In magazines and books, on television and the internet. In your doctor's office and your workplace. As if we didn't know! But admonitions are not enough, so we pay for help. The weight-loss industry consumes about $60 billion per year in the United States alone, about half for products, half for services.[9,10] Pills, diet foods, counselors, clinics, spas, surgery, and exercise programs thrive, to say nothing of thousands of inspirational books, each with its own special secret formula for weight loss. The proven benefits are few. There are so many competing solutions because none works very well.

A better solution depends on finding the cause. Research has been intensive. Thousands of articles offer possible explanations, each based on some possibly broken part in the weight control mechanism.[11] Is it leptin? A genetic abnormality? Deep insecurity? Lack of early love? Trying to fill an empty place in the soul? Idealized images in magazines? Advertising? The microbiome? Lack of access to fresh, healthy food? Just not knowing what to eat? The surfeit of explanations documents the lack of reliable knowledge.

Here is a terse summary of what we know. The brain mechanisms that normally regulate eating are complex in ways that make intervention at any individual component unlikely to provide an easy solution. We cannot accurately predict who will become obese, but both genetic variations and social factors are important. We know the obesity epidemic in the United States took off in about 1980 and that many things changed about that time, including more sedentary jobs, fast food, new processed foods high in fat and sugar, artificial sweeteners, antibiotics, and mass media. It remains unclear if one of those bears primary responsibility, or if some combination explains the obesity epidemic. Whatever changed makes most of us overweight so reliably that the question of causes could be turned on its head: What is different about those peculiar people who maintain a normal weight?

Control systems work only within a certain range. Your laptop computer has systems that cool its circuits, but the fine print in the instructions says, "Use only in temperatures between 40 and 110 degrees Fahrenheit." If you take your computer outside in the summer sun, the cooling system won't keep up, and your computer will soon shut down. If you take your body outside in the summer sun without adequate protection and water, it, too, will soon shut down.

Our bodies are now exposed to fewer temperature extremes than our ancestors' but more extremes of other kinds, especially food (high) and exercise (low). The systems that evolved to regulate eating protect against starvation superbly. When they detect a caloric deficit, they arouse hunger and extreme efforts to get food and eat it. Those who lack such systems are likely to die during even a brief famine.

The systems that protect against excess body weight are feeble by comparison. Genetic variations that made some people too heavy to escape Paleolithic predators have been selected away. However, the risks of predation because of being too heavy were smaller than the risks of being too thin. Even in modern societies, death rates rise faster for every pound underweight than they do for every pound overweight.[12] So the brain mechanisms that protect against obesity are weaker than those that protect against starvation.

The main evolutionary explanation for the obesity epidemic is obvious: the mechanisms that regulate body weight are poorly suited for our modern environments. Taking your body into a modern grocery store is like taking your computer into the summer sun. The environment is outside the range that the control mechanisms can cope with. Our environment is so different from the one we evolved in that it's remarkable that anyone eats normally. Our hunter-gatherer ancestors walked miles each day gathering food and hunting game, eager to satisfy hunger with whatever they could find. The food they found was mainly high-fiber fruits and vegetables and lean fish and meat. That was only a few thousand years ago, less for many populations.

Big changes have happened much faster than new control systems can evolve. The biggest change was the spread of agriculture about ten thousand years ago. Drought, fast-growing populations, and political conflicts still cause intermittent famines, but better storage, transportation, and economic systems have reduced the risk greatly. The next big change was the growth of cities, markets, and transportation, further increasing the amount and reliability of available food. Very recently, in just the past few decades, industrialization of food production has combined with marketing to provide people in many societies with whatever food they want whenever they want it. Finally, the human dream has been fulfilled!

The foodlike substances on grocery store shelves are a product of selection—not natural selection but selection by us. Food engineers combine fat, salt, sugar, carbohydrates, proteins, and chemicals into diverse shapes, colors, and textures. Their concoctions reach store shelves. We select what we want. Whatever we buy gets more shelf space and spurs imitators and variations that target our desires ever more accurately, like a heat-seeking missile homing in on a jet engine. Convenience stores display the results: row after row of potato chips, sugar-glazed nuts, chocolate-covered fruits, and double chocolate brownie premium ice cream. If you would rather not even chew, pick up a large Frozen Caramel Coffee Coolatta with Cream at Dunkin' Donuts to get 990 calories in a single cup. The food products we take for granted are fantasies made real, available for pennies everywhere.

Alas, what we want is not good for us. Ask your doctor for diet advice. You already know what you will hear: you should eat plenty of vegetables and fruits, some complex carbohydrates, limited amounts of fatty meat, and minimal sugar. Or, more succinctly, "Don't eat anything that you really like, eat only foods that don't especially appeal to you." The irony is unbearable. We have ready access to an infinite supply of foods shaped to precisely satisfy our desires, but consuming them makes us unattractive, frustrated, sick, and short lived.

As a result, millions now endure a daily torture worthy of Tantalus, the favored son of the Greek god Zeus. His first sin was, appropriately enough, introducing mere mortals to the god's divine nectar and ambrosia. When the gods found out, they expressed their displeasure. As a spiteful pseudopenance, he invited them to a banquet and served them boiled bits of his son Pelops. The gods devised a diabolically appropriate punishment: Tantalus was chained eternally in a pool of cool, clear water that receded whenever he tried to drink. Figs, pears, and pomegranates dangling tantalizingly over his head were snatched away whenever he reached for them.

The predicament aroused his thirst and hunger to a frenzy, never to be satisfied.

Our environments pose temptations worthy of Tantalus, but no chains restrain us. Willpower binds us as effectively as wisps of thread. So we get momentary pleasure, followed by enduring shame and sickness. Worse yet, dieting resets the weight set point upward.[13,14,15] It also slows down metabolism. For people who lost hundreds of pounds on the television show *The Biggest Loser*, eating a normal number of calories resulted in regaining weight, despite their still huge body mass.[16] A few people, however, are capable of dramatically limiting their eating. Their problems are even worse.

Anorexia and Bulimia

I recall vividly the twenty-year-old woman admitted to our hospital at 70 pounds, headed for death within days because she would not even drink water. She was convinced she was obese and disgusting. In front of a full-length mirror, she saw a fat girl, but she looked to us like a concentration camp victim. For breakfast, she ate a single Cheerio with ostentatious ceremony, while looking condescendingly at those around her who lacked such self-control. I told her she did not have to eat anything right away but that she had to take water as a medicine. She agreed, and that stabilized her. We put her on a behavior therapy program that required regular eating, but she didn't gain weight. Finally, we discovered a large plastic wastebasket in her closet filled with vomit. She survived and got back to a somewhat normal body weight after months of hospitalization, but she still thought about little except her weight, and she continued to gorge and vomit.

Bulimia is anorexia nervosa with less self-control. Like anorexics, bulimics try to restrict their food intake drastically, but they invariably lose control and gorge in feeding frenzies. Then they vomit, take laxatives, or pursue extreme exercise regimes. Bulimia is far more common than anorexia; fewer people have the self-control to not eat while starving.

Anorexia and bulimia usually begin with a resolve to lose weight fast. After a few days of severe dieting, thoughts focus almost exclusively on food. At some point, any food that comes within reach is consumed in a frenzy: a half gallon of ice cream or a whole loaf of bread. Have you ever tried to hold your breath as long as you can? A bulimic's eating binge is as involuntary as the giant inhalation that ends an attempt to stop breathing.

When I was providing consultations on psychiatric patients on the medical and surgical wards, I would occasionally meet a surgeon who refused to operate on an obese patient, even for cancer, until the patient lost weight. Sometimes when a surgeon said, "Eating is voluntary; they just need to stop," I would say, "Would you mind holding your breath for a minute while I explain the regulation of food intake?" Few played along, but I made my point—and a few enemies.

Imagine you are two days into a celery-and-water diet, and you have just polished off a half gallon of ice cream. How would you feel? Nauseated, of course. Making yourself vomit can relieve the nausea and prevent absorbing a few calories. But your emotions are shame, fear, and hopelessness. Your eating is out of control. If it continues like this, you really will become a blimp. What is the natural thing to do? Try harder. Resolve to eat nothing for the next three days. But on the evening of the second day, you suddenly find yourself holding an empty thirty-two-ounce jar of peanut butter. Now what? Laxatives? Vomiting after every meal? Starting an exercise regime that burns 4,000 calories a day?

Many studies have analyzed brain mechanisms or genes to explain why some individuals are more vulnerable to eating disorders than others. Our task is different; it is to figure out why we all have eating regulation mechanisms that are so vulnerable to dysregulation. The starting point is recognizing that selection has shaped powerful mechanisms to protect against starvation. During a famine, those mechanisms motivate animals to get food—any food—eat it quickly, and eat more than usual, because food supplies are obviously erratic. The system also adjusts the body weight set point upward because extra fat stores are valuable when food sources are unreliable. And, as noted already, weight loss slows down metabolism, which is appropriate when a person is starving but the opposite of what is needed when trying to lose weight. Also, intermittent access to food signals unreliable access to food supplies, so it increases food intake and bingeing, even in rats.[17]

Some peculiar behaviors of people with eating disorders fit this picture well. Our anorexic patients were caught stealing candy so often that we got to know the staff at the hospital gift shop all too well. More often, we discovered purloined sweets concealed in bedding or a closet corner. It's terrible to imagine survival depending on stealing food, hiding it, and eating it rapidly in secret. However, concentration camp survivors reported stealing and hiding bits of food whenever they could.[18] We don't know about the behavior of those who didn't survive. Patients with anorexia nervosa and bulimia are surrounded by excess food, but their bodies are aware only of starvation. Their behavior is appropriate for a situation in which getting just a few extra calories might make the difference between life and death.

The psychiatrist Hilde Bruch wrote thoughtfully about the hundreds of patients she treated with eating disorders.[19] She observed that most disorders are initiated by intense efforts to lose weight but that patients' motives are diverse. Some anorexics value appearance highly from their earliest years; others learn from parents that love is contingent on thinness. Some take inordinate pride in their superior ability to control themselves, often with contempt for others with less self-control. Sometimes a battle of wills with intrusive parents seems primary. A few cases are set off by unintentional weight loss due to medical causes.[20] Sometimes an eating disorder begins with a traumatic experience, tragically often sexual abuse in childhood leading to using obesity to avoid sex as an adult. In rare cases, a brain tumor inhibits eating. Combinations of causes are often needed to explain why some individuals get sick and others do not. Overwhelmingly, however, eating disorders are preceded by a fear of obesity that initiates severe dietary restriction.[21,22,23]

Vulnerability to eating disorders is influenced by genetic factors. If one twin has anorexia nervosa, the other twin's risk is much higher if they are identical twins with identical genes rather than fraternal twins from two different eggs. About half of individual differences in vulnerability can be attributed to genetic differences.[24,25] This makes eating disorders seem like a genetic disease caused by abnormal genes, but it actually implicates rapidly changing environments;[26] abnormal genes causing serious eating problems would have been selected out. The alleles that influence the risk for new disorders are mostly genetic quirks that cause problems only in novel environments. For instance, who gets nearsightedness depends overwhelmingly on genes, but the variations are not abnormalities, they are quirks that don't cause the problem in cultures where children live outdoors and don't learn to read.[27] Like nearsightedness, smoking, substance abuse, and obesity, anorexia is a disorder of modern environments, and most alleles that influence it are harmless variations in the natural environment.

However, geneticists know how to look for genes, so they do. More than 100 researchers conducted a study of more than 5,000 people with anorexia and 21,000 controls. They surveyed the entire genome to find locations that increase the risk of anorexia. They did not find a single one.[28] Another recently published study analyzed 10,641,224 genetic variations in 3,495 anorexia nervosa cases and 10,982 controls. It found one location in the entire genome that increases the risk of anorexia, but the finding is not exactly a smoking gun. The allele, on the 12th chromosome, is present in 48 percent of cases but also in 44 percent of controls, and it increases the risk of anorexia by only 20 percent.[29] Eating disorders are not caused by abnormal genes; they are caused by normal genes interacting with abnormal environments.

Evolutionary Psychology and Eating Disorders

Evolutionary psychologists have proposed possible benefits from eating disorders. Michele Surbey noted that the cessation of menstrual cycling in anorexia nervosa could postpone reproduction when times are bad.[30] Like many other species, humans have mechanisms that turn off reproduction when available calories are insufficient to support a successful pregnancy.[31,32,33] The system monitors not only fat stores but changes of energy availability. When weight declines rapidly, or when exercise is as extreme as that by ballet dancers or marathon runners, the mechanism turns off fertility even if body weight is normal.[34] The amenorrhea in anorexics is indeed a product of a useful system, but reproduction turns off all by itself when food is scarce; there is no need to stop eating.

Other evolutionary psychologists suggest that anorexia may be an extreme of a female strategy to compete for mates. If men want thin women, then women get thinner to be the winner.[35,36] Men do generally prefer shapes typical of young, fertile women, but those shapes include substantial breast, thigh, and buttock fat, nothing like the skin and bones of anorexia.[37] More damning for the hypothesis, most anorexics don't seem to be on the hunt for a man, many are not interested in sex, and they don't have very many children.

Those who view anorexia as a product of sexual competition do not all assume that anorexia itself is an adaptation; most note only that extreme competitive strategies to get mates often overshoot. This seems plausible: the rate of anorexia is ten times higher for women than for men. An alternative hypothesis is that women are competing for status, but a study of more than 200 young women found that disordered eating was much more common in those rated high on mate competition rather than on status competition.[38] To those not in psychology it must seem blindingly obvious that women intent on getting the best men are especially concerned about their bodies.

It has even been suggested that restricting food intake is a strategy useful during famine. The "fleeing famine" theory tries to explain the failure to eat available food, and the excess exercise often observed in anorexics, as parts of a strategy to run away from an area where food sources are depleted into some other place.[39] I can't make sense of the idea or the other possibilities except as examples of the error of VDAA—Viewing Diseases as Adaptations. Anorexia nervosa and bulimia are disorders, new ones, without redeeming features.

New Problems

While examples of eating disorders can be found throughout history, they became much more common from the 1960s onward in technologically advanced countries, first in women from the upper classes, then spreading across the socioeconomic spectrum.[40] What in modern environments explains the recent epidemic? Several possibilities are plausible. When humans lived in small bands of thirty to fifty foragers, only a few potential mates were available, and they likely looked rather similar. In modern societies, an individual's appearance can be compared instantly to thousands of others', including fantasies made real. The bodies we see on television are carefully selected one-in-a-thousand specimens that have been further augmented and sculpted by exercise and surgery. Then those rare sculpted shapes are airbrushed to create images as artificial, and as exquisitely tuned to what we want, as candy bars are to our appetites.

No real person can measure up. Some people manage to control their weight and get trim and toned. Most of us keep trying to keep eating under control. But the few unfortunate ones, often those driven the most to be thin, slip into a positive feedback spiral in which increased commitment to weight loss leads to out-of-control eating, more fear of gaining weight, more strenuous dieting, and an increased weight set point, in a spiral that can consume life itself.

When I asked one anorexic patient how many cans of diet soda she drank each day, I was dumbstruck by the reply. "About eighteen," she said. The average number per week for patients who binge and purge is forty, along with one hundred packets of artificial sweetener.[41] This should not be surprising; starving people crave sweets.

Sophisticated mechanisms prepare the body for a sugar load. Sweet tastes release insulin, which lowers blood glucose.[42] If the sweetener is artificial and no real sugar comes in, the insulin surge could lower the blood sugar level and increase appetite, but studies of this phenomenon are tricky and results are inconsistent.[43]

There are taste receptors not just on the tongue but also in the stomach and small bowel,[44] so testing the effects of an artificial sweetener by having people swish a sweet solution in the mouth is different from swallowing it. Also, the effects of artificial sweeteners may be different for obese versus lean subjects, and different artificial sweeteners have different effects.[45]

The increased use of artificial sweeteners by obese people could be a cause or a result or both. A study of 3,682 people in San Antonio, Texas, found that the risk of normal-weight people becoming obese over a six-year period was doubled for those who drank more than three cans of artificially sweetened beverages per day.[46] Were people who worried about their weight especially likely to drink them? Or did they feel that the calorie-free drinks allowed them to eat more? Two review papers found no systematic evidence that the use of artificial sweeteners increases weight,[47,48] while a more recent, larger study suggests that they probably do.[49] The question is contentious, and the evidence is hard to interpret, because some research is supported by artificial sweetener manufacturers with billions of dollars at stake.

Thin Babies Become Heavy Adults

The British physician David Barker observed almost thirty years ago that babies born especially thin often developed obesity later in life.[50] They were also especially prone to developing coronary artery disease and diabetes. These findings pose a classic evolutionary puzzle: Does limited nutrition in utero simply damage metabolic control mechanisms, or are the changes part of an adaptive response?

Sir Peter Gluckman, a physician-scientist who has been the chief science adviser to New Zealand's prime minister, came up with a very interesting idea: he suggested that limited nutrition in utero could signal a harsh environment in which it would be wise to shift metabolism so it stores more calories.[51] He calls this the *predictive adaptive response*. His idea inspired fascinating research showing that early exposure to caloric deprivation in utero adds tiny molecules to DNA that stop some genes from making proteins, a process called *genomic imprinting*.[52] Those changes shift metabolism in ways that cause obesity and atherosclerosis. They can be transmitted to a future generation, so the obesity risk of a child may be influenced by a mother's or grandmother's diet.[53] This finding may turn out to be an example of what are called epigenetic effects, but other mechanisms can also influence future generations, for instance, changes in the mother's behavior.[54]

One enterprising primatologist, Jenny Tung, recognized an opportunity to test the predictive adaptive response theory. She studied baboons who were pregnant during a drought and kept track of their babies in future years. Another drought occurred. Were babies born during a drought better protected from the effects of the subsequent drought? No, they did worse than other baboons.[55] This does not by itself shoot down the predictive adaptive response idea, but it's a fine example of how creative scientists find ways to test hypotheses.

People sometimes think that an evolutionary view implies that everything is genetically determined. Quite the opposite: selection shapes systems that monitor the environment and adjust the body and behavior in useful ways. Sun exposure turns on the protective tanning response. Muscles that are used build up to do what needs to be done. The predictive adaptive response is another possible example. The Simon Fraser University evolutionary biologist Bernard Crespi and the leading British researchers Daniel Nettle and Melissa Bateson have shown why such self-adjusting systems are intrinsically vulnerable to going out of whack: they all require positive feedback to shift the system to a different mode, and controlling positive feedback is always a challenge.[56,57]

An evolutionary view offers no simple way to prevent or cure eating disorders, but it asks and answers new questions. It explains why dieting adjusts the weight set point higher: when food supplies are unreliable, extra stores are worthwhile. It explains how a useful response to famine, gorging, can spiral into bulimia and anorexia. It suggests that the brain mechanisms regulating weight will be hard to influence and that we should not expect to find specific defective genes for eating disorders. It encourages close attention to aspects of modern environments that could influence metabolism, such as artificial sweeteners and antibiotics. Most specific to our topic, an evolutionary perspective explains why severe dieting causes eating disorders and weight gain.

These principles may help to find ways to control the eating disorders epidemic. For those already in the clutches of anorexia or bulimia, recognizing how positive feedback maintains the disorder can be a revelation that changes behavior. For others, it can spur useful discussions with a therapist. Understanding why it is hard to control our eating encourages subtler and sometimes paradoxical strategies to control it. As Weight Watchers and other programs recognize, regular small meals work better than resolutions to not eat for days.

Tantalus in a Candy Store Watching Pornography and Tweeting on a Smartphone

Eating disorders are but one example of how modern environments set up our ancient minds for trouble. As resources of diverse kinds become more readily available, we all face multiple predicaments like that of Tantalus.

Social resources are now as abundant as food. Facebook, Twitter, and Snapchat create new kinds of social connections that are, to human relationships, what candy is to food. Watching others become Facebook royalty or Twitter stars boosts social desires more than it provides ways to satisfy them. Dissatisfaction grows from the gap.

Occupations that require boring, backbreaking labor are vanishing. Thousands of new kinds of jobs provide the satisfaction of using talents to accomplish meaningful work. However, satisfying work that pays well is available to only a few. Others watch with envy from factories, hotels, fast-food restaurants, and big-box stores. Seeing opportunities available only to others arouses envy.

Material wealth beyond what previous kings and queens could imagine is now available to many. Possessions are so plentiful that some people make a living helping others to purchase, organize, and discard a surfeit of things. Our minds were not prepared for such material excess any more than they were prepared for social media or fast food. We can restrain clicking to order things from Amazon about as well as we can restrain taking one more bite of hot fudge sundae.

Attractiveness and abilities don't come in the mail, but we can now compare ourselves to actors, models, musicians, artists, athletes, politicians and performers who are one in a million. We watch movies about aspiring, ambitious young men and women who overcome obstacles to succeed grandly; the 999,999 who fail get little attention.

Birth control and disease prevention have made sex more available to more people more often. However, ads, vibrators, and videos arouse desires that previously were at the edge of imagination. So there is more sex but also greater desire. Opportunities for romantic and sexual relationships are now a world marketplace of desire and deception, from Match.com to Tinder. We hardly know what we should do—except get our bodies in better shape and find someone to take attractive photographs of us.

Tantalus was chained, so he could never satisfy his desires. No such chains bind us, so we construct our own. Some people get their teeth wired shut to reduce eating. Some unplug the internet cable and mail it to themselves to get a few days free from distraction. Many join groups to help to control their desires. Psychotherapy and meditation help many more. There are so many solutions because desires will not be denied. Trying to satisfy desires leads to excess and more frustration. Trying to put a lid on them just increases the pressure in the pot.

The conflict is old. Philosophers in ancient Greece described the possible solutions.[58] Hedonism recommended pursuing pleasure without restraint. Stoicism recommended pursuing virtue, putting up with pain, and practicing restraint to avoid being distracted by desire. Epicureanism recognized that suffering comes from pursuing desires, so it encouraged enjoying pleasures as they are available but keeping desires and social striving at a distance. Living with abundance creates new problems—but they are first-world problems many people would love to have.

CHAPTER 13

GOOD FEELINGS FOR BAD REASONS

Then Noah began farming and planted a vineyard. He drank of the wine and became drunk, and uncovered himself inside his tent.

—Genesis 9:20–21 (New American Standard Bible)

Our team of consulting psychiatrists was making rounds on the medicine ward. The internists asked us to see a forty-five-year-old woman whose liver was failing. They told her she would die if she continued drinking. She told them she didn't care. They thought that was suicidal and decided it was time to invite the shrinks for a visit.

She looked as if she were already dead. Her skin was puffy and yellow, her arms had no muscle, and her abdomen was so swollen she looked pregnant. The senior psychiatrist in our group asked her, very gently, about her use of alcohol. She replied, "I like it. You can't stop me. Nothing can." The psychiatrist pointed out that continuing to drink would cause her death in a matter of weeks and that treatment was available. "So?" she said. "I guess I like liquor better than life."

When he tried to engage her further, she interrupted him, paused, and glared at the half circle of young doctors around the foot of her bed. "I've been to rehab ten times, and I've always gone back to the sauce. It won't be any different now. I don't want to quit. You can't help. No one can. I have made my decision. Leave me alone." Portraying her helplessness as a choice gave her a shred of self-respect, but only that of a prisoner on the gallows tightening the noose around her own neck. The next day she was gone, signed out of the hospital, on her way to becoming one of the 100,000 Americans alcohol kills each year.[1]

Substance abuse takes a staggering toll. In the United States, 30 percent of adults have at some point qualified for a diagnosis of alcohol abuse or alcoholism.[2] In 2015 8.4 percent of men and 4.2 percent of women in the United States had an alcohol use disorder and 10 percent of the population used illicit drugs.[3] Tobacco use is more common and more deadly. Worldwide, more than a billion humans are addicted to nicotine, including more than a third of all men over age fifteen. In the United States the smoking rate has decreased to 20 percent of adults, but smoking still kills 480,000 Americans each year, nearly five times as many as alcohol.[4]

The toll extends far beyond users. Some people recall bringing friends home after school to find a parent drunk and half-naked. Others' lives were changed when a father crashed his car into a tree and was never able to talk right or hold a job again. What would it be like at age eight to wonder, every night, if your father was going to wander into your room and possibly hit you, possibly fondle you, or possibly just ramble on, insisting on close attention? What would it be like to listen to your parents screaming and threatening to kill each other in the night and wake to hear them deny that anything had happened? And what do you do when your roommate tokes up every day, stops working, won't pay rent, and won't move out?

Old Questions, New Questions

The enormity of substance abuse problems has spurred gigantic efforts to find solutions. Most have asked the usual questions: Why do some people get addicted when others don't? What brain mechanisms cause substance abuse? What strategies for prevention and treatment work best? Plenty of knowledge is now available, but it hasn't done much to stem the tide.

Our questions are different, as always.[5] Why are members of our species vulnerable to addiction? Drug, alcohol, and tobacco use cause so much early death, you would think that natural selection would have eliminated the alleles that make some people more vulnerable. But it didn't. Why not? Even aside from natural selection, you would think that people would learn about the dangers of substance use and avoid it. Some do, but most don't.

The root cause of the addiction is our capacity for learning.[6] Eliminate learning, and you eliminate substance abuse. That is not a practical solution. Learning is useful. It gives advantages that rigid preprograming can't. Reinforcement learning works by selection—not natural selection but selection among varying behaviors. Individuals do various things. Actions that are followed by rewards become more frequent. Those that fail or cause pain become less frequent.

There are half a dozen ways to pry the shell off a pistachio nut. Those that break fingernails or leave shells intact are set aside; those that work are repeated and refined. To get fruit from a tree, you can climb up, use a stick, throw a stone, or shake the tree. Whatever works best will be repeated. There are also many ways to entice a potential lover. Whatever works induces a powerful dopamine surge that brings pleasure and a tendency to do it again. Orgasms are powerful reinforcers. Students learn about rats in Skinner boxes and get the idea that learning mechanisms are crude, as if giving people M&M's can cure problems. However, facial expressions, touches, and tones of voice are also reinforcers. Even the tone you get from a clarinet can shape your mouth to make it better. Tiny blips of dopamine gradually pin a coherent version of a sentence to the page.

Hijacked

When the behavior control system operates normally, millions of neurons process dozens of auditory, visual, touch, flavor, and odor cues. If the buzzing electrical pattern in the brain is like patterns that have increased fitness previously, for our ancestors or for the individual, then dopamine blips motivate repeating whatever behavior preceded getting into that good space.

Drugs that increase or imitate dopamine hijack these subtle mechanisms like a terrorist in a pilot's uniform taking over an airplane cockpit.[7] They bypass brain navigation systems and grab the joystick. Cues present just before the drug reached the control center become enticing. Drug users move toward them, and after arriving, they repeat whatever behaviors worked before to get the reward. That cold, dingy room thick with smoke swirling around a single lightbulb has little appeal—unless you shot heroin there. In which case you will be drawn back to the room, and when you get there you will again almost certainly insert the needle that induced a dopamine surge that signaled to your brain that your fitness just increased by the equivalent of having sixteen grandchildren.

The pursuit of normal rewards is automatically regulated. Eating is pleasurable at first, but satiation eventually makes even one more Thin Mint unthinkable. Sex has a wonderful conclusion that downregulates desire for a time. The pleasures of social intercourse last longer, but after a while interest declines and shifts behavior elsewhere. Selection never shaped similar systems to control drug taking. Drugs arouse pleasure, causing increased desire and increased drug use, in a vicious spiral down to death.

None of this was much of a problem for our ancestors. Pure drugs were not reliably available, so they caused no harm that would shape protective systems. That suggests another solution for addiction: turn back the clock ten thousand years, to before the age of agriculture, before pure drugs were available. That is about as practical as eliminating learning. However, substance abuse is a dramatic example of a disease caused by the mismatch between our ancestral brains and our modern environments.

New techniques of drug purification, new routes of administration, such as cigarette papers and hypodermic needles, and new technologies of transport and storage combine with market economies to ensure availability. Laws and police efforts hardly make a dent. Markets emerge to provide what people want, and technologies adapt to changing situations. Interdiction efforts motivate chemists to invent new addictive molecules, ever more potent and easier to smuggle.

Why Plants Make Drugs

Addictive chemicals were present long before chemists, thanks to plants. Why do plants make psychotropic drugs? Not for our pleasure, that's for sure. Cocaine, opium, caffeine, hallucinogens, and nicotine are neurotoxins. Natural selection shaped them because plants containing insect toxins are less likely to be eaten. Few insects can eat a tobacco leaf. Nicotine is such an effective insecticide that a spray of tobacco-infused water protects fruit tree leaves. Caffeine seems innocuous, but a single coffee bean can kill a mouse.

Most chemicals that give humans a buzz evolved to disrupt insect nervous systems. If our brains used different chemicals, we would not be so vulnerable. However, we have common ancestors with insects. It was *long* ago, about 500 million years ago, when our ancestors split off from the arthropod lines that became modern insects. However, our neurochemicals remain about the same as theirs. Fortunately, most plant neurotoxins don't kill us. We have evolved to eat plants, and we are much larger than insects, so low doses are not fatal. But drugs can hijack our motivation mechanisms and take control of our lives.

Some psychologists have suggested that natural selection shaped us to like drugs and alcohol.[8,9] Some such proposals deserve consideration; others strain credulity. For instance, some have wondered if people who liked alcohol might have been more likely to loosen up and have sex, directly increasing fitness. That strikes me as an idea hatched by psychology students getting drunk and hopeful at a pickup bar. Would a tendency to disinhibition give similar reproductive advantages in the ancestral human social environment? I doubt it, but social drug use is common in hunter-gatherer societies, so it is hard to say for sure.

A taste for alcohol, beer in particular, has been said to decrease the risk of infection because fermented beverages are less likely than water to carry bacteria. The idea makes a fine meme, but it gets little support from history or science.[10] A better idea is that alcohol in overripe fruit signals available nutrition.[11] This is plausible, but it is also possible that alcohol's influence on reward mechanisms is an accidental side effect.[12] Whatever the reason, people love booze, and some of the most ancient pots discovered by archeologists have residues from fermentation. One can even make a case for people settling down to the boring work of agriculture in part to get reliable access to grain they could use to make beer.[13]

Our preference for tobacco could have been shaped because nicotine is a good deworming agent; it paralyzes helminths so they lose their grip on our intestines and are expelled.[14,15,16] If this is correct, you would expect tobacco to be used mainly in locations where worms are prevalent, mainly by people with high burdens of worms and mainly orally instead of by smoking. However, diverse species are vulnerable to nicotine addiction; only a few animals in the wild use nicotine-containing plants, and humans don't usually eat those plants.

People living in the Andes have chewed coca leaves for centuries. Especially at high altitudes, it relieves fatigue and gives energy for physical work. But I don't know of evidence that people were shaped to like cocaine. It powerfully reinforces behavior for most animals, not just humans.[17]

This is not to say that humans have not influenced plants because of their drugs. We like them so much that we have bred—selected for— tobacco with a high nicotine concentration and marijuana with a high THC concentration. We plant thousands of acres of tobacco, marijuana, coca, and poppies, giving these domesticated species a big advantage over similar plants that don't offer the same kick. Edward Hagen and his colleagues have suggested that humans have used and benefited from plant psychoactive chemicals long enough for protection against their toxic effects to evolve.[18,19,20]

An Old Problem Escalating

Substance use isn't new. Neither are its problems. Two anthropologist friends, Paul Turke and Laura Betzig, did field research on a small atoll in the Pacific.[21]

The men who live there work a few hours a day fishing with nets. They also make wine by cutting off the tips of young palm trees and bending them over with a string so that the sap drips into a pot. A few days later they return to collect a fermented beverage that gives everyone a good time during evening parties. Pots and string to make palm wine are early drug paraphernalia. Every advance in technology is used to provide ever purer drugs by ever more direct routes of administration.

Fermentation is easy. Distillation is harder, but the necessary knowledge and equipment are now available almost everywhere. The resulting hard liquor is far more prone to cause addiction. Even without addiction, drunks can be dangerous. Trying to control them has been a function and challenge for governments and policing from the beginnings of written records.

Tobacco provides a mild high when chewed and more when smoked in cigars. But the addiction that kills more people than any other was initiated when cigarette papers and mild tobacco allowed deep inhalation that gets nicotine to the brain instantly.

Marijuana is relaxing in the doses available from wild-growing plants. Concentrations have been increased manyfold by breeding and more yet by extracting potent THC concentrates that give hallucinations instead of a gentle high.

Coca leaves have been chewed for centuries as an energizer, but cocaine was first extracted in the mid-1800s. Its use in beverages and tonics grew so fast at the start of the twentieth century that laws were soon passed to control it, not so much because of addiction but because users were likely to get out of control.[22] Freud was a cocaine user, along with many others in the nineteenth century.[23] But the problems then were nothing compared to the epidemic in the 1980s that followed the widespread availability of crack, the crystallized form of cocaine.

Natural opium is addictive when smoked and was a chronic problem in India and China even before new trade routes brought it to Europe in the 1600s. Soon after that, the British East India Company was selling Indian opium in China.[24] The Chinese government tried to ban it in 1799. In 1839, the British sent warships to defend their opium business in China. The active ingredient, morphine, is more addictive. A process to extract it was discovered in 1804, and morphine was first marketed by Merck in 1827. Sales soared after the invention of hypodermic needles in the middle of the nineteenth century. Heroin was marketed by the Bayer Company early in the twentieth century as a nonaddicting form of morphine. Whoops! The Harrison Act of 1914 imposed restrictions, and heroin was banned in the United States in the 1920s, but the trade and addiction continue unabated.[25,26]

The trajectory is clear: our minds have always been vulnerable to capture by alcohol, marijuana, tobacco, coca, and opium, but problems with them have escalated as advances in chemistry, transportation, and technology have increased the diversity, purity, and availability of drugs. The mismatch was bad before; now it's getting much worse.

Some drugs, such as amphetamine, are synthetic from the start, but their effects result from their similarity to neurotransmitters. The rise of easy-to-synthesize methamphetamine has combined with intravenous administration to create a plague that paralyzes whole countries.[27] The invention of new superpotent synthetic narcotics makes interdiction efforts nearly hopeless. Carfentanil is ten thousand times more potent than morphine.[28] Touching it can cause a fatal overdose, so police now need to wear gloves when making drug arrests. One smuggled printer cartridge can contain a million doses.[29] Imagine being the worker who stirs it with powdered milk to dilute it to the right concentration. Slightly inadequate stirring leaves pockets with higher concentrations that will turn into pockets of overdose deaths in the surrounding community.

Withdrawal, Wanting, and Liking

When I first learned about substance abuse, the emphasis was on withdrawal. That is what doctors mainly need to manage; however, this focus left the misimpression that people continue to use drugs mainly to avoid withdrawal. Withdrawal is painful, but learning sustains use even without withdrawal.

Withdrawal syndromes reflect a normal useful regulatory process. Continued stimulation of bodily systems results in opposing shifts that stabilize them. The mellow calm after several evening drinks is countered by arousal at 3 a.m. The excitement and energy induced by amphetamines crash into depression and fatigue a few hours later. Taking fast-acting antianxiety drugs for a few months downregulates the arousal system. When they are stopped suddenly, compensating systems push anxiety levels sky-high. In the years when we psychiatrists were assured by the highest authorities that it was not habit forming, I started many patients on Xanax. The distress many experienced while getting off the drug still makes me feel guilty and stupid for naively trusting experts who turned out to be shills for pharmaceutical companies.

Behavior regulation systems use carefully controlled bursts of positive feedback to shift behavior from one activity to another. Reward for the previous activity plummets while reward for the new one escalates. Supercues, of the sort found in modern environments, can hijack such systems. A potato chip advertisement challenges, "Betcha can't eat just one." The company wins the bet; our diets lose.

Most bouts of activity follow a predictable cycle. Once we start an activity, we continue until we are finished, and woe to anyone who interferes. It's easier to put down the newspaper than a bag of potato chips. And it's much easier to put down a bag of potato chips than to stop in the middle of making love. As for snorting cocaine . . . Whatever the activity, it tends to rev up at the beginning in ways that make it hard to stop.

Why do our behavior regulation mechanisms structure our activities into discrete bouts? The proximate explanation is found in brain mechanisms. The evolutionary reason is that most behaviors have start-up costs. They are like the time spent looking for another raspberry bush. Imagine if you picked berries for five minutes, then went out to build a fence, then talked with friends, and then came back and picked berries for another five minutes. At the end of the day, you would be undernourished, the fence would be unfinished, and your friends would likely be very annoyed.

The problem with abused drugs is not that they arouse pleasure; the problem is that they increase desire. My colleague the psychologist Kent Berridge has shown that this "wanting" system tends to overwhelm and outlast the "liking" system, so that some chronic users desperately want drugs that no longer provide much pleasure.[30] "Wanting" hardly begins to describe the tragedy of people in the trap of spending all their available time, effort, thought, and money getting and taking drugs, even though the high is no longer all that pleasurable.

Why Are Some People Especially Vulnerable?

Not everyone gets addicted. Some people can even use heroin recreationally, setting it aside when they need to. The variation in vulnerability results, as for so many other traits, mainly from genetic variations.[31,32] It might seem that the alleles that make people vulnerable are defects, but they probably didn't influence fitness much in environments where drugs weren't available. They probably did, however, influence behavior. Finding out how should be a high priority.

I suspect that people who are especially vulnerable to addiction may use different foraging strategies from other people. Higher sensitivity to rewards would make them more likely than others to go back to the same places where they found food before. People with brains less vulnerable to addiction would likely wander more widely. It would be well worth watching how children forage for raspberries. Do children from families prone to addiction forage differently from others? If they do, it should be possible to create computer games that would predict, better than any questionnaire, interview, or genetic test, which individuals are especially vulnerable to addiction.

Different populations vary dramatically in substance use, thanks to cultural variations, especially prohibitions enforced by religious teachings and leaders. Within a population, however, people whose lives are going badly are more vulnerable.[33] People who get little pleasure from their daily lives and those plagued by anxiety, low mood, or boredom find the pleasure from drug use more compelling. A huge body of literature describes how personality, experiencing trauma, poverty, and difficult life situations influence vulnerability to addiction.[34] They combine with genetic variations to explain why some people are more vulnerable than others.

Taming the Plague

An evolutionary perspective is no better at suggesting new quick cures for addiction than any other perspective is. It does not even try to explain how drugs change brain mechanisms. It does, however, correct false ideas and provide suggestions for new studies. For public policy, the implications are discouraging. Criminalization and interdiction have filled prisons and corrupted governments in country after country. However, increasingly potent drugs that can be synthesized in any basement make controlling access increasingly impossible. Legalization seems like a good idea but causes more addiction. Our strongest defense is likely to be education, but scare stories make kids want to try drugs. Every child should learn that drugs take over the brain and turn some people into miserable zombies and that we have no way to tell who will get addicted the fastest. They should also learn that the high fades as addiction takes over.

New treatments are desperately needed. Nora Volkow, the leader of the National Institute on Drug Abuse, describes how rapid progress in understanding the brain mechanisms that cause addiction should lead to new drugs to block those mechanisms.[35] This offers a real way forward. The substance abuse epidemic is created by novel environments, but changing social environments is difficult and changing human nature is impossible. Solutions will more likely come from finding ways to change our brains.

CHAPTER 14

MINDS UNBALANCED ON FITNESS CLIFFS

The superiority of the human brain to others . . . is a reason why mental disorders are certainly most conspicuous and probably most common in man . . . the longest chain of effectively operated neuronic chains, is . . . likely to perform a complicated type of behavior efficiently very close to the edge of an overload, [and] will give way in a serious and catastrophic way . . . very possibly amounting to insanity.

—Norbert Wiener,
*Cybernetics; or Control and Communication
in the Animal and the Machine*[1]

Schizophrenia, autism, and bipolar disorder are very different diseases. Schizophrenia is a cognitive collapse in which every event is imbued with excess personal meaning and the inability to separate inner life from outer life gives rise to hallucinations and delusions. Autism is manifested in early childhood by a lack of social connectedness and solitary preoccupation with repeated motions and nonsocial thinking. Bipolar disease is the product of a broken moodostat that causes alternating periods of depression and mania. These are dire diseases.

Despite their differences, these diseases have overlapping features that make an evolutionary perspective especially useful. Each afflicts approximately 1 percent of populations worldwide. Each has milder forms that affect 2 to 5 percent of people. Vulnerability depends overwhelmingly on what genes a person has, but people with schizophrenia or autism have fewer children than other people. The evolutionary question is obvious: Why hasn't natural selection eliminated the genetic variations causing these diseases?

The evidence for genetic causes is strong. Genetic variations explain about 70 percent of the risk of bipolar disorder,[2] 80 percent of schizophrenia,[3] and 50 percent of autism.[4] Having a parent or sibling with one of these diseases increases the risk roughly tenfold.[5,6,7] Having an identical twin with one of these disorders increases the risk to over 50 percent.[8]

Because identical twins do not always have the same diagnosis, some conclude that an environmental factor must also be involved. However, studies of adopted children show that the family in which a child is raised has little influence on the risk. It is more likely that the differences between identical twins result from chance variations influencing brain development, such as which genes are turned on or turned off and when, and the wandering paths of neurons as they grow.

I wish I had known sooner that these are genetic diseases. I recall trying to console a mother who was bereft because her son's doctors would not allow her to visit him during a hospital stay of several months for psychosis. Worse, they said, her early relationship with him had contributed to his schizophrenia. Home videotapes of babies who later developed schizophrenia show parents behaving slightly differently toward them compared to their siblings. However, those differences are not because parental behavior causes schizophrenia; it is because babies with a predisposition to schizophrenia are already slightly different.[9] My patient felt guilty and distraught, but at the time no one knew enough to tell her and her doctors firmly that parenting has nothing to do with causing schizophrenia.

Autism was also blamed on parents, especially women viewed as intellectualized "refrigerator mothers." I saw one such mother, an accomplished academic. She was indeed intellectual, but she was not cold; she was alternately hot with anger about being blamed for her son's illness, then depressed and guilty because of thinking that it might be true. She had a touch of the social awkwardness that characterizes many relatives of people with autism, not surprising since half of her genes were the same as her son's. Such incredibly wrong theories about these diseases caused untold harm. Thank goodness, we know more now and can avoid adding unwarranted guilt to the already huge burden borne by the parents of afflicted children.

Dashed Hopes

At the turn of the millennium, hope was high that the alleles causing these diseases would soon be found. The human genome had just been sequenced. Cheaper ways to get genetic data were coming online. All signs suggested that the genetic causes would be found soon. Different versions of scores of genes had been investigated as suspected causes of schizophrenia at a cost of about $250 million. However, the first really large studies revealed that those early candidate genes were all innocent.[10,11] Whole careers were spent chasing statistical will-o'-the-wisps.

The next stage was to examine the entire genome instead of specific genes. Researchers looked at markers spread over all twenty-three chromosomes to see if variations at certain locations were more common in people with these diseases than they were in other people. Every bit of the genome has been scoured. The conclusion is firm: there are no common genetic variations that substantially increase the risk of schizophrenia, autism, or bipolar disease.[12,13] Some increase the risk, but almost all by less than 1 percent. All the identified loci that influence the risk of schizophrenia together explain only 5 percent of the variation.[14] Furthermore, the alleles that increase the risk of schizophrenia also increase the risk of bipolar disorder.[15]

The disappointment has been crushing. Imagine being one of the scientists who spent years in the lab studying genetic variations that cause these diseases and then discovering that they were all just statistical flukes. We thought we would find specific genetic flaws causing specific diseases. What we found is organic complexity beyond our imagining. It is as if archaeologists using radar sensors were sure they saw a new Rosetta stone deep in a pyramid, but when they finally got to it in person, the first flashlight beam revealed that it was just a pile of sand.

Some genetic disorders are caused by specific genetic mutations with big effects. Huntington's chorea (aka Woody Guthrie's disease) is a good example: if you have the allele, you get the disease. For diseases such as cystic fibrosis caused by recessive genes, you get the disease if you have two copies of a defective allele. However, most common genetic diseases are very different. Instead of a few identifiable genetic variations with big effects, they are caused by thousands of variations spread across the genome, each with only a tiny effect. This is the case not only for schizophrenia, autism, and bipolar disease but also for type II diabetes, high blood pressure, coronary artery disease, migraine headaches, and obesity.

The inability to find specific alleles that cause genetic diseases is called the problem of "missing heritability."[16,17,18] The heritability is not really missing; solid studies document strong effects of genes. What is missing is identification of the specific alleles that account for the heritability. If variations in who gets schizophrenia result mostly from genetic variations, why is it so hard to find the specific responsible alleles?

One possibility is that the responsible variations are rare and so can't be found even if they have big effects. Some very rare variations in the number of copies of a gene do increase the risk of major mental disorders by five times or more. However, even they don't cause disease reliably on their own. For autism, only 5 percent of the heritable variation arises from rare mutations.[19] Also, rare variations are unlikely to account for very many cases. One study that looked at both common genetic variations in genes and rare variations in the numbers of copies of genes influencing schizophrenia found that each identified variation explained almost exactly the same proportion of the overall variation in risk: 0.04 percent, that is, 4 parts out of 10,000.[20] Hardly any. How curious that they all have the same effect size, albeit tiny.

Despite the challenges, the search for genetic causes of mental disorders is nonetheless proceeding fast. The current hope is that combinations of genes will be found to have potent effects that identify the brain circuits causing the problems. Such advances could emerge even before this book is published; that would be wonderful. However, it is now seeming likely that what we have been looking for is not there. A leader in this research area, Kenneth Kendler, says, "The most pessimistic prediction that we will observe only a mess is unlikely. But discovering a highly coherent single pathway to illness also seems improbable . . . despite our wishing so, individual gene variants of large effect appear to have a small to non-existent role in the etiology of major psychiatric disorders."[21] In hindsight, this should not have been surprising; natural selection tends to eliminate alleles that cause dire illnesses.

The mystery of missing heritability is becoming a bit less mysterious. New studies show that even though specific alleles have tiny influences, most effects can be explained by very complex interactions of many alleles.[22] However, no combination of three or ten specific alleles causes disease reliably. Instead, disease risk is influenced by variations in thousands of genes with tiny effects interacting with one another and the environment. One recent report discovered that the number of genetic variations on each chromosome that increase the risk for schizophrenia is proportional to the size of the chromosome.[23] They are spread randomly over the entire genome like tiny beads on twenty-three strings, with more beads on the longer strings. Another important finding is that most of the alleles influencing the risk of schizophrenia also influence the risk of bipolar disorder.[24]

The discovery that the risk of schizophrenia and autism increases with the age of the father but not the mother suggested that new mutations were responsible. This is because a woman's lifetime supply of eggs is formed about the time of birth but sperm are formed continuously by multiple cell divisions prone to errors.[25,26] However, new studies show that the risk comes not from the age a father had a child but from the age at which he had his first child.[27,28] Men who start families late in life are different from other men in ways that increase the risk of schizophrenia in their children. Nonetheless, 75 percent of new mutations come from fathers, and this accounts for 10 to 20 percent of cases of schizophrenia in the offspring of older fathers.

The mountain of new facts is revealing the limits of the standard schema. A mechanic's model assumes that the brain is constructed of discrete circuits with specific functions. It assumes specific disorders that can be defined by specific identifiable brain pathology with specific genetic causes. It assumes that normal brains are made by normal genomes and abnormal brains are products of abnormal genes. But many alleles that influence risk are not abnormal, and many of them influence multiple disorders. A deeper evolutionary perspective suggests the need to embrace the reality of organic complexity and look for causes not just in mechanisms but in trade-offs that cause intrinsic vulnerabilities.

Instead of just looking for broken parts and the causes of disease in some individuals, we can also ask why all members of our species are vulnerable.

Many US readers will have listened to *Car Talk*, the wonderful public radio show in which Click and Clack, the Tappet Brothers, diagnosed automotive problems with their thick Boston accents and uproarious laughter.

Callers describe arcane problems. Sally in Dallas has an MG that won't start again after being driven on a hot day. Click and Clack first diagnose her car's problem: vapor lock. They then describe the mechanism that causes the problem: the fuel pump can move only liquid, so when the gasoline in a hot fuel line vaporizes, the car won't start again until it cools down. Click and Clack then go into engineering mode. They describe the design flaw that makes the problem common for that specific car model: MGs from that year have a fuel line near the hot exhaust manifold, so they are especially prone to vapor lock. Finally they explain why vapor lock is an inherent problem for all cars with carburetors. When I was a teenager, I listened to an automotive engineer neighbor talk about his work trying to prevent vapor lock. I said, "Well, if it is just too much heat, that should be easy to solve." He said, "Oh, yeah? It is hot above an engine. Where would you put the fuel pump and carburetor?" After spending years creating strategies to minimize the problem, he had little patience for a kid who did not understand that vapor lock is an intrinsic vulnerability with no easy solution.

Could schizophrenia, autism, and bipolar disorder result from similar intrinsic vulnerabilities in human minds? If so, genetic variations that influence risk are related to the cause only in the same distant way that different auto models differ in their vulnerability to vapor lock. An evolutionary approach suggests looking for inherent constraints in the brain's information-processing systems.

The Evolutionary Genetics of Dire Disorders

People with schizophrenia or autism have far fewer offspring than unaffected siblings, with the reduction stronger for men than for women.[29,30] Sisters of affected individuals tend to have very slightly increased numbers of children, perhaps in compensation, but brothers have fewer.[31] Selection against these disorders should be strong.

The most probable evolutionary explanation is that there are limits to what selection can do. In an influential review paper Matthew Keller and Geoffrey Miller discounted the role of environmental mismatch and expressed skepticism about the idea that alleles for mental disorders give advantages.[32] They concluded that the most plausible explanation is that new mutations are continually created and only slowly selected out. That is certainly correct and a major cause of mental disorders. They went on to suggest that the brain is especially vulnerable because so many genes are involved in constructing it. This is more questionable. Even more genes influence height, but height abnormalities are uncommon. Machines malfunction if even one part fails, but bodies usually work just fine despite many mutations and minor bits of damage.

A model based only on mutation implies that some combination of normal genes could prevent disease completely while maximizing fitness. However, this may be incorrect. Vulnerability to dire disorders could persist even if all mutations could be eliminated. Several possibilities deserve consideration.

One is the intriguing idea, developed by the evolutionary biologist Bernard Crespi and colleagues, that schizophrenia and autism are genetic flip sides of the same coin and that they result from genes that benefit their own transmission despite the cost to the host.[33,34] The logic is based on an observation by Robert Trivers, further developed by the Harvard biologist David Haig, that chemical tags placed on chromosomes early in development inhibit the expression of certain genes.[35] The relevance of this imprinting process for obesity was described in chapter 13. Imprinting can also turn off genes selectively, depending on whether they come from the mother or from the father.[36]

Genes that come from mothers get an advantage by keeping a fetus a bit smaller to conserve the mother's resources for a future pregnancy with her same genes and to ensure safe childbirth. Genes from the paternal line get an advantage if they make a baby a bit bigger and use more of the mother's stored calories, since her subsequent offspring may have a different father.[37] The details get complex fast, but Crespi has assembled evidence that excess dominance of paternal alleles may increase the risk of autism, while excess unopposed activity of maternal alleles may increase the risk of schizophrenia.[38,39,40,41]

This predicts that babies born a bit larger than average will be more likely to get autism because of expression of genes from the father, while those born smaller will be more vulnerable to schizophrenia. Remarkably, the prediction is supported by a study of the medical records of 5 million Danes.[42] I am unsure if this hypothesis will turn out to be correct, but it is a fine example of creative thinking and research inspired by an evolutionary perspective.

Boys are many times more vulnerable to autism than girls are.[43] Even for rats, females are better at social tasks and males are better at systematizing. This suggested to Simon Baron-Cohen and colleagues that autism is a product of an extremely male brain.[44] Does the sex difference in rates of autism result from testosterone, genomic imprinting, the effects of genes on the X and Y chromosomes, or what? The answer to this question may provide the key to understanding autism.

The huge fitness costs of these diseases have inspired suggestions that their symptoms, or the alleles that cause them, must offer selective advantages.[45] Such ideas have spurred creative flights. One idea is that schizophrenics become shamans or charismatic leaders, and the resulting status gets them extra matings.[46,47] This is inconsistent with data showing that people with these diseases have reduced numbers of children, although a recent report suggests that people with creative traits related to schizophrenia may have increased mating opportunities.[48]

A more plausible possibility is that the same genetic tendencies that make a disorder likely also give other advantages. The association of creativity and intelligence with bipolar disorder has spurred enormous interest and many studies.[49,50] My exceptionally creative academic friends seem especially likely to have children with major mental disorders, and the relatives of my patients with severe disorders also seem likely to be exceptionally creative. But this could be an illusion. Practice in a university setting gives increased exposure to creative people, and extraordinarily successful patients and their relatives are easier to remember because they fit the pattern. Also, people with dire disorders may choose creative occupations because they have a hard time getting and keeping other kinds of jobs. Or perhaps people with special abilities are especially likely to get social validation that encourages grand pursuits that escalate to mania. Some traits associated with bipolar disorder may give advantages, but I am unconvinced that creativity is a major influence; it may instead be a some-times fortunate side effect of mood dysregulation and its complications.

Several new studies support the idea that associated benefits preserve alleles that increase vulnerability. A study of twins found that the like-lihood of developing bipolar disorder is associated with higher-than-average levels of sociality and verbal skills.[51] A just-published article by Yale geneticists Renato Polimanti and Joel Gelernter found that alleles that increase the risk of autism spectrum disorder have been subject to positive selection, presumably because they give cognitive benefits.[52] Another study found that the amount of a protein made by genes related to schizophrenia was related to verbal learning ability.[53] As for why so many alleles with tiny effects can't be added together to create big effects, it appears that brain development is influenced by their complex interactions.[54] However, scores of suggestions about possible benefits from traits or genes associated with these diseases have been proposed without confirmation, so skepticism is warranted.

New methods make it possible to estimate when genetic variations that influence vulnerability to schizophrenia first appeared. Most seem to have emerged sometime after our last common ancestor with chimpanzees, about 5 million years ago.[55] A study of bits of DNA that enhance the ex-pression of certain genes has found that the ones that influence brain de-velopment are evolving five times faster than others and that these variations also increase the risk of late-life diseases such as Alzheimer's disease.[56] This is a fine example of how alleles that cause disease late in life can be selected for because they give advantages earlier. Stephen Corbett, Stephen Stearns, and their colleagues argue that this phenomenon, called *antagonistic plei-otropy*, imposes much higher costs for organisms, such as humans, living in environments vastly different from those they evolved in.[57]

If alleles that increase vulnerability to bipolar disorder really have offered a selective advantage across the course of human evolution, those alleles should have spread and become universal. Maybe they have. The psychia-trist Hagop Akiskal and colleagues have conducted a series of wonderful studies showing that full-fledged bipolar illness is just the tip of a spectrum of mood instability disorders.[58,59] Mild versions of mood instability may be common because they increase reproductive success on average over the long run, despite their malign effects on health for some people. This could be because of productivity during bursts of manic energy or because such individuals get more sex partners.[60] Mood disorders may offer another tragic example of how we were shaped for reproductive success at the cost of health.

Another possibility is that the responsible genetic variations are not defects but genetic quirks, normal variations like those that cause eating disorders and substance abuse only in modern environments. The possibility that schizophrenia is more common in modern environments has been advanced several times in recent decades, but evidence to support it is limited.[61,62] The prevailing view that schizophrenia rates are the same everywhere has been challenged by new studies showing slightly higher rates for immigrants and city dwellers.[63,64,65] However, the evolutionary psychiatrist Jay Feierman tells me that he has seen many cases of clear-cut psychoses in his travels to cultures based on subsistence hunting and agriculture. More cross-cultural data would be useful, but these disorders are not diseases like eating disorders and substance abuse that are mainly products of modern environments.

Infection offers another possible evolutionary explanation. Could dire disorders result from infections that influence brain development? The risk of schizophrenia is increased by infection during pregnancy with *Toxoplasma gondii*, a parasite associated with cats.[66] Rates of schizophrenia are also increased in children whose mothers had influenza during the second trimester.[67,68,69] The influence of such infections on brain development may help to explain some variations in rates across time and location, but such infections during pregnancy are rare, so their contribution to the total causation is small. They do, however, offer crucial evidence that the disruption of neural development due to diverse causes can cause similar syndromes.

Many of the suggestions for why schizophrenia alleles persist consider the general idea that they were selected for in the process that shaped human cognition and language.[70,71,72] This has long seemed plausible but untestable, but it is finding support in new genetic evidence for the effects of schizophrenia-associated alleles on cognition.[73,74,75,76,77,78,79,80,81,82,83]

Minds Unbalanced on Fitness Cliffs

The discussed ideas all help to explain the persistence of alleles that cause dreaded diseases, but I found myself still wondering why natural selection did not greatly reduce the risk of such devastating disorders. Each occurs with a frequency of about 1 percent. If they were 0.001 percent, that would be different, but 1 percent is relatively common. Linkage with helpful alleles before our progenitors left Africa seemed to offer a potential explanation,[84] but the process of genetic recombination would have split such pairings long ago.[85] I also found it mysterious that tiny effects from so many different genes could cause relatively consistent syndromes.

After racking my brain on the problem for weeks, I finally found inspiration by rereading early studies by the British ornithologist David Lack.[86,87] He wondered why birds didn't lay more eggs in order to have more offspring and suspected that additional eggs would sometimes pay off but would sometimes result in fewer total surviving offspring. To test the idea, he moved eggs from some nests to others. As he suspected, adding one egg to a nest increased the number of fledglings somewhat on average, but beyond a certain number, added eggs decreased the total number of chicks fledged. His insight inspired me to wonder if a similar "cliff-edged fitness landscape" might explain vulnerability to schizophrenia.[88]

Biologists use the metaphor of a "fitness landscape" to think about how variations in a trait influence Darwinian fitness. For instance, birds that have wings that are longer or shorter than average are less likely to survive a storm,[89] so the fitness landscape for wing length is shaped like a hill, with a fitness peak in the middle at average lengths and smooth downward slopes on either side as fitness decreases for birds with shorter or longer wings. Long wings have both advantages and disadvantages; short wings have opposite advantages and disadvantages. The result is inevitable trade-offs, many of which are relevant to disease. Bernard Crespi has written profoundly about pairs of "diametric disorders" resulting from deviations to one side or the other.[90,91]

The figure on the next page illustrates the standard model for genetic vulnerability to disease. Trade-offs are central. For example, risk-taking rabbits are at high risk of predation, but they have plenty of time to eat. Cautious rabbits are protected from predation, but they have too little time to eat. Rabbits with medium levels of cautiousness have the highest fitness, so selection shapes the population mean to the peak, where fitness for genes and individuals coincides with maximum health. Mutations spread out the distribution, resulting in some individuals having trait values far from the mean and lower fitness. Stabilizing selection eliminates such mutations, narrowing the distribution.

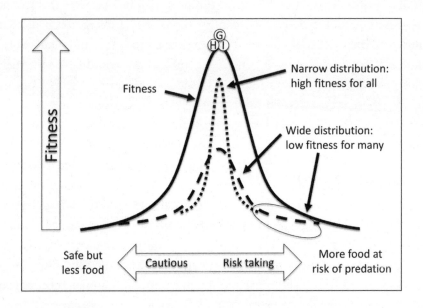

The Standard Model

The solid line is the fitness at each level of cautiousness. The points that maximize fitness for an individual (I) and a gene (G) and health (H) all coincide at the peak of the fitness landscape. If the distribution of degrees of cautiousness is narrow (the tall dotted curve), most individuals will have high fitness and good health. If the distribution is wide (the dashed curve), some will be at high risk of predation and others will be at a high risk of starvation.

However, fitness landscapes can be asymmetrical. Sometimes fitness increases as a trait is pushed in one direction, but going one step too far results in going off the cliff, just like the bird nest that had one egg too many. Racehorses are prone to breaking the cannon bone in their legs. Why didn't natural selection make it thicker? It did; wild horses are unlikely to break their legs. However, breeding only the fastest horses made their leg bones longer and longer, thinner and thinner, and lighter and lighter. Successive generations of racehorses have become faster and faster but also more and more vulnerable to breaking a leg, something that now happens about once every thousand times a racehorse starts a race.[92]

Because all racehorses have been selected for speed, horses that break their legs and their relatives will not be much faster than other horses. The same logic may explain why it has been hard to find advantages experienced by the relatives of people who have serious mental disorders. Strong selection for extreme mental capacities may have given us all minds like the legs of racehorses, fast but vulnerable to catastrophic failures. This model fits well with the idea that schizophrenia is intimately related to language and cognitive ability.[93] It also fits well with the observation that schizophrenia may be intimately related to the human capacity for "theory of mind," our ability to intuit other people's motives and cognitive abilities in general.[94,95]

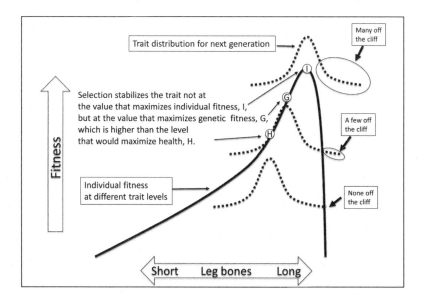

How Cliff-Edged Fitness Functions Make Disease Inevitable

Traits with asymmetrical fitness functions are stabilized not at the level that maximizes individual fitness (I) or at the level that maximizes health (H), but at the level that maximizes gene transmission (G), despite dire outcomes for a few individuals.

An individual at point I will have the maximum number of offspring, but inevitable variations among those offspring (the dotted curve above point I) will leave many off the fitness cliff with a high vulnerability to disease. An individual at point G will have almost as many offspring but only a few of them will have values off the cliff. Natural selection will stabilize the trait at this point. An individual at point H will have healthy offspring but fewer, so overall fitness will be lower.

A mathematical model I created shows that whenever fitness for a trait peaks at a cliff edge, selection will shape the average trait mean to be a bit below what would maximize an individual's reproductive success but above the level that would maximize health. A few percent of a population with that average trait value will have values off the cliff that put them at high risk of disease.[96]

Diseases resulting from cliff-edged fitness functions should be highly heritable, observed in a few percent of the population, and the risk will be influenced by the complex interactions of many normal alleles that all have about the same small influence on disease risk. This matches the data for many diseases.

Many traits are subject to catastrophic failure. Babies with larger brains and heads have advantages, but in environments without obstetric surgery, just one centimeter too large is fatal for both mother and baby.[97] High uric acid levels protect against aging, but just a bit too high causes gout when uric acid crystals precipitate in joints.[98] Having more stem cells slows aging, but increased numbers make cancer more likely.[99] Some aspect of neuronal transmission may have been pushed to a cliff edge,[100] making brains vulnerable to epilepsy from many causes, including mutations, infection, tumors, injury, and drugs.

Competition between hosts and pathogens are especially likely to create steep cliffs.[101] The price of not being able to defend adequately against an infection is death. In order to ensure the ability to counter such threats, the immune system is shaped to a level of aggressiveness that sometimes attacks normal tissues, causing rheumatic fever, OCD, rheumatoid arthritis, multiple sclerosis, and other autoimmune disorders.[102] This makes the finding that many alleles with effects on schizophrenia are involved in immune responses especially salient.[103]

A trade-off with immune benefits may also be involved in Alzheimer's disease. Dying and dead neurons are usually surrounded by a protein called amyloid beta. Scientists have often assumed that this protein is a toxic by-product of metabolism. However, in a deep disappointment, drugs that prevent the synthesis of amyloid beta don't slow progression of the disease.[104] Furthermore, amyloid beta turns out to be a potent antimicrobial agent,[105] and the system that prunes connections between neurons relies on a part of the immune system.[106] Herpes virus remnants have just been discovered to be more common in the brains of people with Alzheimer's disease.[107] Our vulnerability to Alzheimer's disease may be related to a trade-off involving immune system costs and several kinds of benefits.[108]

These diseases all may result from natural selection stabilizing traits at the point close to a cliff edge that maximizes genetic fitness despite the dire outcomes for a few individuals. This idea is by no means widely accepted or even recognized, but I suggest it anyhow because it offers a potential explanation for why we have been unable to find specific genetic causes for specific mental disorders. In cliff-edge models, the problem results not from defective genes but from steep slopes on fitness landscapes that result from intrinsic trade-offs, like those that cause vapor lock. A two-dimensional landscape offers only a crude model; actual fitness landscapes are likely to be rugged in multiple dimensions. For some diseases vulnerability may turn out to result from the equivalent of sinkholes in a fitness landscape. If it accomplishes nothing else, however, considering cliff-edged fitness landscapes encourages looking for traits and trade-offs that may be crucial for explaining dire diseases.

Information Devices Fail in Special Ways

Mental disorders are often thought to be fundamentally different from other medical disorders. Their vulnerability results from the same six evolutionary reasons that explain other medical disorders, but the brain is different from other organs in one important respect: it is a very general information-processing device. It receives information from many internal and external sources, uses chemical and electrical mechanisms to process the information, and produces output that adjusts physiology and guides behavior. Such systems fail in special ways.

The analogy of brain as computer is easy to take too far. Engineers design computers with discrete components that serve specific functions. One part translates keystrokes into digital signals; another creates images on a screen; another allocates memory; another ensures that long strings of zeros and ones calculate what should be calculated. Airplanes and space shuttles have backup computers in case the primary one fails. We don't have backup minds, but because our brains are organically complex integrated systems they carry on relatively well despite mutations and minor bits of damage.

Software failures are somewhat different, but they provide a useful analogy for the different ways organic information systems can fail. Failure to receive adequate signals from the environment is serious, as you know if you have ever tried to log on to your computer when your keyboard is not working. Decreased sensory input in medical patients can cause delirium and hallucinations in similar ways. Software programs can reach a dead end. This is very much like the "thought blocking" experienced by some schizophrenics, who report that their train of thought sometimes just stops.

Software designers work hard to avoid infinite loops, a problem that often requires rebooting. The ruminations and obsessions that plague many patients with paranoia or obsessive-compulsive disorder seem similar. Information can also feed back into the same loop, filling memory and shutting down the system. This is like the escalation of manic or depressive episodes to extremes that then get stuck. It is also reminiscent of the human tendency to what psychologists call "confirmation bias," which makes us attend preferentially to all information that confirms a prior belief and ignore information that does not fit. Asking a patient with schizophrenia to describe concerns about spying by the secret police can result in some patients concluding that your questions prove that you are part of the conspiracy.

In his profound book *Cybernetics*, Norbert Wiener, the father of information theory, suggested that dysregulated feedback control systems might be responsible for some mental disorders. His idea is especially germane to bipolar disorder.[109] Most people who experience life reverses slow down and invest less effort, but bipolar patients sometimes do the opposite. After a setback, most of us gradually recover our optimism and carry on, but patients who are vulnerable to mood disorders can slide into feedback spirals that trap them in isolation and depression.

Conversely, after a grand success most of us tend to find ourselves unaccountably feeling down a few days later. Psychologists note that this "opponent process" is a general characteristic of human motivation systems.[110] One evolution-minded author has even suggested that extreme happiness itself provokes extreme depression as a stabilizing measure.[111] Some system like this that helps to stabilize mood may be absent in people with bipolar disorder.

An evolutionary perspective on dire mental diseases encourages new perspectives that shift attention away from the easy assumption that because they are influenced by genes, they are caused by defective genes. It calls new attention to traits, fitness landscapes, and control systems that may result in vulnerability. What such traits might be is a very good question. They are unlikely to be things as obvious as creativity or intelligence. Instead, they may be things such as rates of neuron growth in early development, rates of neuron pruning in adolescence, and rates of transmission in neural networks. On a higher level, attributing meaning to tiny gestures by others may be increasingly useful up to some peak beyond which it crashes into sustained paranoia. I am all too aware that these are mere speculations and that the actual systems are likely to be complex in ways that make them hard to grasp. Nonetheless, investigating how selection shapes traits that maximize fitness but leave some individuals vulnerable offers opportunities to look for causes that are not underneath the streetlamps of population genetics and neuroscience.

EVOLUTIONARY PSYCHIATRY: A BRIDGE, NOT AN ISLAND

If at first the idea is not absurd, then there is no hope for it.
—Albert Einstein

Ideas won't keep. Something must be done about them.
—Alfred North Whitehead

Why did natural selection leave us so vulnerable to so many mental disorders? The question is a good one, and attempts to answer it will deepen our understanding of mental disorders. That is the simple thesis of this book. Its aim is to encourage taking the question seriously and searching for answers. That requires constructing a bridge across the canyon that separates evolutionary biology from psychiatry, a project that is just getting started.

In the middle of the nineteenth century, tourists packed the shores of Niagara Falls. It was obvious that a bridge connecting Canada and the United States would be popular and profitable. Other engineers said it would be impossible, but Charles Ellet, Jr., took on the challenge. The first task was to get a cable across. Boats, rockets, and cannons were ruled out in favor of the kite contest Ellet announced in January 1848. A fifteen-year-old American boy, Homan Walsh, crossed to the Canadian side and flew his kite named "Union" all day and into the night, when the string went slack, severed by sharp rocks on the far shore. It was eight days until the ferry could get through the ice so he could retrieve and repair his kite and cross the border to try again. Finally, on one of the last days in, his kite spanned the gap. The thin string pulled across a stronger string that pulled a rope that pulled a cable that made possible the first bridge across the Niagara gorge.[1]

The canyon between evolutionary biology and psychiatry is also deep, wide, and filled with rough waters. Many strings have been severed by sharp rocks at the edges. This book floats another string across the gap in hopes that it will join existing strings to encourage pulling across successively stronger ropes and cables. Evolutionary biology is the foundational science for medicine and all studies of behavior. Bringing it to bear on mental disorders offers a new perspective that will lead to new advances.

The explanations suggested here for our vulnerability to mental disorders illustrate the opportunity; they don't provide definitive answers. Each one requires full investigation by many scientists. I have tried to show how some are inconsistent with theory and others are contradicted by facts, but the remaining ones are not necessarily true; they are just those that best fit what we know now. Every hypothesis about evolution and mental disorders needs testing.

That is often difficult. Unfortunately, it seems easy. Human minds carve experience into categories defined by functions. Chairs are for sitting. Hammers are for pounding. Eyes are for seeing. So it seems natural to ask what schizophrenia is for and how anorexia nervosa is useful. But disorders don't have functions. VDAA (Viewing Diseases As Adaptations) is the most serious error in evolutionary psychiatry. The error of thinking that most everything is an adaptation comes naturally to human minds. My favorite outlandish hypothesis is the suggestion that flamingos are pink so they will be camouflaged when viewed against a sunset. Physiologists and behavioral ecologists are more circumspect, but because their everyday work is about adaptations, they tend to start with the assumption that most traits are there because they offer benefits—along with inevitable trade-offs.

Other scientists are skeptical, even hostile, to suggestions about how traits are useful. Geneticists and paleontologists see the effects of random factors in their everyday work, so some tend to assume that most genes and traits are products of random events, sometimes dismissing viable hypotheses as just-so stories without even considering the evidence or alternatives. A remarkable number think that proximate or phylogenetic explanations are sufficient.

The battle between these tribes has created a scientific brouhaha.[2,3,4,5,6,7] Those on one side are likely to wrongly accuse evolutionary psychiatry of "adaptationism," despite my efforts to emphasize that nothing about the body can be perfect and plenty of problems are plain old diseases with no redeeming features. On the other side, some evolutionary psychologists will view my perspective as too slow to acknowledge adaptive functions. Battles between these groups resemble tribal warfare, with stereotyping, prejudice, and global attacks on unfortunate display. However, generalized arguments are counterproductive. Progress will come from testing specific hypotheses. Many deserve to be put on the table. Most will be knocked off by the onslaught of facts. That will take time and resources. Best strategies for testing hypotheses about disease vulnerability are still developing, but experiments, naturalistic observations, and the comparative method all can help. No simple cookbook approach will suffice.[8]

These challenges should not slow efforts to use our understanding of normal behavior to understand abnormal behavior. Eating disorders were not shaped by selection, but mechanisms that regulate eating during famines were. ADHD was not shaped by selection, but mechanisms that regulate attention were. Serious depression was not shaped by natural selection, but capacities for normal low and high mood were. The rest of medicine uses its understanding of normal functioning as the foundation for understanding pathology. This allows it to distinguish symptoms from diseases and to recognize syndromes such as heart failure that can have many causes. An evolutionary framework provides psychiatry with a foundation like the one physiology and biochemistry provides for the rest of medicine.

What Good Is Evolutionary Psychiatry?

Patients want help now. Practitioners want more effective treatments. If someone you love is hospitalized with a manic episode, your only concern is that the doctors have made an accurate diagnosis and are providing the most effective treatment possible. Speculation about why we are all vulnerable to mania seems frivolous. If your spouse is headed for death from alcoholism, if your child has schizophrenia, if you have depression or obsessive-compulsive disorder that is not responding to treatment, then ideas about why evolution left us vulnerable can't help but seem irrelevant. In the face of such urgent clinical needs, it is understandable that some people will ask, "If evolutionary psychiatry doesn't provide better treatment, why bother?"

There are two reasons. In the long term, an evolutionary perspective will transform our understanding of mental disorders in ways that lead to better treatments. In the short term, evolutionary perspectives can be somewhat helpful even now.

An evolutionary foundation will advance research and resolve some enduring controversies. If I met Ms. A again today and she again asked if I realized that psychiatry was deeply confused, I would tell her that much confusion can be resolved. There are good reasons for bad feelings. Anxiety and depression are often excessive because they benefit genes at our expense, because of the Smoke Detector Principle, because we live in modern environments, and because regulation mechanisms are intrinsically vulnerable. Looking for problems in the brain is worthwhile, but because it is an information-processing mechanism, specific causes and brain abnormalities may be found for only some disorders. Others will turn out to be syndromes similar to kidney failure or heart failure that can have many causes. Some causes come from below, via genes and brain mechanisms; others come from above, via information and information processing. Top-down and bottom-up causes interact to create tangled webs, but this is not confusion, it is just reality. An evolutionary framework helps make sense of mental illness.

Several changes will be needed to reap the benefits of an evolutionary perspective. All health professionals and researchers should learn the basic principles of evolutionary biology. Mental health professionals should also learn how natural selection shapes brains and behavior. This cannot happen fast, because few health education professionals know enough evolutionary biology to teach it or even enough to insist that it be included in curricula. Creating new education resources and curricular guidelines will speed progress. While education is essential, funding priorities also need reform. The search for specific genetic and brain abnormalities responsible for specific diseases has gotten nearly all research funding. Some would say that this paradigm has come to a dead end. I hope that is wrong, but there is no need to put all bets on the same horse. The moment of discovery may be, as Jonas Salk suggested, the moment when we find a new question. Funding to answer new questions will open up new directions for psychiatry. Finding out how life situations influence emotions is crucial. Studies of how normal low mood is regulated and useful are needed, along with investigations of how drugs disrupt mood mechanisms in ways that relieve symptoms. Studies of persistence need to be revisited in light of the adaptive value of stopping useless effort. Foraging patterns of people vulnerable to drug abuse will be fascinating. Integration of cybernetic approaches with evolution, psychology, and neuroscience offers great promise. Dozens of studies are ready to go as soon as sponsors recognize the opportunity.

Improving treatment is the goal, but much will be lost if evolutionary psychiatry becomes just another brand of therapy. Different treatments tend to become isolated islands of shared beliefs. Such beliefs influence what people do. Or, more often, what they don't do. Early in my career I saw many patients with severe anxiety or depression who refused medications, saying something like "Drugs will just cover over the symptoms, I need to find the cause." The prevailing psychodynamic schema prevented them from accepting available help from medications. As the years passed and more drug ads appeared on television, the prevailing schema flipped. I provided a consultation for a desperately depressed twenty-two-year-old man whose symptoms had not responded to five different medications. He was living in the basement of his parents' house, mostly staring at a wall, but sometimes watching television or playing video games. When I asked what he wanted to do in life, he said, "I have to get over my depression before I can do anything." When I asked how he would do that, he said, "It is a brain disease, so I just have to wait until they find a medication that works."

Schemas about mental disorders also limit the perspectives of clinicians and researchers. Some doctors who attribute problems to brain disorders feel little need to get a detailed history; they are satisfied with making a diagnosis and administering a treatment approved for the disorder. Conversely, clinicians who attribute problems to mental conflicts provoked by early experiences put enormous effort into dredging up memories and connecting them to current behaviors, sometimes to the detriment of considering brain problems and current life situations. Evolutionary psychiatry builds bridges between such diverse views. It gives substance and structure to George Engel's biopsychosocial model. Instead of blaming a person's problems on one or another specific cause, it encourages consideration of how multiple factors interact to cause this individual's problem, and how various treatments can help to resolve it.

In the Clinic Now

My friend and colleague Alfonso Troisi, the psychiatrist at the University of Rome who coauthored *Darwinian Psychiatry*, has convinced me that learning about evolution can make clinicians more effective now.[9,10] Those who study evolution can better understand motivations and emotions that arise in response to difficulties pursuing goals. Their understanding of relationships helps them to understand why conflicts are inevitable and how to reduce them. Martin Brüne, a German evolutionary psychiatrist and author of *Evolutionary Psychiatry*, has also advocated bringing evolutionary views to the clinic.[11] The UK psychiatrists Riadh Abed and Paul St. John-Smith have organized hundreds of their peers in the Royal College of Psychiatry who share these interests. Clinical psychologists including Paul Gilbert and Leif Kennair are using evolutionary thinking to make cognitive behavioral therapies more effective.[12,13,14,15] Clinician-researchers like these will inspire the next generation.

Despite my reluctance to claim quick benefits now, learning about evolution and behavior has transformed my treatment of many conditions. Treatment of panic disorder is improved if clinicians recognize that panic attacks are false alarms in the fight-or-flight system and that the Smoke Detector Principle explains why false alarms are common. Treatment of eating disorders is improved by the recognition that strenuous dieting arouses famine protection mechanisms that are prone to initiate a positive feedback spiral. Addiction treatment is improved by recognizing that addiction results when learning mechanisms encounter substances and routes of delivery that our ancestors never imagined. And the psychiatry residents I have trained tell me they find it invaluable to ask their depressed patients, "Is there something very important that you are trying to do that you can't succeed at and can't give up?"

Understanding social selection provides a foundation for understanding committed relationships and the prevalence of guilt and social anxiety. Recognizing the tension between relationships based on exchange and those based on commitment facilitates discussion with patients about what a therapeutic relationship can and cannot offer. Realizing that long hours of intimate conversation automatically create feelings of intimate connection can help keep therapeutic relationships professional.

These insights from the frontier of evolutionary psychiatry are useful now, but they should not be viewed as "evolutionary psychotherapy." Bridges will accomplish much more than constructing a new island.

Why Is Life So Full of Suffering?

We come full circle to the largest question. For those of us who have been fortunate, life began the way it did for Siddhartha, the boy who became the Buddha. While not as perfectly cosseted as he was, we spend our early years in secure cocoons, protected by loving parents from even knowing about suffering in the larger world. When he was finally allowed to go into the city, Siddhartha confronted life's pain and sadness with a searing abruptness that fueled his search for the cause and a solution. He concluded that suffering has its origins in desire. That seems right. If Siddhartha lived today, he would likely ask why natural selection shaped desires and the painful and pleasurable emotions aroused by their pursuit.

The general answer is simple: our brains were shaped to maximize transmission of our genes. Emotions are specialized modes of operation that are useful in certain situations. But a subtler perspective provides an escape from cynicism and determinism. We are capable of genuine goodness and caring. They make life worthwhile at the price of guilt and grief. We have built-in mechanisms for controlling desire. They are not always reliable, but they allow most of us to carry on with good humor and good relationships, little concerned about what we don't have. All this comes at the price of caring inordinately about what others think about us. Together, these products of natural selection make life happy and meaningful for many, even most, people. All of this encourages turning one more question on its head. Instead of being appalled at life's suffering, we should be astounded and awed by the miracle of mental health for so many.

FURTHER READING

Alcock J. *The triumph of sociobiology.* New York: Oxford University Press, 2001.

Archer J. *The nature of grief.* New York: Oxford University Press, 1999.

Baron-Cohen S (ed). *The maladapted mind: classic readings in evolutionary psychopathology.* East Sussex: Psychology Press, 1997.

Brüne M. *Textbook of evolutionary psychiatry: the origins of psychopathology.* 2nd ed. Oxford: Oxford University Press, 2016.

Dugatkin LA. *The altruism equation: seven scientists search for the origins of goodness.* Princeton, NJ: Princeton University Press, 2006.

Gilbert P, Bailey KG. *Genes on the couch: explorations in evolutionary psychotherapy.* Philadelphia: Taylor & Francis, 2000.

Horwitz AV, Wakefield JC. *The loss of sadness: how psychiatry transformed normal sorrow into depressive disorder.* New York: Oxford University Press, 2007.

Hrdy SB. *Mothers and others: the evolutionary origins of mutual understanding.* Cambridge, MA: Belknap Press of Harvard University Press, 2009.

Konner M. *The tangled wing: biological constraints on the human spirit.* 2nd ed. New York: Times Books, 2002.

Low BS. *Why sex matters: a Darwinian look at human behavior.* Princeton, NJ: Princeton University Press, 2015.

McGuire MT, Troisi A. *Darwinian psychiatry.* New York: Oxford University Press, 1998.

Natterson-Horowitz B, Bowers K. *Zoobiquity: the astonishing connection between human and animal health.* New York: Vintage, 2013.

Nesse RM, Williams GC. *Why we get sick: the new science of Darwinian medicine.* New York: Vintage Books, 1994.

Pinker S. *The blank slate: the modern denial of human nature.* New York: Viking, 2002.

Ridley M. *The origins of virtue: human instincts and the evolution of cooperation.* New York: Viking, 1996.

Rottenberg J. *The depths: the evolutionary origins of the depression epidemic.* New York: Basic Books, 2014.

Taylor J. *Body by Darwin: how evolution shapes our health and transforms medicine.* Chicago: University of Chicago Press, 2015.

Wenegrat B. *Sociobiological psychiatry: a new conceptual framework.* Lexington, MS: Lexington, 1990.

Zimmer C. *Evolution: the triumph of an idea.* New York: Random House, 2011.

NOTES

PREFACE

1. Darwin C. The descent of man and selection in relation to sex. London: Murray; 1888. p. 390.

CHAPTER 1 | A NEW QUESTION

1. Engel G. The need for a new medical model: a challenge for biomedicine. Science. 1977 Apr 8;196(4286):129–36.

2. American Psychiatric Association. Diagnostic and statistical manual of mental disorders: DSM-IV. 4th ed. Washington (DC): American Psychiatric Association; 1994.

3. Frances A. Saving normal: an insider's revolt against out-of-control psychiatric diagnosis, *DSM-5*, big pharma, and the medicalization of ordinary life. New York: William Morrow; 2013.

4. Insel T, Cuthbert B, Garvey M, Heinssen R, Pine DS, Quinn K, et al. Research domain criteria (RDoC): toward a new classification framework for research on mental disorders. Am J Psychiatry. 2010 Jul;167(7):748–51.

5. Insel TR, Wang PS. Rethinking mental illness. JAMA. 2010 May 19;303(19):1970–1.

6. Gatt JM, Burton KLO, Williams LM, Schofield PR. Specific and common genes implicated across major mental disorders: a review of meta-analysis studies. J Psychiatr Res. 2015 Jan;60:1–13.

7. Consortium C-DG of the PG. Identification of risk loci with shared

effects on five major psychiatric disorders: a genome-wide analysis. The Lancet. 2013 Apr 26;381(9875):1371–9.

8. Akil H, Brenner S, Kandel E, Kendler KS, King M-C, Scolnick E, et al. The future of psychiatric research: genomes and neural circuits. Science. 2010;327(5973):1580–1.

9. Greenberg G. The rats of N.I.M.H. The New Yorker [Internet]. 2013 May 16 [cited 2018 Jun 13]. Available from: https://www.newyorker.com/tech/elements/the-rats-of-n-i-m-h.

10. Brüne M, Belsky J, Fabrega H, Feierman HR, Gilbert P, Glantz K, et al. The crisis of psychiatry—insights and prospects from evolutionary theory. World Psychiatry. 2012;11(1):55–7.

11. Williams GC. Pleiotropy, natural selection, and the evolution of senescence. Evolution. 1957;11(4):398–411.

12. Gaillard J-M, Lemaître J-F. The Williams' legacy: a critical reappraisal of his nine predictions about the evolution of senescence. Evolution [Internet]. 2017 Oct 20 [cited 2017 Oct 30]. Available from: http://doi.wiley.com/10.1111/evo.13379.

13. Alcock J, Sherman P. The utility of the proximate ultimate dichotomy in ethology. Ethology. 1994;96(1):58–62.

14. Dewsbury DA. The proximate and the ultimate: past, present and future. Behav Process. 1999;46:189–99.

15. Mayr E. Cause and effect in biology. Science. 1961;134(3489):1501–6.

16. Nesse RM. Evolutionary and proximate explanations. In: Scherer K, Sander D, editors. The Oxford companion to emotion and the affective sciences. Oxford (UK): Oxford University Press; 2009. pp. 158–9.

17. Tinbergen N. On the aims and methods of ethology. Z für Tierpsychol. 1963;20:410–63.

18. Nesse RM. Tinbergen's four questions, organized: a response to Bateson and Laland. Trends Ecol Evol. 2013;28(12):681–2.

19. Sternbach RA. Congenital insensitivity to pain. Psychol Bull. 1963;60(3):252–64.

20. Nesse RM. Life table tests of evolutionary theories of senescence. Exp Gerontol. 1988;23(6):445–53.

21. Kirkwood TB. Understanding the odd science of aging. Cell. 2005 Feb 25;120(4):437–47.

22. Rose M, Charlesworth B. A test of evolutionary theories of senescence. Nature. 1980 Sep 287(5778):141–2.

23. Kirkwood TB, Austad SN. Why do we age? Nature. 2000;408(6809):233–8.

24. Peterson ML. The problem of evil: selected readings. 2nd ed. Notre Dame (IN): University of Notre Dame Press; 2016.

25. Southgate C. God and evolutionary evil: theodicy in the light of Darwinism. Zygon. 2002;37(4):803–24.

26. Tooley M. The problem of evil. In: Zalta EN, editor. The Stanford Encyclopedia of Philosophy [Internet]. Fall 2015. Metaphysics Research Lab, Stanford University; 2015 [cited 2018 Jun 4]. Available from: https://plato.stanford.edu/archives/fall2015/entries/evil.

27. Hume D. Dialogues concerning natural religion. Whithorn (UK): CreateSpace Independent Publishing Platform:Anodos Books; 1779 [2017]. p. 52.

28. Peterson ML. The problem of evil.

29. Barash DP. Buddhist biology: ancient Eastern wisdom meets modern Western science. New York: Oxford University Press; 2014.

30. Ekman P, Davidson RJ, Ricard M, Wallace BA. Buddhist and psychological perspectives on emotions and well-being. Curr Dir Psychol Sci. 2005;14(2):59–63.

31. Barash DP. Buddhist biology.

32. Dawkins R. The selfish gene. Oxford (UK): Oxford University Press; 1976.

33. Williams GC. Natural selection, the costs of reproduction, and a refinement of Lack's principle. Am Nat. 1966 Nov–Dec; 100(916):687–90.

CHAPTER 2 | ARE MENTAL DISORDERS DISEASES?

1. Grebb JA, Carlsson A. Introduction and considerations for a brain-based diagnostic system in psychiatry. In: Sadock BJ, Sadock VA, Ruiz P, Kaplan HI, editors. Kaplan & Sadock's comprehensive textbook of psychiatry.

9th ed. Philadelphia: Wolters Kluwer Health/Lippincott Williams & Wilkins; 2009. pp. 1–4.

2. Kendell RE, Cooper JE, Gourlay AJ, Copeland JRM, Sharpe L, Gurland BJ. Diagnostic criteria of American and British psychiatrists. Arch Gen Psychiatry. 1971 Aug 1;25(2):123–30.

3. Rosenhan DL. On being sane in insane places. Science. 1973;179 (4070):250–8.

4. American Psychiatric Association. Diagnostic and statistical manual of mental disorders. 2nd ed. Washington (DC): American Psychiatric Association; 1968.

5. American Psychiatric Association. Diagnostic and statistical manual of mental disorders. 3rd ed. Washington (DC): American Psychiatric Association; 1980.

6. Wilson M. DSM-III and the transformation of American psychiatry: a history. Am J Psychiatry [Internet]. 1993 Mar 1;150(3):399–410. Available from: http://ajp.psychiatryonline.org/cgi/content/abstract/150/3/399.

7. Spitzer RL, Williams JB, Gibbon M, First MB. The structured clinical interview for DSM-III-R (SCID). I: History, rationale, and description. Arch Gen Psychiatry. 1992 Aug;49(8):624 9.

8. Andreasen NC. DSM and the death of phenomenology in America: an example of unintended consequences. Schizophr Bull. 2007 Jan 1;33(1):108–12.

9. Hyman SE. Can neuroscience be integrated into the DSM-V? Nat Rev Neurosci. 2007 Sep;8(9):725–32.

10. Andreasen NC. DSM and the death of phenomenology in America.

11. Kessler RC, Anthony JC, Blazer DG, Bromet E, Eaton WW, Kendler K, et al. The US National Comorbidity Survey: overview and future directions. Epidemiol Psichiatr Soc. 1997 Jan;6(1):4–16.

12. Angst J, Vollrath M, Merikangas KR, Ernst C. Comorbidity of anxiety and depression in the Zurich Cohort Study of Young Adults. In: Maser JD, Cloninger CR, editors. Comorbidity of mood and anxiety disorders. Arlington (VA): American Psychiatric Association; 1990. pp. 123–37.

13. Gorman JM. Comorbid depression and anxiety spectrum disorders. Depress Anxiety. 1996;4(4):160–8.

14.   Kessler RC, Berglund P, Demler O, Jin R, Koretz D, Merikangas KR, et al. The epidemiology of major depressive disorder: results from the National Comorbidity Survey Replication (NCS-R). JAMA. 2003;289(23):3095–105.

15.   Sartorius N, Üstün TB, Lecrubier Y, Wittchen H-U. Depression comorbid with anxiety: results from the WHO study on psychological disorders in primary health care. Br J Psychiatry. 1996 Jun;30:38–43.

16.   Frances A, Egger HL. Whither psychiatric diagnosis. Aust N Z J Psychiatry. 1999;33:161–5.

17.   Insel TR, Wang PS. Rethinking mental illness. JAMA. 2010 May 19;303(19):1970–1.

18.   Greenberg G. Inside the battle to define mental illness. Wired [Internet]. 2010 Dec 27. Available from: http://www.wired.com/magazine/2010/12/ff_dsmv/all/1.

19.   Frances A. A warning sign on the road to DSM-V: beware of its unintended consequences. Psychiatric Times [Internet]. 2009 Jun 27 [cited 2017 May 9]. Available from: http://www.psychiatrictimes.com/articles/warning-sign-road-dsm-v-beware-its-unintended-consequences.

20.   Ibid.

21.   Kupfer DJ, First MB, Regier DA. A research agenda for DSM-V [Internet]. Washington (DC): American Psychiatric Association; 2002. xxiii, 307. Available from: http://www.loc.gov/catdir/toc/fy033/2002021556.html.

22.   Mezzich JE. Culture and psychiatric diagnosis: a DSM-IV perspective. Washington (DC): American Psychiatric Press; 1996.

23.   Phillips KA, First MB, Pincus HA. Advancing DSM: dilemmas in psychiatric diagnosis. Washington (DC): American Psychiatric Association; 2003.

24.   American Psychiatric Association. Diagnostic and statistical manual of mental disorders: DSM-5 [Internet]. 5th ed. Arlington (VA): American Psychiatric Association; 2013. Available from: http://dsm.psychiatry online.org/book.aspx?bookid=556.

25.   Akil H, et al. The future of psychiatric research.

26.   Wakefield JC. Disorder as harmful dysfunction: a conceptual critique of DSM-III-R's definition of mental disorder. Psychol Rev. 1992; 99(2):232–47.

27.   First M, Wakefield JC. Defining "mental disorder" in DSM-V. Psychol Med. 2010;40(11):1779–82.

28.   Wakefield JC. The concept of mental disorder: diagnostic implications of the harmful dysfunction analysis. World Psychiatry. 2007;6(3):149.

29.   Ibid.

CHAPTER 3 | WHY ARE MINDS SO VULNERABLE?

1.   Schopenhauer A, Hollingdale RJ. Essays and aphorisms. Harmondsworth (UK): Penguin Books; 2004. p. 41.

2.   Dunbar RI. The social brain: mind, language, and society in evolutionary perspective. Annu Rev Anthropol. 2003;32:163–81.

3.   Hamilton WD. The genetical evolution of social behaviour. I and II. J Theoret Biol. 1964;7:1–52.

4.   Ibid.

5.   Alcock J. The triumph of sociobiology. New York: Oxford University Press; 2001.

6.   Crespi B, Foster K, Úbeda F. First principles of Hamiltonian medicine. Philos Trans R Soc B Biol Sci [Internet]. 2014 May 19 [cited 2018 Jan 2];369(1642). Available from: https://www.ncbi.nlm.nih.gov/pmc/articles/PMC3982667.

7.   Segerstrale U, Segerstrale UCO. Nature's oracle: the life and work of W. D. Hamilton. Oxford (UK): Oxford University Press; 2013.

8.   Williams GC. Adaptation and natural selection: a critique of some current evolutionary thought. Princeton (NJ): Princeton University Press; 1966.

9.   Wynne-Edwards VC. Animal dispersion in relation to social behavior. Edinburgh: Oliver and Boyd; 1962.

10.   Marschall LA. Do lemmings commit suicide? The Sciences. 1996; 36(6):39–41.

11.   Crespi BJ. The evolution of maladaptation. Hered Edinb. 2000 Jun;84 (Pt 6):623–9.

12.   Gluckman PD, Low FM, Buklijas T, Hanson MA, Beedle AS. How evolutionary principles improve the understanding of human health and

disease: evolutionary principles and human health. Evol Appl. 2011 Mar;4(2):249–63.

13.   Kennair LEO, Kleppestø TH, Jørgensen BEG, Larsen SM. Evolutionary clinical psychology. In: Shackelford TK, Weekes-Shackelford VA, editors. Encyclopedia of evolutionary psychological science. Cham (Switzerland): Springer International Publishing; 2018. pp. 1–14.

14.   Nesse RM. Maladaptation and natural selection. Q Rev Biol. 2005 Mar;80(1):62–70.

15.   Nesse RM, Williams GC. Why we get sick: the new science of Darwinian medicine. New York: Vintage Books; 1994.

16.   Corbett S, Courtiol A, Lummaa V, Moorad J, Stearns S. The transition to modernity and chronic disease: mismatch and natural selection. Nat Rev Genet. 2018 May 9;19:419–30.

17.   Gluckman PD, Hanson M. Mismatch: why our world no longer fits our bodies. New York: Oxford University Press; 2006.

18.   Li NP, van Vugt M, Colarelli SM. The evolutionary mismatch hypothesis: implications for psychological science. Curr Dir Psychol Sci. 2018 Feb 1;27(1):38–44.

19.   Spinella M. Evolutionary mismatch, neural reward circuits, and pathological gambling. Int J Neurosci. 2003;113(4):503–12.

20.   Corbett, et al. The transition to modernity and chronic disease.

21.   Gluckman PD, Hanson M. Mismatch.

22.   Eaton SB, Shostak M, Konner M. The Paleolithic prescription. New York: Harper & Row; 1988.

23.   Gluckman PD, Hanson MA. The fetal matrix: evolution, development, and disease. New York: Cambridge University Press; 2005.

24.   Konner M. The tangled wing: biological constraints on the human spirit. New York: Harper Colophon; 1983.

25.   Gluckman PD, Hanson M. Mismatch.

26.   Eaton SB, Eaton SB III. Breast cancer in evolutionary context. In: Trevathan WR, Smith EO, McKenna JJ, editors. Evolutionary medicine. New York: Oxford University Press; 1999. pp. 429–42.

27.   Jasieńska G, Thune I. Lifestyle, hormones, and risk of breast cancer. BMJ. 2001;322(7286):586–7.

28. Blaser MJ. Missing microbes: how the overuse of antibiotics is fueling our modern plagues. New York: Macmillan; 2014.

29. Rook G, editor. The hygiene hypothesis and Darwinian medicine. Boston: Birkhauser; 2009.

30. Eaton SB, Shostak M, Konner M. The Paleolithic prescription.

31. Bellisari A. Evolutionary origins of obesity. Obes Rev. 2008 Mar 1;9(2):165–80.

32. Flegal KM, Carroll MD, Ogden CL, Johnson CL. Prevalence and trends in obesity among US adults, 1999–2000. JAMA. 2002 Oct 9; 288(14):1723–7.

33. Konner M, Eaton SB. Paleolithic nutrition twenty-five years later. Nutr Clin Pract. 2010;25(6):594–602.

34. Pontzer H, Raichlen DA, Wood BM, Mabulla AZP, Racette SB, Marlowe FW. Hunter-gatherer energetics and human obesity. PLOS ONE. 2012;7(7):e40503.

35. Power ML, Schulkin J. The evolution of obesity. Baltimore: Johns Hopkins University Press; 2009.

36. Nesse RM. An evolutionary perspective on substance abuse. Ethol Sociobiol. 1994;15(5–6):339–48.

37. Nesse RM, Berridge KC. Psychoactive drug use in evolutionary perspective. Science. 1997;278(5335):63–6.

38. Pomerleau OF, Pomerleau CS. A biobehavioral view of substance abuse and addiction. J Drug Issues. 1987;17(1):111–31.

39. Smith EO. Evolution, substance abuse, and addiction. In: Trevathan WR, Smith EO, McKenna JJ, editors. Evolutionary medicine. New York: Oxford University Press; 1999. pp. 375–405.

40. St. John-Smith P, McQueen D, Edwards L, Schifano F. Classical and novel psychoactive substances: rethinking drug misuse from an evolutionary psychiatric perspective. Hum Psychopharmacol Clin Exp. 2013 Jul 1;28(4):394–401.

41. Soliman A, De Sanctis V, Elalaily R. Nutrition and pubertal development. Indian J Endocrinol Metab. 2014 Nov;18(7):39–47.

42. Blask DE. Melatonin, sleep disturbance and cancer risk. Sleep Med Rev. 2009;13(4):257–64.

43. Strassmann BI. Menstrual cycling and breast cancer: an evolutionary perspective. J Womens Health. 1999 Mar;8(2):193–202.

44. Antonovics J, Abbate JL, Baker CH, Daley D, Hood ME, Jenkins CE, et al. Evolution by any other name: antibiotic resistance and avoidance of the e-word. PLOS Biol. 2007;5(2):e30.

45. Bergstrom CT, Lo M, Lipsitch M. Ecological theory suggests that antimicrobial cycling will not reduce antimicrobial resistance in hospitals. Proc Natl Acad Sci. 2004 Sep 7;101(36):13285–90.

46. Llewelyn MJ, Fitzpatrick JM, Darwin E, Tonkin-Crine S, Gorton C, Paul J, et al. The antibiotic course has had its day. BMJ. 2017 Jul 26;358:j3418.

47. Read AF, Woods RJ. Antibiotic resistance management. Evol Med Public Health. 2014 Jan 1;2014(1):147.

48. Goodenough UW. Deception by pathogens. Am Sci. 1991;79(4): 344–55.

49. Leonard HL, Swedo SE. Pediatric autoimmune neuropsychiatric disorders associated with streptococcal infection (PANDAS). Int J Neuropsychopharmacol. 2001;4(2):191–8.

50. Blaser MJ. The microbiome revolution. J Clin Invest. 2014 Oct 1;124(10):4162–5.

51. Pepper JW, Rosenfeld S. The emerging medical ecology of the human gut microbiome. Trends Ecol Evol. 2012 Jul;27(7):381–4.

52. Warinner C, Lewis CM. Microbiome and health in past and present human populations. Am Anthropol. 2015 Dec 1;117(4):740–1.

53. Blaser MJ. Missing microbes.

54. Kahneman D. Thinking, fast and slow. New York: Macmillan; 2011.

55. Nisbett R, Ross L. Human inference: strategies and shortcomings of social judgment. Englewood Cliffs (NJ): Prentice-Hall; 1980.

56. Ellison PT. Evolutionary tradeoffs. Evol Med Public Health. 2014 Jan 1;2014(1):93.

57. Garland T. Trade-offs. Curr Biol. 2014;24(2):R60–1.

58. Stearns S. Trade-offs in life-history evolution. Funct Ecol. 1989;- 3:259–68.

59. Summers K, Crespi BJ. Xmrks the spot: life history tradeoffs, sexual

selection and the evolutionary ecology of oncogenesis. Mol Ecol. 2010 Aug;19(15):3022–4.

60. Zuk M, Bryant MJ, Kolluru GR, Mirmovitch V. Trade-offs in parasitology, evolution and behavior. Parasitol Today. 1996;12(2):46–7.

61. Wilson M, Daly M. Competitiveness, risk taking, and violence: the young male syndrome. Ethol Sociobiol. 1985;6:59–73.

62. Kruger DJ, Nesse RM. Sexual selection and the male: female mortality ratio. Evol Psychol. 2004;2:66–85.

63. Kruger DJ, Nesse RM. An evolutionary life-history framework for understanding sex differences in human mortality rates. Hum Nat. 2006;17(1):74–97.

64. Nesse RM. The Smoke Detector Principle: natural selection and the regulation of defensive responses. Ann N Y Acad Sci. 2001 May;935:75–85.

65. Nesse RM. Natural selection and the regulation of defenses: a signal detection analysis of the Smoke Detector Principle. Evol Hum Behav. 2005;26:88–105.

CHAPTER 4 | GOOD REASONS FOR BAD FEELINGS

1. Ross L, Nisbett RE. The person and the situation: perspectives of social psychology. London: Pinter & Martin Publishers; 2011.

2. Wakefield JC, Schmitz MF, First MB, Horwitz AV. Extending the bereavement exclusion for major depression to other losses: evidence from the National Comorbidity Survey. Arch Gen Psychiatry. 2007 Apr 1;64(4):433.

3. Wakefield JC. The loss of grief: science and pseudoscience in the debate over DSM-5's elimination of the bereavement exclusion. In: Demazeux S, Singy P, editors. The DSM-5 in perspective [Internet]. Springer Netherlands; 2015 [cited 2015 Nov 27]. pp. 157–78. (History, Philosophy and Theory of the Life Sciences). Available from: http://link.springer.com /chapter/10.1007/978-94-017-9765-8_10.

4. Nesse RM, Williams GC. Evolution and the origins of disease. Sci Am. 1998 Nov:86–93.

5. Keltner D, Gross JJ. Functional accounts of emotions. Cogn Emot. 1999;13(5):467–80.

6. Nesse RM. Evolutionary explanations of emotions. Hum Nat. 1990; 1(3):261–89.

7. Nesse RM, Ellsworth PC. Evolution, emotions, and emotional disorders. Am Psychol. 2009 Feb;64(2):129–39.

8. Bateson P, Gluckman P. Plasticity, robustness, development and evolution. Cambridge (UK): Cambridge University Press; 2011.

9. Stearns SC. The evolutionary significance of phenotypic plasticity. Bio-Science. 1989;39(7):436–45.

10. West-Eberhard MJ. Developmental plasticity and evolution. New York: Oxford University Press; 2003.

11. Ellison P, Jasienska G. Adaptation, health, and the temporal domain of human reproductive physiology. In: Panter-Brick C, Fuentes A, editors. Health, risk and adversity: a contextual view from anthropology. Oxford (UK): Berghahn Books; 2008. pp. 108–28.

12. Schmidt-Nielsen K. Animal physiology: adaptation and environment. Cambridge (UK): Cambridge University Press; 1990.

13. Schulkin J. Rethinking homeostasis: allostatic regulation in physiology and pathophysiology. Cambridge (MA): MIT Press; 2003.

14. Alcock J. Animal behavior: an evolutionary approach. 10th ed. Sunderland (MA): Sinauer Associates; 2013.

15. Krebs J, Davies N. Behavioral ecology: an evolutionary approach. 3rd ed. Oxford (UK): Blackwell; 1991.

16. Westneat DF, Fox CW. Evolutionary behavioral ecology. New York: Oxford University Press; 2010.

17. Lench HC, editor. The function of emotions: when and why emotions help us. New York: Springer Science+Business Media; 2018.

18. Wilson EO. Sociobiology: a new synthesis. Cambridge (MA): Harvard University Press; 1975. p. 4.

19. Buss DM. The dangerous passion: why jealousy is as necessary as love or sex. New York: Free Press; 2000.

20. Sadock BJ, Sadock VA, Ruiz P, Kaplan HI, editors. Kaplan & Sadock's comprehensive textbook of psychiatry. 9th ed. Philadelphia: Wolters Kluwer Health/Lippincott Williams & Wilkins; 2009.

21. Clore G, Ketelaar T. Minding our emotions: on the role of automatic,

unconscious affect. In: Wyer RS, editor. The automaticity of everyday life: advances in social cognition. Mahwah (NJ): Lawrence Erlbaum Associates; 1997. pp. 105–20.

22. Ekman P. Emotions inside out: 130 years after Darwin's *The expression of the emotions in man and animals.* New York: New York Academy of Sciences; 2003.

23. Frijda NH. The emotions. Cambridge (UK): Cambridge University Press; 1986.

24. Frijda NH. Emotions and hedonic experience. In: Kahneman D, Diener E, Schwartz N, editors. Well-being. New York: Russell Sage Foundation; 1999. pp. 190–210.

25. Griffiths PE. What emotions really are: the problem of psychological categories. Chicago: University of Chicago Press; 1997.

26. Haselton MG, Ketelaar T. Irrational emotions or emotional wisdom?: The evolutionary psychology of emotions and behavior. In: Forgas J, editor. Hearts and minds: affective influences on social cognition and behavior. New York: Psychology Press, 2006.

27. Oatley K. Best laid schemes: the psychology of emotions. Cambridge (UK): Cambridge University Press; 1992.

28. Panksepp J. Affective neuroscience: the foundations of human and animal emotions. London: Oxford University Press; 1998.

29. Rorty AO. Explaining emotions. Berkeley: University of California Press; 1980.

30. Scherer KR. What are emotions? And how can they be measured? Soc Sci Inf. 2005 Dec 1;44(4):695–729.

31. Tooby J, Cosmides L. The past explains the present: emotional adaptations and the structure of ancestral environments. Ethol Sociobiol. 1990;11(4/5):375–424.

32. James W. The principles of psychology. New York: Collier Books; 1962 [1890]. p. 377.

33. Darwin C. The expression of the emotions in man and animals. New York: St. Martin's Press; 1979.

34. Ekman P. Emotions inside out.

35. Fridlund AJ. Darwin's anti-Darwinism in *The expression of the emotions*

in man and animals. In: Strongman KT, editor. International review of studies on emotions. New York: John Wiley & Sons; 1992. pp. 117–37.

36. Bell SC, Shaw A. The anatomy and philosophy of expression as connected with the fine arts. London: George Bell & Sons; 1904.

37. Loudon IS. Sir Charles Bell and the anatomy of expression. Br Med J Clin Res Ed. 1982 Dec 18;285(6357):1794–6.

38. MacLean PD. The triune brain in evolution. New York: Plenum; 1990.

39. LeDoux JE. Evolution of human emotion. Prog Brain Res. 2012; 195:431–42.

40. Ibid.

41. BPD & the function of anger. OnLine CEUCredit. [Internet]. [cited 2018 Aug 15]. Available from: http://www.mftonlineceus.com/ceus-online /bpicabb-borderline-schema/secBPICAbb10.html.

42. Stosny S. Anger problems: how words make them worse. Psychology Today [Internet]. 2009 Feb 1 [cited 2017 May 31]. Available from: http://www .psychologytoday.com/blog/anger-in-the-age-entitlement/200902 /anger-problems-how-words-make-them-worse.

43. Izard CE, Ackerman BP. Motivational, organizational, and regulatory functions of discrete emotions. In: Lewis M, Haviland-Jones JM, Barrett LF, editors. Handbook of emotions. 2nd ed. New York: Guilford Press; 2000. pp. 253–64.

44. Ibid.

45. Ibid., p. 259.

46. Ibid., p. 260.

47. Lench HC, Bench SW, Darbor KE, Moore M. A functionalist manifesto: goal-related emotions from an evolutionary perspective. Emotion Review. 2015 Jan;7(1):90–8.

48. Nesse RM. Evolutionary explanations of emotions.

49. Nesse RM. Computer emotions and mental software. Soc Neurosci. 1994;7(2):36–7.

50. Tooby J, Cosmides L. The evolutionary psychology of the emotions and their relationship to internal regulatory variables. In: Lewis M, Haviland-Jones JM, Barrett LF, editors. Handbook of emotions. 3rd ed. New York: Guilford Press; 2010. pp. 114–37.

51. Plutchik R. Emotions and life: perspectives from psychology, biology, and evolution. Washington (DC): American Psychological Association; 2003.

52. Nesse RM. Evolutionary explanations of emotions.

53. Ekman P. An argument for basic emotions. Cogn Emot. 1992;6(3/4): 169–200.

54. Izard CE. Basic emotions, natural kinds, emotion schemas, and a new paradigm. Perspect Psychol Sci. 2007 Sep 1;2(3):260–80.

55. Plutchik R. Emotion: a psychoevolutionary synthesis. New York: Harper and Row; 1980.

56. Tomkins SS. Affect as amplification: some modifications in theory. Emot Theory Res Exp. 1980;1:141–64.

57. Eibl-Eibesfeldt I. Human ethology. New York: Aldine de Gruyter; 1983.

58. Ekman P. Strong evidence for universals in facial expressions. Psychol Bull. 1994;115(2):268–87.

59. Russell JA. Culture and the categorization of emotions. Psychol Bull. 1991;110(3):426–50.

60. Clore GL, Ortony A. What more is there to emotion concepts than prototypes? J Pers Soc Psychol. 1991;60(1):48–50.

61. Nesse RM. Natural selection and the elusiveness of happiness. Philos Trans R Soc Lond B Biol Sci. 2004 Sep 29;359(1449):1333–47.

62. Clore G, Ketelaar T. Minding our emotions.

63. Taylor GJ, Bagby RM. An overview of the alexithymia construct. In: Bar-On R, Parker JDA, editors. The handbook of emotional intelligence: theory, development, assessment, and application at home, school, and in the workplace. San Francisco: Jossey-Bass; 2000. pp. 40–67.

64. Lyon P. The cognitive cell: bacterial behavior reconsidered. Front Microbiol [Internet]. 2015 Apr 14 [cited 2018 Jun 13];6. Available from: http://journal.frontiersin.org/article/10.3389/fmicb.2015.00264 /abstract.

65. Ibid.

66. Koshland DE. Bacterial chemotaxis as a model behavioral system. New York: Raven Press; 1980.

67. Adler J. Chemotaxis in bacteria. Annu Rev Biochem. 1975;44(1):341–56.

68. Hu B, Tu Y. Behaviors and strategies of bacterial navigation in chemical and nonchemical gradients. PLOS Comput Biol [Internet]. 2014 Jun 19 [cited 2017 Oct 27];10(6). Available from: https://www.ncbi.nlm.nih.gov/pmc/articles/PMC4063634.

69. Kirby JR. Chemotaxis-like regulatory systems: unique roles in diverse bacteria. Annu Rev Microbiol. 2009;63:45–59.

70. Kitayama S, Markus H. Emotion and culture: empirical studies of mutual influence. Washington (DC): American Psychological Association; 1994.

71. Izard CE. The psychology of emotions. New York: Plenum Press; 1991.

72. Eibl-Eibesfeldt I. Human ethology. Hawthorne (NY): Aldine De Gruyter; 1989.

73. Ekman P. An argument for basic emotions.

74. Russell JA. Is there universal recognition of emotion from facial expression?: a review of the cross-cultural studies. Psychol Bull. 1994;115(1): 102–41.

75. Russell JA. Facial expressions of emotion: what lies beyond minimal universality? Psychol Bull. 1995;118(3):379–91.

76. Wierzbicka A. Emotions across languages and cultures: diversity and universals. New York: Cambridge University Press; 1999.

77. Barrett LF. Psychological construction: the Darwinian approach to the science of emotion. Emot Rev. 2013;5(4):379–89.

78. Barrett LF, Russell JA. The psychological construction of emotion. New York: Guilford Press; 2014.

79. Barrett LF. How emotions are made: the secret life of the brain. New York: Houghton Mifflin Harcourt; 2017.

80. Plato. Phaedrus [Internet]. c. 370 BC. Available from: http://www.gutenberg.org/ebooks/1636.

81. Mineka S, Ohman A. Born to fear: non-associative vs. associative factors in the etiology of phobias. Behav Res Ther. 2002 Feb;40(2):173–84.

82. Mineka S, Keir R, Price V. Fear of snakes in wild- and laboratory-reared rhesus monkeys (Macaca mulatta). Anim Learn Behav. 1980;8(4):653–63.

83. Öhman A, Dimberg U, Ost L. Animal and social phobias: biological constraints on learned fear responses. In: Reiss S, Bootzin RR, editors.

Theoretical issues in behavioral therapy. Orlando (FL): Academic Press; 1985. pp. 123–75.

84. Poulton R, Menzies RG. Fears born and bred: toward a more inclusive theory of fear acquisition. Behav Res Ther. 2002 Feb;40(2):197–208.

85. Gibbard A. Wise choices, apt feelings: a theory of normative judgment. Oxford (UK): Oxford University Press; 1990.

86. Atkinson JW, Bastian JR, Earl JW, Litwin GH. The achievement motive, goal setting, and probability preferences. J Abnorm Soc Psychol. 1960;60:27–36.

87. Cantor N, Fleeson W. Social intelligence and intelligent goal pursuit: a cognitive slice of motivation. In: Spaulding WD, editor. Nebraska symposium on motivation. Vol. 41. Integrative views of motivation, cognition, and emotion. Lincoln: University of Nebraska Press; 1994. pp. 125–79.

88. Carver CS, Scheier MF. Goals and emotion. In: Robinson MD, Watkins ER, Harmon-Jones E, editors. Guilford handbook of cognition and emotion. New York: Guilford Press; 2013. pp. 176–94.

89. Deci EL, Ryan RM. The "what" and "why" of goal pursuits: human needs and the self-determination of behavior. Psychol Inq. 2000 Oct 1;11(4):227–68.

90. Emmons RA. Striving and feeling: personal goals and subjective well-being. In: Gollwitzer PM, editor. The psychology of action: linking cognition and motivation to behavior. New York: Guilford Press; 1996. pp. 313–37.

91. Fleeson W, Cantor N. Goal relevance and the affective experience of daily life: ruling out situational explanations. Motiv Emot. 1995;19(1):25–57.

92. Higgins ET, Shah J, Friedman R. Emotional responses to goal attainment: strength of regulatory focus as moderator. J Pers Soc Psychol. 1997;72(3):515–25.

93. Wrosch C, Amir E, Miller GE. Goal adjustment capacities, coping, and subjective well-being: the sample case of caregiving for a family member with mental illness. J Pers Soc Psychol. 2011;100(5):934–46.

94. Dennett DC, Weiner P. Consciousness explained. Paperback ed. Boston: Back Bay Books; 1991.

95. Humphrey N. A history of the mind: evolution and the birth of consciousness. New York: Springer Science+Business Media; 1999.

96. Tannenbaum AS. The sense of consciousness. J Theor Biol. 2001 Aug;211(4):377–91.

97. Dunbar RI. Coevolution of neocortical size, group size and language in humans. Behav Brain Sci. 1993;16(4):681–94.

98. Ellsworth PC. Appraisals, emotions, and adaptation. In: Forgas JP, Haselton MG, von Hippel W, editors. Evolution and the social mind. New York: Psychology Press; 2007. pp. 71–88.

99. Ellsworth PC. Appraisal theory: old and new questions. Emot Rev. 2013;5(2):125–31.

100. Scherer KR, Schorr A, Johnstone T. Appraisal processes in emotion: theory, methods, research. New York: Oxford University Press; 2001.

101. Gross JJ, Feldman Barrett L. Emotion generation and emotion regulation: one or two depends on your point of view. Emot Rev. 2011;3(1): 8–16.

102. Brickman P, Coates D, Janoff-Bulman R. Lottery winners and accident victims: is happiness relative? J Pers Soc Psychol. 1978;36(8):917–27.

103. Gilbert DT, Pinel EC, Wilson TD, Blumberg SJ, Wheatley TP. Immune neglect: a source of durability bias in affective forecasting. J Pers Soc Psychol. 1998;75(3):617–38.

104. Seligman ME, Csikszentmihalyi M. Positive psychology. an introduction. Am Psychol. 2000 Jan;55(1):5–14.

105. Andrews PW, Thompson JA. The bright side of being blue: depression as an adaptation for analyzing complex problems. Psychol Rev. 2009;116(3):620–54.

106. Bank C, Ewing GB, Ferrer-Admettla A, Foll M, Jensen JD. Thinking too positive?: revisiting current methods of population genetic selection inference. Trends Genet. 2014 Dec;30(12):540–6.

107. Bastian B, Jetten J, Hornsey MJ, Leknes S. The positive consequences of pain: a biopsychosocial approach. Pers Soc Psychol Rev. 2014 Aug;18(3):256–79.

108. Keller PA, Lipkus IM, Rimer BK. Depressive realism and health risk accuracy: the negative consequences of positive mood. J Consum Res. 2002 Jun 1;29(1):57–69.

109. Stein DJ. Positive mental health: a note of caution. World Psychiatry. 2012;11(2):107–9.

110. Keltner D, Gross JJ. Functional accounts of emotions. Cogn Emot. 1999;13(5):467–80.

111. Frijda NH. The emotions.

112. Haselton MG, Ketelaar T. Irrational emotions or emotional wisdom?

113. Izard CE, Ackerman B. Motivational, organizational, and regulatory functions of discrete emotions.

114. Gibbard A. Wise choices, apt feelings.

115. Scherer KR. When and why are emotions disturbed?: suggestions based on theory and data from emotion research. Emot Rev. 2015 Jul 1;7(3):238–49.

CHAPTER 5 | ANXIETY AND SMOKE DETECTORS

1. Kierkegaard S. The concept of anxiety. Trans. Reidar Thomte. Princeton (NJ): Princeton University Press; 1980. p. 1.

2. Kessler RC, Aguilar-Gaxiola S, Alonso J, Chatterji S, Lee S, Ormel J, et al. The global burden of mental disorders: an update from the WHO World Mental Health (WMH) surveys. Epidemiol Psichiatr Soc. 2009;18(1):23–33.

3. Kessler RC, Berglund P, Demler O, Jin R, Merikangas KR, Walters EE. Lifetime prevalence and age-of-onset distributions of *DSM-IV* disorders in the National Comorbidity Survey Replication. Arch Gen Psychiatry. 2005 Jun 1;62(6):593–602.

4. Curtis GC, Nesse RM, Buxton M, Wright J, Lippman D. Flooding in vivo as research tool and treatment method for phobias: a preliminary report. Compr Psychiatry. 1976 Jan–Feb;17(1):153–60.

5. Nesse RM, Curtis GC, Thyer BA, McCann DS, Huber SMJ, Knopf RF. Endocrine and cardiovascular responses during phobic anxiety. Psychosom Med. 1985;47(4):320–32.

6. Kennair LEO. Fear and fitness revisited. J Evol Psychol. 2007;5(1):105–17.

7. Marks IM, Nesse RM. Fear and fitness: an evolutionary analysis of anxiety disorders. Ethol Sociobiol. 1994;15(5–6):247–61.

8.   Poulton R, Davies S, Menzies RG, Langley JD, Silva PA. Evidence for a non-associative model of the acquisition of a fear of heights. Behav Res Ther. 1998 May;36(5):537–44.

9.   Ibid.

10.   Cannon WB. The wisdom of the body. New York: W. W. Norton; 1939.

11.   Green DM, Swets JA. Signal detection theory and psycho-physics. New York: Wiley; 1966.

12.   Hacking I. The logic of Pascal's wager. Am Philos Q. 1972;9(2):186–92.

13.   Nesse RM, Williams GC. Why we get sick.

14.   Nesse RM. The Smoke Detector Principle.

15.   Nesse RM. Natural selection and the regulation of defenses.

16.   Marks IM, Nesse RM. Fear and fitness.

17.   Öhman A. Face the beast and fear the face: animal and social fears as prototypes for evolutionary analyses of emotion. Psychophysiology. 1986;23(2):123–45.

18.   Mineka S, Keir R, Price V. Fear of snakes in wild- and laboratory-reared rhesus monkeys (*Macaca mulatta*).

19.   Curio E, Ernst U, Vieth W. The adaptive significance of avian mobbing. Z für Tierpsychol. 1978 Jan 12;48(2):184–202.

20.   Kochanek KD, Murphy SL, Xu J, Tejada-Vera B. National vital statistics reports 2014 [Internet]. 2016 Jun 30;65(4). Available from: https://www.cdc.gov/nchs/data/nvsr/nvsr65/nvsr65_04.pdf.

21.   World Health Organization. Global status report on road safety 2015 [Internet]. Geneva: World Health Organization; 2015. Available from: http://apps.who.int/iris/bitstream/handle/10665/44122/97892415 63840_eng.pdf;jsessionid=5C79BDD3A583A50B85E7FF6978536B16? sequence=1.

22.   Schulkin J. The CRF signal: uncovering an information molecule. New York: Oxford University Press; 2017.

23.   Sara SJ. The locus coeruleus and noradrenergic modulation of cognition. Nat Rev Neurosci. 2009 Mar;10(3):211–23.

24.   Lima SL, Dill LM. Behavioral decisions made under the risk of predation: a review and prospectus. Can J Zool. 1990;68(4):619–40.

25.   Nesse RM. An evolutionary perspective on panic disorder and agora-phobia. Ethol Sociobiol. 1987;8:73S–83S.

26.   Breslau N, Kessler RC, Chilcoat HD, Schultz LR, Davis GC, Andreski P. Trauma and posttraumatic stress disorder in the community: the 1996 Detroit Area Survey of Trauma. Arch Gen Psychiatry. 1998 Jul 1;55(7):626–32.

27.   Breslau N, Davis GC, Andreski P. Risk factors for PTSD-related traumatic events: a prospective analysis. Am J Psychiatry. 1995 Apr;152(4):529–35.

28.   Ibid.

29.   Breslau N et al. Trauma and posttraumatic stress disorder in the community.

30.   Cantor C. Evolution and posttraumatic stress: disorders of vigilance and defence. New York: Routledge; 2005.

31.   Middeldorp CM, Cath DC, Van Dyck R, Boomsma DI. The co-morbidity of anxiety and depression in the perspective of genetic epidemiology: a review of twin and family studies. Psychol Med. 2005;35(5):611–24.

32.   Bateson M, Brilot B, Nettle D. Anxiety: an evolutionary approach. Can J Psychiatry Rev Can Psychiatr. 2011;56(12):707–15.

33.   Milad MR, Rauch SL, Pitman RK, Quirk GJ. Fear extinction in rats: implications for human brain imaging and anxiety disorders. Biol Psychol. 2006 Jul;73(1):61–71.

34.   Streatfeild D. Brainwash: the secret history of mind control. New York: Macmillan; 2008.

35.   Nettle D, Bateson M. The evolutionary origins of mood and its disorders. Curr Biol. 2012;22(17):R712–21.

CHAPTER 6 | LOW MOOD AND THE ART OF GIVING UP

1.   Darwin C. The life and letters of Charles Darwin, including an autobiographical chapter. Darwin F, editor. 3rd ed. London: J. Murray; 1887.

2.   Whiteford HA, Degenhardt L, Rehm J, Baxter AJ, Ferrari AJ, Erskine HE, et al. Global burden of disease attributable to mental and substance use disorders: findings from the Global Burden of Disease Study 2010. The Lancet. 2013 Nov 15;382(9904):1575–86.

3. Curtin SC, Warner M, Hedegaard, H. Increase in suicide in the United States, 1999–2014 [Internet]. NCHS data brief, no. 241. Hyattsville (MD): National Center for Health Statistics; 2016 [cited 2017 Dec 10]. Available from: https://www.cdc.gov/nchs/products /databriefs/db241.htm.

4. Zachar P, First MB, Kendler KS. The bereavement exclusion debate in the *DSM-5*: a history. Clin Psychol Sci. 2017 Sep 1;5(5):890–906.

5. Bowlby J. Attachment and loss. Vol. 3. Loss: sadness and depression. New York: Basic Books; 1980.

6. Ibid.

7. Ainsworth MD, Blehar MC, Waters E, Wall S. Patterns of attachment: a psychological study of the strange situation. Hillsdale (NJ): Erlbaum; 1978.

8. Cassidy J, Shaver PR. Handbook of attachment: theory, research, and clinical applications. New York: Guilford Press; 1999.

9. Belsky J. Developmental origins of attachment styles. Attach Hum Dev. 2002 Sep;4(2):166–70.

10. Chisholm JS. The evolutionary ecology of attachment organization. Hum Nat. 1996 Mar 1;7(1):1–37.

11. Crespi BJ. The strategies of the genes: genomic conflicts, attachment theory, and development of the social brain. In: Petronas A, Mill J, editors. Brain, behavior and epigenetics. Berlin: Springer-Verlag; 2011. pp. 143–67.

12. Engel G, Schmale A. Conservation-withdrawal: a primary regulatory process for organismic homeostasis. In: Porter R, Night J, editors. Physiology, emotion, and psychosomatic illness. Amsterdam: CIBA; 1972. pp. 57–85.

13. Schmale A, Engel GL. The role of conservation-withdrawal in depressive reactions. In: Benedek T, Anthony EJ, editors. Depression and human existence. Boston: Little, Brown; 1975. pp. 183–98.

14. Lewis AJ. Melancholia: a clinical survey of depressive states. J Ment Sci. 1934;80:277–378.

15. Hamburg D, Hamburg B, Barchas J. Anger and depression in perspective of behavioral biology. In: Levi L, editor. Emotions: their parameters and measurement. New York: Raven Press; 1975. pp. 235–78.

16. Hagen EH. The functions of postpartum depression. Evol Hum Behav. 1999;20:325–59.

17. Hagen EH. Depression as bargaining: the case postpartum. Evol Hum Behav. 2002;23(5):323–36.

18. Coyne JC, Kessler RC, Tal M, Turnbull J. Living with a depressed person. J Consult Clin Psychol. 1987;55(3):347–52.

19. deCatanzaro D. Human suicide: a biological perspective. Behav Brain Sci. 1980;3(2):265–90.

20. Price JS. The dominance hierarchy and the evolution of mental illness. The Lancet. 1967;290(7509):243–6.

21. Price JS, Sloman L. Depression as yielding behavior: an animal model based on Schjelderup-Ebbe's pecking order. Ethol Sociobiol. 1987; 8:85S–98S.

22. Ibid.

23. Zuroff DC, Fournier MA, Moskowitz DS. Depression, perceived inferiority, and interpersonal behavior: evidence for the involuntary defeat strategy. J Soc Clin Psychol. 2007;26(7):751–78.

24. Sloman L, Price J, Gilbert P, Gardner R. Adaptive function of depression: psychotherapeutic implications. Am J Psychother. 1994; 48:1–16.

25. Price J, Sloman L, Gardner R, Gilbert P, Rohde P. The social competition hypothesis of depression. Br J Psychiatry. 1994;164(3):309–15.

26. Hartung J. Deceiving down. In: Lockard JS, Paulhus D, editors. Self-deception: an adaptive mechanism? Englewood Cliffs (NJ): Prentice Hall; 1988. pp. 170–85.

27. Brown GW, Harris T. Social origins of depression: a study of psychiatric disorder in women. London: Tavistock Publications; 1979.

28. Bifulco A, Brown GW, Moran P, Ball C, Campbell C. Predicting depression in women: the role of past and present vulnerability. Psychol Med. 1998;28(1):39–50.

29. Hammen C. Stress and depression. Annu Rev Clin Psychol. 2005; 1(1):293–319.

30. Kendler KS, Karkowski LM, Prescott CA. Causal relationship between stressful life events and the onset of major depression. Am J Psychiatry. 1999;156(6):837–41.

31.   Kessler RC. The effects of stressful life events on depression. Annu Rev Psychol. 1997;48(1):191–214.

32.   Lloyd C. Life events and depressive disorders reviewed. Arch Gen Psychiatry. 1980;37(5):529–35.

33.   Monroe SM, Reid MW. Life stress and major depression. Curr Dir Psychol Sci. 2009 Apr 1;18(2):68–72.

34.   Monroe SM, Rohde P, Seeley JR, Lewinsohn PM. Life events and depression in adolescence: relationship loss as a prospective risk factor for first onset of major depressive disorder. J Abnorm Psychol. 1999;108(4):606.

35.   Paykel ES. The evolution of life events research in psychiatry. J Affect Disord. 2001;62(3):141–9.

36.   Paykel ES, Myers JK, Dienelt MN, Klerman GL, Lidenthal JJ, Pepper MP. Life events and depression: a controlled study. Arch Gen Psychiatry. 1969 Dec 1;21(6):753–60.

37.   Troisi A, McGuire MT. Evolutionary biology and life-events research. Arch Gen Psychiatry. 1992 Jun;49(6):501–2.

38.   Brown GW, Harris TO, Hepworth C. Loss, humiliation and entrapment among women developing depression: a patient and non-patient comparison. Psychol Med. 1995;25(1):7–21.

39.   Fried EI, Nesse RM, Guille C, Sen S. The differential influence of life stress on individual symptoms of depression. Acta Psychiatr Scand. 2015 Jun;131(6):465–71.

40.   Fried EI, Nesse RM. Depression is not a consistent syndrome: an investigation of unique symptom patterns in the STAR*D study. J Affect Disord. 2015 Feb 1;172:96–102.

41.   Fried EI, Nesse RM. Depression sum-scores don't add up: why analyzing specific depression symptoms is essential. BMC Med. 2015;13(1):72.

42.   Nolen-Hoeksema S, Wisco BE, Lyubomirsky S. Rethinking rumination. Perspect Psychol Sci. 2008;3(5):400–24.

43.   Nolen-Hoeksema S, Morrow J. A prospective study of depression and posttraumatic stress symptoms after a natural disaster: the 1989 Loma Prieta earthquake. J Pers Soc Psychol. 1991;61(1):115–21.

44.   Andrews PW, Thomson JA. The bright side of being blue: depression as an adaptation for analyzing complex problems. Psychol Rev. 2009; 116(3):620–54.

45. Watson PJ, Andrews PW. Toward a revised evolutionary adaptationist analysis of depression: the social navigation hypothesis. J Affect Disord. 2002;72(1):1–14.

46. Nettle D. Evolutionary origins of depression: a review and reformulation. J Affect Disord. 2004;81:91–102.

47. Kennair LEO, Kleppestø TH, Larsen SM, Jørgensen BEG. Depression: is rumination really adaptive? In: The evolution of psychopathology [Internet]. Cham (Switzerland): Springer; 2017 [cited 2017 Nov 18]. pp. 73–92. Available from: https://link.springer.com/chapter/10.1007/978-3-319 -60576-0_3.

48. Gut E. Productive and unproductive depression: its functions and failures. New York: Basic Books; 1989.

49. Nesse RM. Is depression an adaptation? Arch Gen Psychiatry. 2000;57(1):14–20.

50. Kramer PD. Should you leave? New York: Scribner; 1997.

51. Sinervo B. Optimal foraging theory [Internet]. 1997. Available from: http://bio.research.ucsc.edu/~barrylab/classes/animal_behavior /FORAGING.HTM.

52. Charnov EL. Optimal foraging: the marginal value theorem. Theor Popul Biol. 1976;9(2):129–36.

53. Rosetti MF, Ulloa RE, Vargas-Vargas IL, Reyes-Zamorano E, Palacios-Cruz L, de la Peña F, et al. Evaluation of children with ADHD on the Ball-Search Field Task. Sci Rep [Internet]. 2016 Jan 25 [cited 2018 Jan 14];6. Available from: https://www.ncbi.nlm.nih.gov/pmc/articles /PMC4726146.

54. Heinrich B. Bumblebee economics. Cambridge (MA): Harvard University Press; 1979.

55. Körtner G, Geiser F. The key to winter survival: daily torpor in a small arid-zone marsupial. Naturwissenschaften. 2009 Apr 1;96(4):525.

56. Caraco T, Blanckenhorn WU, Gregory GM, Newman JA, Recer GM, Zwicker SM. Risk-sensitivity: ambient temperature affects foraging choice. Anim Behav. 1990;39(2):338–45.

57. Porsolt RD, Le Pichon M, Jalfre M. Depression: a new animal model sensitive to antidepressant treatments. Nature. 1977;266(5604):730–2.

58. Molendijk ML, de Kloet ER. Immobility in the forced swim test is

adaptive and does not reflect depression. Psychoneuroendocrinology. 2015 Dec 1;62(Suppl C):389–91.

59.   Seligman ME. Depression and learned helplessness. New York: John Wiley & Sons; 1974.

60.   Nesse RM. Is depression an adaptation?

61.   Lasker GW. The effects of partial starvation on somatotype: an analysis of material from the Minnesota Starvation Experiment. Am J Phys Anthropol. 1947;5(3):323–42.

62.   Müller MJ, Enderle J, Pourhassan M, Braun W, Eggeling B, Lagerpusch M, et al. Metabolic adaptation to caloric restriction and subsequent refeeding: the Minnesota Starvation Experiment revisited. Am J Clin Nutr. 2015;102(4):807–19.

63.   Davis C, Levitan RD. Seasonality and seasonal affective disorder (SAD): an evolutionary viewpoint tied to energy conservation and reproductive cycles. J Affect Disord. 2005;87(1):3–10.

64.   Oren D, Rosenthal N. Seasonal affective disorder. In: Paykel E, editor. Handbook of affective disorders. New York: Churchill Livingstone; 1992.

65.   Rosenthal NE, Sack DA, Gillin JC, Lewy AJ, Goodwin FK, Davenport Y, et al. Seasonal affective disorder: a description of the syndrome and preliminary findings with light therapy. Arch Gen Psychiatry. 1984; 41(1):72–80.

66.   Hart BL. Biological basis of the behavior of sick animals. Neurosci Biobehav Rev. 1988;12(2):123–37.

67.   Johnson RW. The concept of sickness behavior: a brief chronological account of four key discoveries. Vet Immunol Immunopathol. 2002; 87(3):443–50.

68.   Raison CL, Capuron L, Miller AH. Cytokines sing the blues: inflammation and the pathogenesis of depression. Trends Immunol. 2006; 27(1):24–31.

69.   Loftis JM, Socherman RE, Howell CD, Whitehead AJ, Hill JA, Dominitz JA, et al. Association of interferon-[alpha]-induced depression and improved treatment response in patients with hepatitis C. Neurosci Lett. 2004;365(2):87–91.

70.   Raison CL, Miller AH. The evolutionary significance of depression

in pathogen host defense (PATHOS-D). Mol Psychiatry. 2013;18(1):-15–37.

71. Dantzer R, O'Connor JC, Freund GG, Johnson RW, Kelley KW. From inflammation to sickness and depression: when the immune system subjugates the brain. Nat Rev Neurosci. 2008 Jan;9(1):46–56.

72. Miller AH, Raison CL. The role of inflammation in depression: from evolutionary imperative to modern treatment target. Nat Rev Immunol. 2016 Jan;16(1):22–34.

73. Musselman DL, Evans DL, Nemeroff CB. The relationship of depression to cardiovascular disease: epidemiology, biology, and treatment. Arch Gen Psychiatry. 1998;55(7):580–92.

74. Stewart JC, Rand KL, Muldoon MF, Kamarck TW. A prospective evaluation of the directionality of the depression-inflammation relationship. Brain Behav Immun. 2009 Oct 1;23(7):936–44.

75. Shakespeare W. Julius Caesar, act 4, scene 3. 1599.

76. Fredrickson BL. The role of positive emotions in positive psychology: the broaden-and-build theory of positive emotions. Am Psychol. 2001; 56(3):218–26.

77. Tennov D. Love and limerence: the experience of being in love [Internet]. 1999 [cited 2017 Dec 17]. Available from: http://site.ebrary .com/id/10895438.

78. Taylor GJ. Recent developments in alexithymia theory and research. Can J Psychiatry. 2000;45(2):134–42.

79. Galbraith JK, Purcell G. The butterfly effect. In: Unbearable cost [Internet]. London: Palgrave Macmillan; 2006 [cited 2017 Dec 10]. pp. 129–32. Available from: https://link.springer.com/chapter/10.1057 /9780230236721_37.

80. Klinger E. Consequences of commitment to and disengagement from incentives. Psychol Rev. 1975;82(1):1–25.

81. Heckhausen J, Wrosch C, Fleeson W. Developmental regulation before and after a developmental deadline: the sample case of "biological clock" for childbearing. Psychol Aging. 2001 Sep;16(3):400–13.

82. Wrosch C, Scheier MF, Miller GE. Goal adjustment capacities, subjective well-being, and physical health. Soc Personal Psychol Compass. 2013; 7(12):847–60.

83.   Wrosch C, Scheier MF, Miller GE, Schulz R, Carver CS. Adaptive self-regulation of unattainable goals: goal disengagement, goal re-engagement, and subjective well-being. Personal Soc Psychol Bull Menn Clin. 2003; 29(12):1494–508.

84.   Carver CS, Scheier MF. On the self-regulation of behavior. New York: Cambridge University Press; 1998.

85.   Lawrence JW, Carver CS, Scheier MF. Velocity toward goal attainment in immediate experience as a determinant of affect. J Appl Soc Psychol. 2002;32(4):788–802.

86.   Carver CS, Scheier MF. On the self-regulation of behavior.

87.   Carver CS, Scheier MF. Origins and functions of positive and negative affect: a control-process view. Psychol Rev. 1990;97(1):19–35.

88.   Hoagland T. What narcissism means to me. Saint Paul (MN): Graywolf Press; 2003.

89.   Carver CS, Scheier MF. Dispositional optimism. Trends Cogn Sci. 2014;18(6):293–99.

90.   Giltay EJ, Kamphuis MH, Kalmijn S, Zitman FG, Kromhout D. Dispositional optimism and the risk of cardiovascular death: the Zutphen Elderly Study. Arch Intern Med. 2006 Feb 27;166(4):431–6.

91.   Alloy LB, Abramson LY. Depressive realism: four theoretical perspectives. In: Cognitive processes in depression. New York: Guilford Press; 1988.

92.   Taylor SE, Brown JD. Positive illusions and well-being revisited: separating fact from fiction [Internet]. 1994 [cited 2017 May 15]. Available from: http://psycnet.apa.org/journals/bul/116/1/21.

93.   Moore MT, Fresco DM. Depressive realism: a meta-analytic review. Clin Psychol Rev. 2012 Aug;32(6):496–509.

94.   Taylor SE, Brown JD. Positive illusions and well-being revisited.

95.   Schwarz N. Emotion, cognition, and decision making. Cogn Emot. 2000;14(4):433–40.

96.   Taylor SE, Brown JD. Illusion and well-being: a social psychological perspective on mental health. Psychol Bull. 1988;103(2):193–210.

97.   Moore MT, Fresco DM. Depressive realism: a meta-analytic review. Clin Psychol Rev. 2012 Aug;32(6):496–509.

98. Keller MC, Nesse RM. Is low mood an adaptation?: evidence for subtypes with symptoms that match precipitants. J Affect Disord. 2005; 86(1):27–35.

99. Fried EI, Nesse RM, Zivin K, Guille C, Sen S. Depression is more than the sum score of its parts: individual DSM symptoms have different risk factors. Psychol Med. 2014 Jul; 44(10): 2067–76.

CHAPTER 7 | BAD FEELINGS FOR NO REASON: WHEN THE MOODOSTAT FAILS

1. Wolpert L. Malignant sadness: the anatomy of depression. New York: Free Press; 1999. p. 79.

2. Smith K. Mental health: a world of depression. Nature. 2014 Nov 12;515(7526):180–1.

3. Greenberg PE, Fournier A-A, Sisitsky T, Pike CT, Kessler RC. The economic burden of adults with major depressive disorder in the United States (2005 and 2010). J Clin Psychiatry. 2015 Feb;76(2):155–62.

4. Ledford H. Medical research: if depression were cancer. Nature. 2014 Nov 12;515(7526):182–4.

5. Lewin K. Principles of topological psychology. New York: McGraw-Hill; 1936.

6. Nisbett R, Ross L. Human inference: strategies and shortcomings of social judgment. Englewood Cliffs (NJ): Prentice-Hall; 1980.

7. Ross LD, Amabile TM, Steinmetz JL. Social roles, social control, and biases in social-perception processes. J Pers Soc Psychol. 1977; 35(7):485–94.

8. Gopnik A. How an 18th-century philosopher helped solve my midlife crisis. The Atlantic [Internet]. 2015 Oct. Available from: https://www.theatlantic.com/magazine/archive/2015/10/how-david-hume-helped-me-solve-my-midlife-crisis/403195.

9. Hume D. A treatise of human nature. London: Penguin Classics; 1985 [1738].

10. Barash DP. Buddhist biology: ancient Eastern wisdom meets modern Western science. New York: Oxford University Press; 2014.

11. Ekman P, Davidson RJ, Ricard M, Wallace BA. Buddhist and psychological perspectives on emotions and well-being. Curr Dir Psychol Sci. 2005;14(2):59–63.

12. Miller T. How to want what you have: discovering the magic and grandeur of ordinary existence. New York: H. Holt; 1995.

13. Lewis AJ. Melancholia.

14. Kessler RC. The effects of stressful life events on depression. Annu Rev Psychol. 1997;48(1):191–214.

15. Charney DS, Manji HK. Life stress, genes, and depression: multiple pathways lead to increased risk and new opportunities for intervention. Sci STKE. 2004 Mar 23;2004(225):re5.

16. Monroe SM, Kupfer DJ, Frank E. Life stress and treatment course of recurrent depression: 1. Response during index episode. J Consult Clin Psychol. 1992 Oct;60(5):718–24.

17. Monroe SM, Simons AD, Thase ME. Onset of depression and time to treatment entry: roles of life stress. J Consult Clin Psychol. 1991; 59(4):566–73.

18. Hlastala SA, Frank E, Kowalski J, Sherrill JT, Tu XM, Anderson B, et al. Stressful life events, bipolar disorder, and the "kindling model." J Abnorm Psychol. 2000;109(4):777–86.

19. Kupfer DJ, Frank E. Role of psychosocial factors in the onset of major depression. Ann N Y Acad Sci. 1997;807(1):429–39.

20. Monroe SM, Harkness KL. Life stress, the "kindling" hypothesis, and the recurrence of depression: considerations from a life stress perspective. Psychol Rev. 2005;112(2):417–45.

21. Akiskal HS, McKinney WT Jr. Depressive disorders: toward a unified hypothesis: clinical, experimental, genetic, biochemical, and neurophysiological data are integrated. Science. 1973 Oct 5;182(4107):20–9.

22. Klein DF. Endogenomorphic depression: a conceptual and terminological revision. Arch Gen Psychiatry. 1974 Oct 1;31(4):447–54.

23. Wakefield JC, Schmitz MF. Uncomplicated depression is normal sadness, not depressive disorder: further evidence from the NESARC. World Psychiatry. 2014 Oct;13(3):317–9.

24. Carr D. Methodological issues in studying bereavement. In: Carr D,

Nesse R, Wortman CB, editors. Late-life widowhood in the United States. New York: Springer; 2005.

25. Nesse RM. An evolutionary framework for understanding grief. Spousal Bereave Late Life. 2005;195–226.

26. Miller T. How to want what you have.

27. Hidaka BH. Depression as a disease of modernity: explanations for increasing prevalence. J Affect Disord. 2012;140(3):205–14.

28. Baxter AJ, Scott KM, Ferrari AJ, Norman RE, Vos T, Whiteford HA. Challenging the myth of an "epidemic" of common mental disorders: trends in the global prevalence of anxiety and depression between 1990 and 2010. Depress Anxiety. 2014 Jun;31(6):506–16.

29. Cross-National Collaborative Group. The changing rate of major depression: cross-national comparisons. J Am Med Assoc. 1992;268(21): 3098–105.

30. Jorm AF, Duncan-Jones P, Scott R. An analysis of the re-test artefact in longitudinal studies of psychiatric symptoms and personality. Psychol Med. 1989 May;19(2):487–93.

31. Wells JE, Horwood LJ. How accurate is recall of key symptoms of depression?: a comparison of recall and longitudinal reports. Psychol Med. 2004;34(6):1001–11.

32. Centers for Disease Control and Prevention (CDC). Current depression among adults—United States, 2006 and 2008. Morb Mortal Wkly Rep. 2010 Oct 1;59(38):1229–35.

33. Steel Z, Marnane C, Iranpour C, Chey T, Jackson JW, Patel V, et al. The global prevalence of common mental disorders: a systematic review and meta-analysis 1980–2013. Int J Epidemiol. 2014 Apr 1;43(2):- 476–93.

34. Salk RH, Petersen JL, Abramson LY, Hyde JS. The contemporary face of gender differences and similarities in depression throughout adolescence: development and chronicity. J Affect Disord. 2016 Nov 15; 205:28–35.

35. Rao U, Hammen C, Daley SE. Continuity of depression during the transition to adulthood: a 5-year longitudinal study of young women. J Am Acad Child Adolesc Psychiatry. 1999 Jul;38(7):908–15.

36. Ibrahim AK, Kelly SJ, Adams CE, Glazebrook C. A systematic review

of studies of depression prevalence in university students. J Psychiatr Res. 2013 Mar 1;47(3):391–400.

37. Weissman MM, Bland RC, Canino GJ, Faravelli C, Greenwald S, Hwu H-G, et al. Cross-national epidemiology of major depression and bipolar disorder. JAMA. 1996;276(4):293–99.

38. Andrade L, Caraveo-Anduaga JJ, Berglund P, Bijl RV, De Graff RD, Vollebergh W, et al. The epidemiology of major depressive episodes: results from the International Consortium of Psychiatric Epidemiology (ICPE) surveys. Int J Methods Psychiatr Res. 2003 Feb;12(1):3–21.

39. Simon GE, Goldberg DP, Korff MV, Üstün TB. Understanding cross-national differences in depression prevalence. Psychol Med. 2002 May;32(4):585–94.

40. Taylor SE, Lobel M. Social comparison activity under threat: downward evaluation and upward contacts. Psychol Rev. 1989;96(4):569–75.

41. Vogel EA, Rose JP, Roberts LR, Eckles K. Social comparison, social media, and self-esteem. Psychol Pop Media Cult. 2014;3(4):206–22.

42. Gibbons FX, Gerrard M. Effects of upward and downward social comparison on mood states. J Soc Clin Psychol. 1989 Mar 1;8(1):14–31.

43. Gilbert P. An evolutionary approach to emotion in mental health with a focus on affiliative emotions. Emot Rev. 2015 Jul 1;7(3):230–7.

44. Gilbert P, Price J, Allen S. Social comparison, social attractiveness and evolution: how might they be related? New Ideas Psychol. 1995; 13(2):149–65.

45. Appel H, Gerlach AL, Crusius J. The interplay between Facebook use, social comparison, envy, and depression. Curr Opin Psychol. 2016 Jun 1;9:44–9.

46. Blease CR. Too many "friends," too few "likes"?: evolutionary psychology and "Facebook depression." Rev Gen Psychol. 2015;19(1):1–13.

47. Lee H, Lee IS, Choue R. Obesity, inflammation and diet. Pediatr Gastroenterol Hepatol Nutr. 2013 Sep;16(3):143–52.

48. Patterson E, Wall R, Fitzgerald GF, Ross RP, Stanton C. Health implications of high dietary omega-6 polyunsaturated fatty acids. J Nutr Metab [Internet]. 2012. Available from: http://www.ncbi.nlm.nih.gov/pmc/articles/PMC3335257.

49. Craft LL, Perna FM. The benefits of exercise for the clinically depressed. Prim Care Companion J Clin Psychiatry. 2004;6(3):104–11.

50. Schuch FB, Deslandes AC, Stubbs B, Gosmann NP, da Silva CTB, de Almeida Fleck MP. Neurobiological effects of exercise on major depressive disorder: a systematic review. Neurosci Biobehav Rev. 2016;61:1–11.

51. Cooney G, Dwan K, Mead G. Exercise for depression. JAMA. 2014 Jun 18;311(23):2432–3.

52. Sullivan PF, Neale MC, Kendler KS. Genetic epidemiology of major depression: review and meta-analysis. Am J Psychiatry. 2000 Oct 1; 157(10):1552–62.

53. Ripke S, Wray NR, Lewis CM, Hamilton SP, Weissman MM, Breen G, et al. A mega-analysis of genome-wide association studies for major depressive disorder. Mol Psychiatry. 2013 Apr;18(4):497–511.

54. Cai N, Bigdeli TB, Kretzschmar W, Li Y, Liang J, Song L, et al. Sparse whole-genome sequencing identifies two loci for major depressive disorder. Nature. 2015 Jul 15;523(7562):588–91.

55. Peterson RE, Cai N, Bigdeli TB, Li Y, Reimers M, Nikulova A, et al. The genetic architecture of major depressive disorder in Han Chinese women. JAMA Psychiatry. 2017 Feb 1;74(2):162–8.

56. Salfati E, Morrison AC, Boerwinkle E, Chakravarti A. Direct estimates of the genomic contributions to blood pressure heritability within a population-based cohort (ARIC). PLOS ONE. 2015 Jul 10;10(7): e0133031.

57. Weedon MN, Lango H, Lindgren CM, Wallace C, Evans DM, Mangino M, et al. Genome-wide association analysis identifies 20 loci that influence adult height. Nat Genet. 2008 May;40(5):575–83.

58. Wood AR, Esko T, Yang J, Vedantam S, Pers TH, Gustafsson S, et al. Defining the role of common variation in the genomic and biological architecture of adult human height. Nat Genet. 2014 Nov;46(11):1173–86.

59. Wiener N. Cybernetics: control and communication in the animal and the machine. New York: Wiley; 1948.

60. Beck AT, Alford BA. Depression: causes and treatment. 2nd ed. Philadelphia: University of Pennsylvania Press; 2009.

61. Cuijpers P, van Straten A, Warmerdam L. Behavioral activation treatments of depression: a meta-analysis. Clin Psychol Rev. 2007;27(3):318–26.

62. Mazzucchelli T, Kane R, Rees C. Behavioral activation treatments for depression in adults: a meta-analysis and review. Clin Psychol Sci Pract. 2009 Dec 1;16(4):383–411.

63. Post RM. Transduction of psychosocial stress into the neurobiology. Am J Psychiatry. 1992;149:999–1010.

64. Monroe SM, Harkness KL. Life stress, the "kindling" hypothesis, and the recurrence of depression.

65. Post RM, Weiss SR. Sensitization and kindling phenomena in mood, anxiety, and obsessive-compulsive disorders: the role of serotonergic mechanisms in illness progression. Biol Psychiatry. 1998 Aug 1;44(3):193–206.

66. Nettle D. An evolutionary model of low mood states. J Theor Biol. 2009;257(1):100–3.

67. Trimmer PC, Higginson AD, Fawcett TW, McNamara JM, Houston AI. Adaptive learning can result in a failure to profit from good conditions: implications for understanding depression. Evol Med Public Health. 2015 May 29;2015(1):123–35.

68. Goodwin FK, Jamison KR. Manic-depressive illness. New York: Oxford University Press; 1990.

69. Ferrell JE. Self-perpetuating states in signal transduction: positive feedback, double-negative feedback and bistability. Curr Opin Cell Biol. 2002 Apr 1;14(2):140–8.

70. Monod J, Jacob F. General conclusions: teleonomic mechanisms in cellular metabolism, growth, and differentiation. Cold Spring Harb Symp Quant Biol. 1961;26:389–401.

71. Low BS. Why sex matters: a Darwinian look at human behavior. Princeton (NJ): Princeton University Press; 2015.

72. Goldbeter A. A model for the dynamics of bipolar disorders. Prog Biophys Mol Biol. 2011 Mar 1;105(1):119–27.

73. James W. The principles of psychology. New York: H. Holt and Company; 1890.

74. Akiskal HS, Bourgeois ML, Angst J, Post R, Möller H-J, Hirschfeld R. Re-evaluating the prevalence of and diagnostic composition within the broad clinical spectrum of bipolar disorders. J Affect Disord. 2000 Sep;59(Suppl 1):S5–30.

75. Angst J, Azorin J-M, Bowden CL, Perugi G, Vieta E, Gamma A, et al.

Prevalence and characteristics of undiagnosed bipolar disorders in patients with a major depressive episode: the BRIDGE Study. Arch Gen Psychiatry. 2011 Aug 1;68(8):791–9.

76. Grande I, Berk M, Birmaher B, Vieta E. Bipolar disorder. The Lancet. 2016;387(10027):1561–72.

77. Kieseppä T, Partonen T, Haukka J, Kaprio J, Lönnqvist J. High concordance of bipolar I disorder in a nationwide sample of twins. Am J Psychiatry. 2004 Oct 1;161(10):1814–21.

78. Rao AR, Yourshaw M, Christensen B, Nelson SF, Kerner B. Rare deleterious mutations are associated with disease in bipolar disorder families. Mol Psychiatry. 2017 Jul;22(7):1009–14.

79. Kendler KS. The dappled nature of causes of psychiatric illness: replacing the organic-functional/hardware-software dichotomy with empirically based pluralism. Mol Psychiatry. 2012 Apr;17(4):377–88.

80. Abramson LY, Metalsky GI, Alloy LB. Hopelessness depression: a theory-based subtype of depression. Psychol Rev. 1989;96(2):358–72.

81. Cross JG, Guyer MJ. Social traps. Ann Arbor: University of Michigan Press; 1980.

82. Kennedy SH, Rizvi S. Sexual dysfunction, depression, and the impact of antidepressants. J Clin Psychopharmacol. 2009 Apr;29(2):157–64.

83. Montejo AL, Llorca G, Izquierdo JA, Rico-Villademoros F. Incidence of sexual dysfunction associated with antidepressant agents: a prospective multicenter study of 1022 outpatients. J Clin Psychiatry. 2001;62(Suppl 3):10–21.

84. Hjemdal O, Hagen R, Solem S, Nordahl H, Kennair LEO, Ryum T, et al. Metacognitive therapy in major depression: an open trial of comorbid cases. Cogn Behav Pract. 2017 Aug 1;24(3):312–8.

85. Gilbert P. Evolution and depression: issues and implications. Psychol Med. 2006;36(3):287–97.

86. Gilbert P. Introducing compassion-focused therapy. Adv Psychiatr Treat. 2009;15(3):199–208.

87. Gilbert P. The origins and nature of compassion focused therapy. Br J Clin Psychol. 2014;53(1):6–41.

88. Hammen C. Stress and depression. Annu Rev Clin Psychol. 2005; 1(1):293–319.

89. Baumeister D, Akhtar R, Ciufolini S, Pariante CM, Mondelli V. Childhood trauma and adulthood inflammation: a meta-analysis of peripheral C-reactive protein, interleukin-6 and tumour necrosis factor-α. Mol Psychiatry. 2016 May;21(5):642–9.

90. Belsky J, Jonassaint C, Pluess M, Stanton M, Brummett B, Williams R. Vulnerability genes or plasticity genes? Mol Psychiatry. 2009 Aug;14 (8):746–54.

91. Labonté B, Suderman M, Maussion G, Navaro L, Yerko V, Mahar I, et al. Genome-wide epigenetic regulation by early-life trauma. Arch Gen Psychiatry [Internet]. 2012 Jul 1 [cited 2018 Jun 22];69(7). Available from: http://archpsyc.jamanetwork.com/article.aspx?doi=10.1001/arch genpsychiatry.2011.2287.

92. Monroe SM, Reid MW. Life stress and major depression. Curr Dir Psychol Sci. 2009;18(2):68–72.

93. Sieff DF. Understanding and healing emotional trauma: conversations with pioneering clinicians and researchers. London: Routledge; 2015.

CHAPTER 8 | HOW TO UNDERSTAND AN INDIVIDUAL HUMAN BEING

1. Vaillant G. Lifting the field's "repression" of defenses. Am J Psychiatry. 2012 Sep;169(9):885–7.

2. Windelband W. Rectorial address, Strasbourg, 1894. Hist Theory. 1980;19(2):169–85.

3. Hurlburt RT, Knapp TJ. Münsterberg in 1898, not Allport in 1937, introduced the terms "idiographic" and "nomothetic" to American psychology. Theory Psychol. 2006 Apr 1;16(2):287–93.

4. Ibid., p. 22.

5. Ćuk M, Stewart ST. Making the moon from a fast-spinning Earth: a giant impact followed by resonant despinning. Science. 2012;338(6110): 1047–52.

6. Rahe RH, Meyer M, Smith M, Kjaer G, Holmes TH. Social stress and illness onset. J Psychosom Res. 1964 Jul 1;8(1):35–44.

7. Brown GW, Harris T. Social origins of depression. New York: Free Press; 1978.

8. Monroe SM, Simons AD. Diathesis-stress theories in the context of life stress research: implications for the depressive disorders. Psychol Bull. 1991;110(3):406–25.

9. Oatley K, Bolton W. A social-cognitive theory of depression in reaction to life events. Psychol Rev. 1985;92(3):372–88.

10. Monroe SM. Modern approaches to conceptualizing and measuring human life stress. Annu Rev Clin Psychol. 2008;4(1):33–52.

11. Brown GW, Harris TO, Hepworth C. Loss, humiliation and entrapment among women developing depression: a patient and non-patient comparison. Psychol Med. 1995;25(1):7–21.

12. Kendler KS, Hettema JM, Butera F, Gardner CO, Prescott CA. Life event dimensions of loss, humiliation, entrapment, and danger in the prediction of onsets of major depression and generalized anxiety. Arch Gen Psychiatry. 2003 Aug;60(8):789–96.

13. Ellsworth PC. Appraisal theory: old and new questions. Emot Rev. 2013;5(2):125–31.

14. Scherer KR, Schorr A, Johnstone T. Appraisal processes in emotion: theory, methods, research. New York: Oxford University Press; 2001.

15. Diener E, Fujita F. Resources, personal strivings, and subjective well-being: a nomothetic and idiographic approach. J Pers Soc Psychol. 1995; 68(5):926–35.

16. Apgar V. A proposal for a new method of evaluation of the newborn infant. Anesth Analg. 1953 Jan;32(1):260–7.

17. Klinger E. The interview questionnaire technique: reliability and validity of a mixed idiographic-nomothetic measure of motivation. Adv Personal Assess. 1987;6:31–48.

18. Grice JW. Bridging the idiographic-nomothetic divide in ratings of self and others on the big five. J Pers. 2004;72(2):203–41.

19. Zevon MA, Tellegen A. The structure of mood change: an idiographic /nomothetic analysis. J Pers Soc Psychol. 1982;43(1):111–22.

20. Tufts Center for the Study of Drug Development. PR Tufts CSDD 2014 Cost Study [Internet]. 2014 [cited 2017 Jun 15]. (No longer available.)

21. Monroe SM, Simons AD. Diathesis-stress theories in the context of life stress research.

22. Belsky J, Pluess M. Beyond diathesis stress: differential susceptibility to environmental influences. Psychol Bull. 2009;135(6):885–908.

23. Diener E, Fujita F. Resources, personal strivings, and subjective well-being.

CHAPTER 9 | GUILT AND GRIEF: THE PRICE OF GOODNESS AND LOVE

1. Smith A. The theory of moral sentiments. Oxford (UK): Clarendon Press; 1976 [1759]. p. 136.

2. Dawkins R. The selfish gene. Oxford (UK): Oxford University Press; 1976.

3. Midgley M. The solitary self: Darwin and the selfish gene. London: Routledge; 2014.

4. Segerstrale U. Colleagues in conflict: an "in vivo" analysis of the sociobiology controversy. Biol Philos. 1986;1(1):53–87.

5. Sterelny K. Dawkins vs. Gould: survival of the fittest. New ed., expanded and updated. Cambridge (UK): Icon Books; 2007.

6. Nesse RM. Why so many people with selfish genes are pretty nice—except for their hatred of *The selfish gene*. In: Grafen A, Ridley M, editors. London: Oxford University Press; 2006. pp. 203–12.

7. Ridley M. The origins of virtue: human instincts and the evolution of cooperation. New York: Viking; 1996.

8. Frank RH. Passions within reason: the strategic role of the emotions. New York: W. W. Norton; 1988.

9. Frank RH, Gilovich T, Regan DT. Does studying economics inhibit cooperation? J Econ Perspect. 1993 Jun;7(2):159–71.

10. Alexander RD. The biology of moral systems. New York: Aldine de Gruyter; 1987.

11. Didyoung J, Charles E, Rowland NJ. Non-theists are no less moral than theists: some preliminary results. Secularism & nonreligion [Internet]. 2013 Mar 2 [cited 2017 Dec 14];2. Available from: http://www.secularismandnonreligion.org/articles/abstract/10.5334/snr.ai.

12. Hofmann W, Wisneski DC, Brandt MJ, Skitka LJ. Morality in everyday life. Science. 2014 Sep 12;345(6202):1340–3.

13. Zuckerman P. Atheism, secularity, and well-being: how the findings of social science counter negative stereotypes and assumptions. Sociol Compass. 2009;3(6):949–71.

14. Williams GC. Huxley's evolution and ethics in sociobiological perspective. Zygon. 1988;23(4):383–407.

15. Williams GC, Williams DC. Natural selection of individually harmful social adaptations among sibs with special reference to social insects. Evolution. 1957;11:249–53.

16. Paradis JG, Huxley TH, Williams GC. Evolution & ethics: T. H. Huxley's evolution and ethics with new essays on its Victorian and sociobiological context. Princeton (NJ): Princeton University Press; 1989.

17. Wilson DS, Sober E. Reintroducing group selection to the human behavioral sciences. Behav Brain Sci. 1994;17(4):585–607.

18. Smith JM. Group selection and kin selection. Nature [Internet]. 1964 Mar [cited 2017 Dec 14];201(4924):1145. Available from: https://www-nature-com.proxy.lib.umich.edu/articles/2011145a0.

19. West SA, Griffin AS, Gardner A. Social semantics: how useful has group selection been? J Evol Biol. 2008;21(1):374–85.

20. Pinker S. The false allure of group selection. Edge [Internet]. 2012 Jun 18. Available from: https://www.edge.org/conversation/steven_pinker-the-false-allure-of-group-selection.

21. Dugatkin LA, Reeve HK. Behavioral ecology and levels of selection: dissolving the group selection controversy. Adv Study Behav. 1994; 23:101–33.

22. Reeve HK, Holldobler B. The emergence of a superorganism through intergroup competition. Proc Natl Acad Sci. 2007 Jun 5;104(23): 9736–40.

23. West SA, Griffin AS, Gardner A. Social semantics.

24. Nowak MA, McAvoy A, Allen B, Wilson EO. The general form of Hamilton's rule makes no predictions and cannot be tested empirically. Proc Natl Acad Sci. 2017 May 30;114(22):5665–70.

25. Nowak MA, Tarnita CE, Wilson EO. The evolution of eusociality. Nature. 2010;466(7310):1057–62.

26. Abbot P, Abe J, Alcock J, Alizon S, Alpedrinha JAC, Andersson M,

et al. Inclusive fitness theory and eusociality. Nature. 2011 Mar;471 (7339):E1–E4.

27. Muir WM. Group selection for adaptation to multiple-hen cages: selection program and direct responses. Poult Sci. 1996 Apr;75(4):447–58.

28. Ortman LL, Craig JV. Social dominance in chickens modified by genetic selection—physiological mechanisms. Anim Behav. 1968 Feb;16(1):33–7.

29. Fisher RA. The genetical theory of natural selection: a complete variorum edition. New York: Oxford University Press; 1999.

30. Nesse RM. Five evolutionary principles for understanding cancer. In: Ujvari B, Roche B, Thomas F, editors. Ecology and evolution of cancer. New York: Academic Press; 2017. pp. xv–xxi.

31. Segerstrale U. Nature's oracle: the life and work of W. D. Hamilton. New York: Oxford University Press; 2013.

32. Hamilton WD. The evolution of altruistic behavior. Am Nat. 1963 Sep 1;97(896):354–6.

33. Smith JM. Group selection and kin selection. Nature [Internet]. 1964 Mar [cited 2017 Dec 14];201(4924):1145. Available from: https://www-nature-com.proxy.lib.umich.edu/articles/2011145a0.

34. Nowak MA et al. The general form of Hamilton's rule makes no predictions and cannot be tested empirically.

35. West SA, El Mouden C, Gardner A. Sixteen common misconceptions about the evolution of cooperation in humans. Evol Hum Behav. 2011;32(4):231–62.

36. West SA, Griffin AS, Gardner A. Social semantics: altruism, cooperation, mutualism, strong reciprocity and group selection. J Evol Biol. 2007; 20(2):415–32.

37. Bergstrom CT, Bronstein JL, Bshary R, Connor RC, Daly M, Frank SA, et al. Interspecific mutualism: puzzles and predictions. In: Hammerstein P, editor. Genetical and cultural evolution of cooperation. Cambridge (MA): MIT Press; 2003. pp. 241–56.

38. Clutton-Brock T. Breeding together: kin selection and mutualism in cooperative vertebrates. Science. 2002 Apr 5;296(5565):69–72.

39. Connor RC. The benefits of mutualism: a conceptual framework. Biol Rev. 1995;70(3):427–57.

40. Dugatkin LA. Cooperation among animals: an evolutionary perspective. New York: Oxford University Press; 1997.

41. Trivers RL. The evolution of reciprocal altruism. Q Rev Biol. 1971; 46(1):35–57.

42. Axelrod R, Hamilton W. The evolution of cooperation. Science. 1981;211:1390–6.

43. Axelrod RM. The evolution of cooperation. New York: Basic Books; 1984.

44. Axelrod R, Dion D. The further evolution of cooperation. Science. 1988;242:1385–90.

45. Mengel F. Risk and temptation: a meta-study on prisoner's dilemma games. Econ J. 2017 Sep 18.

46. Pepper JW, Smuts BB. The evolution of cooperation in an ecological context: an agent-based model. In: Kohler TA, Gumerman GJ, editors. Dynamics of human and primate societies: agent-based modelling of social and spatial processes. New York: Oxford University Press; 1999. pp. 44–76.

47. Nesse RM. Evolutionary explanations of emotions. Hum Nat. 1990; 1(3):261–89.

48. Forgas JP, editor. Affect in social thinking and behavior. New York: Psychology Press; 2006.

49. Ketelaar T. Ancestral emotions, current decisions: using evolutionary game theory to explore the role of emotions in decision making. In: Crawford CB, Salmon C, editors. Evolutionary psychology, public policy and personal decisions. Mahwah (NJ): Lawrence Erlbaum; 2004. pp. 145–168.

50. Ketelaar T. Evolutionary psychology and emotion: a brief history. In: Zeigler-Hill V, Welling LLM, Shackelford TK, editors. Evolutionary perspectives on social psychology [Internet]. Cham (Switzerland): Springer International Publishing; 2015 [cited 2018 Jun 13]. pp. 51–67. Available from: http://link.springer.com/10.1007/978-3 -319-12697-5_5.

51. Nesse RM. Evolutionary explanations of emotions.

52. Ibid.

53. Keltner D, Busswell B. Evidence for the distinctness of embarrassment, shame, and guilt: a study of recalled antecedents and facial expressions of emotion. Cogn Emot. 1996;10(2):155–72.

54. Haselton MG, Ketelaar T. Affect in social thinking and behavior. In: Forgas JP, editor. Frontiers of social psychology. New York: Psychology Press; 2006. pp. 21–40.

55. Ketelaar T. Ancestral emotions, current decisions.

56. Ketelaar T. Evolutionary psychology and emotion.

57. Ridley M. The origins of virtue.

58. Boyd R, Richerson PJ. Culture and the evolution of human cooperation. Philos Trans R Soc B Biol Sci. 2009 Nov 12;364(1533):3281–8.

59. Crespi B. Cooperation: close friends and common enemies. Curr Biol. 2006 Jun 6;16(11):R414–5.

60. Dugatkin LA. The altruism equation: seven scientists search for the origins of goodness. Princeton (NJ): Princeton University Press; 2006.

61. Hammerstein P. Genetic and cultural evolution of cooperation. Cambridge (MA): MIT Press; 2003.

62. Henrich J, Henrich N. Culture, evolution and the puzzle of human cooperation. Cogn Syst Res. 2006;7(2–3):220–45.

63. Kurzban R, Burton-Chellew MN, West SA. The evolution of altruism in humans. Annu Rev Psychol. 2015;66(1):575–99.

64. Ridley M. The origins of virtue.

65. Dugatkin LA. Cooperation among animals.

66. Dugatkin LA. The altruism equation.

67. Binmore K. Bargaining and morality. In: Gauthier DP, Sugden R, editors. Rationality, justice and the social contract: themes from morals by agreement. Ann Arbor: University of Michigan Press; 1993. pp. 131–56.

68. Boehm C. Moral origins: the evolution of virtue, altruism, and shame. New York: Basic Books; 2012.

69. Chisholm JS. Death, hope and sex: steps to an evolutionary ecology of mind and morality. New York: Cambridge University Press; 1999.

70. de Waal FBM, Macedo S, Ober J, Wright R. Primates and philosophers: how morality evolved. Princeton (NJ): Princeton University Press; 2006.

71. Fehr E, Gachter S. Altruistic punishment in humans. Nature. 2002 Jan 10;415(6868):137–40.

72. Gintis H, Bowles S, Boyd R, Fehr E. Explaining altruistic behavior in humans. Evol Hum Behav. 2003;24(3):153–72.

73. Irons W. Morality, religion and human evolution. In: Richardson WM, Wildman WJ, editors. Religion and science: history, methods, dialogue. New York: Routledge; 1996.

74. Katz L, editor. Evolutionary origins of morality: cross disciplinary perspectives. Thorverton (UK): Imprint Academic; 2000.

75. Krebs DL. The evolution of moral dispositions in the human species. Ann N Y Acad Sci. 2000 Apr;907:132–48.

76. Lieberman D, Tooby J, Cosmides L. Does morality have a biological basis?: an empirical test of the factors governing moral sentiments relating to incest. Proc R Soc B Biol. 2003 Apr 22;270(1517):819–26.

77. Midgley M. The ethical primate: humans, freedom, and morality. London: Routledge; 1994.

78. Nitecki M, Nitecki D. Evolutionary ethics. Albany: State University of New York Press; 1993.

79. Pepper JW, Smuts BB. A mechanism for the evolution of altruism among nonkin: positive assortment through environmental feedback. Am Nat. 2002;160(2):205–13.

80. van Veelen M. Does it pay to be good?: competing evolutionary explanations of pro-social behaviour. In: Verplaetse J, De Schrijver J, Braeckman J, Vanneste S, editors. The moral brain: essays on the evolutionary and neuroscientific aspects of morality. Dordrecht (Netherlands): Springer Science+Business Media; 2009. pp. 185–200.

81. Foster KR, Kokko H. Cheating can stabilize cooperation in mutualisms. Proc R Soc B Biol. 2006 Sep 7;273(1598):2233–9.

82. Foster KR, Wenseleers T, Ratnieks FLW, Queller DC. There is nothing wrong with inclusive fitness. Trends Ecol Evol. 2006 Nov;21(11):599–600.

83. Aktipis, C. Athena. Know when to walk away: contingent movement and the evolution of cooperation. J Theor Biol. 2004;231(2):249–60.

84. Dunbar RIM. Grooming, gossip, and the evolution of language. Cambridge (MA): Harvard University Press; 1996.

85. West SA, Griffin AS, Gardner A. Social semantics: altruism, cooperation, mutualism, strong reciprocity and group selection. J Evol Biol. 2007 Mar;20(2):415–32.

86. Boyd R, Richerson PJ. Culture and the evolution of human cooperation. Philos Trans R Soc B Biol Sci. 2009 Nov 12;364(1533):3281–8.

87. Richerson P, Baldini R, Bell A, Demps K, Frost K, Hillis V, et al. Cultural group selection plays an essential role in explaining human cooperation: a sketch of the evidence. Behav Brain Sci. 2015;1–71.

88. Nesse RM. Social selection is a powerful explanation for prosociality. Behav Brain Sci. 2016 Jan;39:e47.

89. Brickman P, Sorrentino RM, Wortman CB. Commitment, conflict, and caring. Englewood Cliffs (NJ): Prentice-Hall; 1987.

90. Hirshleifer J. On the emotions as guarantors of threats and promises. In: Dupré J, editor. The latest on the best: essays on evolution and optimality. Cambridge (MA): MIT Press; 1987. pp. 307–26.

91. Nesse RM, editor. Evolution and the capacity for commitment. New York: Russell Sage Foundation; 2001.

92. Schelling TC. The strategy of conflict. Cambridge (MA): Harvard University Press; 1960.

93. Tooby J, Cosmides L. Friendship and the banker's paradox: other pathways to the evolution of adaptations for altruism. In: Runciman WG, Smith JM, Dunbar RIM, editors. Proceedings of the British Academy. Vol. 88. Evolution of social behavior patterns in primates and man. New York: Oxford University Press; 1996. pp. 119–43.

94. Nesse RM. Natural selection and the capacity for subjective commitment. In: Nesse RM, editor. Evolution and the capacity for commitment. New York: Russell Sage Foundation; 2001. pp. 1–44. (The Russell Sage Foundation series on trust. Vol. 3).

95. Mills J, Clark MS. Communal and exchange relationships: controversies and research. In: Erber R, Gilmour R, editors. Theoretical frameworks for personal relationships. Hillsdale (NJ): Lawrence Erlbaum; 1994. pp. 29–42.

96. West-Eberhard MJ. The evolution of social behavior by kin selection. Q Rev Biol. 1975;50(1):1–33.

97.   West-Eberhard MJ. Sexual selection, social competition, and evolution. Proc Am Philos Soc. 1979;123(4):222–34.

98.   Miller GF. The mating mind: how sexual choice shaped the evolution of human nature. New York: Doubleday; 2000.

99.   Boehm C. Moral origins.

100.   Noë R, Hammerstein P. Biological markets: supply and demand determine the effect of partner choice in cooperation, mutualism and mating. Trends Ecol Evol. 1995;10(8):336–9.

101.   Nesse RM. Runaway social selection for displays of partner value and altruism. Biol Theory. 2007;2(2):143–55.

102.   Nesse RM. Social selection and the origins of culture. In: Schaller M, Heine SJ, Norenzayan A, Yamagishi T, Kameda T, editors. Evolution, culture, and the human mind. Philadelphia: Psychology Press; 2010. pp. 137–50.

103.   Barclay P, Willer R. Partner choice creates competitive altruism in humans. Proc R Soc B Biol. 2007;274(1610):749–53.

104.   Hardy CL, Van Vugt M. Nice guys finish first: the competitive altruism hypothesis. Soc Psychol Bull. 2006 Oct 1;32(10):1402–13.

105.   Pleasant A, Barclay P. Why hate the good guy?: antisocial punishment of high cooperators is greater when people compete to be chosen. Psychol Sci. 2018 Jun;29(6):868–76.

106.   Hrdy SB. Mothers and others: the evolutionary origins of mutual understanding. Cambridge (MA): Belknap Press of Harvard University Press; 2009.

107.   Wilson DS. Social semantics: toward a genuine pluralism in the study of social behaviour. J Evol Biol. 2008;21(1):368–73.

108.   Noë R, Hammerstein P. Biological markets.

109.   Kiers ET, Duhamel M, Beesetty Y, Mensah JA, Franken O, Verbruggen E, et al. Reciprocal rewards stabilize cooperation in the mycorrhizal symbiosis. Science. 2011 Aug 12;333(6044):880–2.

110.   Wyatt GAK, Kiers ET, Gardner A, West SA. A biological market analysis of the plant-mycorrhizal symbiosis: mycorrhizal symbiosis as a biological market. Evolution. 2014 Sep;68(9):2603–18.

111.   Nesse RM. Social selection and the origins of culture.

112. Hobbes T. Leviathan. Cambridge (UK): Cambridge University Press; 1996. p. 120.

113. Veblen T. The theory of the leisure class: an economic study in the evolution of institutions. New York: Macmillan; 1899.

114. Kirkpatrick LA, Ellis BJ. An evolutionary-psychological approach to self-esteem: multiple domains and multiple functions. In: Fletcher JGO, Clark MS, editors. Blackwell handbook of social psychology: interpersonal processes. Oxford(UK): Blackwell; 2001. pp. 409–36.

115. Leary MR, Baumeister RF. The nature and function of self-esteem: sociometer theory. In: Zanna MP, editor. Advances in experimental social psychology. San Diego (CA): Academic Press; 2000. pp. 2–51.

116. Mealey L. Sociopathy. Behav Brain Sci. 1995;18(3):523–99.

117. Boehm C. Moral origins.

118. Demirel OF, Demirel A, Kadak MT, Emül M, Duran A. Neurological soft signs in antisocial men and relation with psychopathy. Psychiatry Res. 2016 Jun 30;240:248–52.

119. Smuts B. Encounters with animal minds. J Conscious Stud. 2001; 8(5–7):293–309.

120. Brüne M. On human self-domestication, psychiatry, and eugenics. Philos Ethics Humanit Med. 2007 Oct 5;2(1):21.

121. Hare B, Wobber V, Wrangham R. The self-domestication hypothesis: evolution of bonobo psychology is due to selection against aggression. Anim Behav. 2012 Mar 1;83(3):573–85.

122. Gregory TR. Artificial selection and domestication: modern lessons from Darwin's enduring analogy. Evol Educ Outreach. 2009;2(1):5–27.

123. Henrich J. The secret of our success: how culture is driving human evolution, domesticating our species, and making us smarter. Princeton (NJ): Princeton University Press; 2015.

124. West SA, Griffin AS, Gardner A. Social semantics: altruism, cooperation, mutualism, strong reciprocity and group selection. J Evol Biol. 2007 Mar;20(2):415–32.

125. Carr D, Nesse RM, Wortman CB, editors. Late life widowhood in the United States.

126. Ibid.

127.   Archer J. The nature of grief. New York: Oxford University Press; 2001. pp. 263–83.

128.   Horowitz MJ, Siegel B, Holen A, Bonanno GA. Diagnostic criteria for complicated grief disorder. Am J Psychiatry. 1997;154(7):904–10.

129.   Prigerson HG, Frank EF, Kasl SV, Reynolds CF III, Anderson B, Zubenko GS, et al. Complicated grief and bereavement-related depression as distinct disorders: preliminary empirical validation in elderly bereaved spouses. Am J Psychiatry. 1995;152(1):22–30.

130.   Shear MK, Reynolds CF, Simon NM, Zisook S, Wang Y, Mauro C, et al. Optimizing treatment of complicated grief: a randomized clinical trial. JAMA Psychiatry. 2016 Jul 1;73(7):685–94.

131.   Nesse RM. Evolutionary framework for understanding grief. In: Carr D, Nesse RM, Wortman CB, editors. Spousal bereavement in late life. New York: Springer; 2006. pp. 195–226.

CHAPTER 10 | KNOW THYSELF—*NOT!*

1.   Belsky J. Psychopathology in life history perspective. Psychol Inq. 2014 Oct 2;25(3–4):307–10.

2.   Del Giudice M. An evolutionary life history framework for psychopathology. Psychol Inq. 2014 Oct 2;25(3–4):261–300.

3.   Kaplan HS, Hill K, Lancaster JB, Hurtado AM. A theory of human life history evolution: diet, intelligence, and longevity. Evol Anthropol. 2000; 9(4):1–30.

4.   Bradbury JW, Vehrencamp SL. Principles of animal communication. Sunderland (MA): Sinauer Associates; 1998.

5.   de Crespigny FE, Hosken DJ. Sexual selection: signals to die for. Curr Biol. 2007 Oct 9;17(19):R853–5.

6.   Alexander RD. The search for a general theory of behavior. Behav Sci. 1975;20(2):77–100.

7.   Trivers R. Foreword to The selfish gene. Oxford (UK): Oxford University Press; 1976. pp. vii–ix

8.   Trivers RL. The folly of fools: the logic of deceit and self-deception in human life. New York: Basic Books; 2011.

9. Hartmann H. Ego psychology and the problem of adaptation. 14th ed. New York: International Universities Press; 1958.

10. Boag S. Freudian repression, the common view, and pathological science. Rev Gen Psychol. 2006;10(1):74–80.

11. Dennett DC, Weiner P. Consciousness explained. Boston: Back Bay Books; 1991.

12. Humphrey N. A history of the mind: evolution and the birth of consciousness. New York: Copernicus; 1999.

13. Tannenbaum AS. The sense of consciousness. J Theor Biol. 2001 Aug; 211(4):377–91.

14. Eccles JC. The evolution of consciousness. In: How the SELF controls its BRAIN. Berlin, Heidelberg: Springer; 1994. pp. 113–24.

15. Dunbar RIM. The social brain hypothesis. Evol Anthropol. 1998; 6(5):178–90.

16. Flinn MV, Ward CV. Ontogeny and evolution of the social child. In: Ellis BJ, Bjorklund DF, editors. Origins of the social mind: evolutionary psychology and child development. New York: Guilford Press; 2005. pp. 19–44.

17. Ronson J. How one stupid tweet blew up Justine Sacco's life. The New York Times [Internet]. 2015 Feb 12 [cited 2017 Oct 29]. Available from: https://www.nytimes.com/2015/02/15/magazine/how-one-stupid -tweet-ruined-justine-saccos-life.html.

18. Brakel LAW. Philosophy, psychoanalysis, and the a-rational mind. Oxford (UK): Oxford University Press; 2009.

19. Wilson TD. Strangers to ourselves: discovering the adaptive unconscious. Cambridge (MA): Belknap Press of Harvard University Press; 2002.

20. Nisbett RE, Wilson TD. Telling more than we can know: verbal reports on mental processes. Psychol Rev. 1977;84(3):231–59.

21. Bargh JA, Chartrand TL. The unbearable automaticity of being. Am Psychol. 1999;54(7):462–79.

22. Bargh JA, Williams LE. The nonconscious regulation of emotion. Handb Emot Regul. 2007;1:429–45.

23. Huang JY, Bargh JA. The selfish goal: autonomously operating moti-

vational structures as the proximate cause of human judgment and behavior. Behav Brain Sci. 2014 Apr;37(2):121–35.

24. Gazzaniga MS. Right hemisphere language following brain bisection: a 20-year perspective. Am Psychol. 1983;38(5):525–37.

25. Zimmer C. A career spent learning how the mind emerges from the brain. The New York Times [Internet]. 2005 May 10 [cited 2017 Jul 14]. Available from: https://www.nytimes.com/2005/05/10/science/a-career-spent-learning-how-the-mind-emerges-from-the-brain.html.

26. Gazzaniga MS. The split brain revisited. Sci Am. 1998;279(1):50–5.

27. Greenwald AG, McGhee DE, Schwartz JLK. Measuring individual differences in implicit cognition: the implicit association test. J Pers Soc Psychol. 1998;74(6):1464–80.

28. Scherer LD, Lambert AJ. Implicit race bias revisited: on the utility of task context in assessing implicit attitude strength. J Exp Soc Psychol. 2012 Jan 1;48(1):366–70.

29. Ghiselin MT. The economy of nature and the evolution of sex. Berkeley (CA): University of California Press; 1969. p. 247.

30. Nesse RM, Lloyd AT. The evolution of psychodynamic mechanisms. In: Barkow JH, Cosmides L, Tooby J, editors. The adapted mind: evolutionary psychology and the generation of culture. New York: Oxford University Press; 1992. pp. 601–24.

31. Brüne M. The evolutionary psychology of obsessive-compulsive disorder: the role of cognitive metarepresentation. Perspect Biol Med. 2006;49(3):317–29.

32. Feygin DL, Swain JE, Leckman JF. The normalcy of neurosis: evolutionary origins of obsessive-compulsive disorder and related behaviors. Prog Neuropsychopharmacol Biol Psychiatry. 2006;30(5):854–64.

33. Goodman WK, Price LH, Rasmussen SA, Mazure C, Fleischmann RL, Hill CL, et al. The Yale-Brown obsessive compulsive scale. I. Development, use, and reliability. Arch Gen Psychiatry. 1989;46(11):1006–11.

34. Stein DJ. Obsessive-compulsive disorder. The Lancet. 2002;360 (9330):397–405.

35. Attwells S, Setiawan E, Wilson AA, Rusjan PM, Mizrahi R, Miler L, et al. Inflammation in the neurocircuitry of obsessive-compulsive disorder. JAMA Psychiatry. 2017;74(8):833–40.

36. Brennan BP, Rauch SL, Jensen JE, Pope HG. A critical review of magnetic resonance spectroscopy studies of obsessive-compulsive disorder. Biol Psychiatry. 2013 Jan 1;73(1):24–31.

37. Robinson D, Wu H, Munne RA, Ashtari M, Alvir JMJ, Lerner G, et al. Reduced caudate nucleus volume in obsessive-compulsive disorder. Arch Gen Psychiatry. 1995;52(5):393–98.

38. Suñol M, Contreras-Rodríguez O, Macià D, Martínez-Vilavella G, Martínez-Zalacaín I, Subirà M, et al. Brain structural correlates of subclinical obsessive-compulsive symptoms in healthy children. J Am Acad Child Adolesc Psychiatry [Internet]. 2017 Nov 10 [cited 2017 Dec 15]. Available from: http://www.sciencedirect.com/science/article/pii/S089085671731835X.

39. Mell LK, Davis RL, Owens D. Association between streptococcal infection and obsessive-compulsive disorder, Tourette's syndrome, and tic disorder. Pediatrics. 2005;116(1):56–60.

40. Swedo SE, Leonard HL, Rapoport JL. The pediatric autoimmune neuropsychiatric disorders associated with streptococcal infection (PANDAS) subgroup: separating fact from fiction. Pediatrics. 2004; 113(4):907–11.

41. Diaferia G, Bianchi I, Bianchi ML, Cavedini P, Erzegovesi S, Bellodi L. Relationship between obsessive-compulsive personality disorder and obsessive-compulsive disorder. Compr Psychiatry. 1997 Jan 1;38(1):38–42.

42. Haselton MG, Nettle D. The paranoid optimist: an integrative evolutionary model of cognitive biases. Soc Psychol Rev. 2006;10(1):47–66.

43. Morewedge CK, Shu LL, Gilbert DT, Wilson TD. Bad riddance or good rubbish?: ownership and not loss aversion causes the endowment effect. J Exp Soc Psychol. 2009 Jul;45(4):947–51.

44. Kendler KS, Gardner CO, Prescott CA. Toward a comprehensive developmental model for major depression in men. Am J Psychiatry. 2006 Jan 1;163(1):115–24.

45. Kendler KS, Prescott CA, Myers J, Neale MC. The structure of genetic and environmental risk factors for common psychiatric and substance use disorders in men and women. Arch Gen Psychiatry. 2003 Sep 1;60(9):929–37.

46. Del Giudice M, Ellis BJ. Evolutionary foundations of developmental

psychopathology. In: Cicchetti D, editor. Developmental psychopathology [Internet]. Hoboken (NJ): John Wiley & Sons; 2016 [cited 2018 Jul 12]. pp. 1–58. Available from: http://doi.wiley.com/10.1002/9781119125556 .devpsy201.

47.   Belsky J. Psychopathology in life history perspective.

48.   Ellis BJ, Del Giudice M, Dishion TJ, Figueredo AJ, Gray P, Griskevicius V, et al. The evolutionary basis of risky adolescent behavior: implications for science, policy, and practice. Dev Psychol. 2012;48(3):598–623.

49.   Ellis BJ, Del Giudice M, Shirtcliff EA. Beyond allostatic load: the stress response system as a mechanism of conditional adaptation. In: Beauchaine TP, Hinshaw SP, editors. Child and adolescent psychopathology. 2nd ed. New York: Wiley; 2013. pp. 251–84.

50.   Brüne M. Borderline personality disorder: why "fast and furious"? Evol Med Public Health. 2016;2016(1):52–66.

51.   Pinker S. Enlightenment now: the case for reason, science, humanism, and progress. New York: Viking; 2018.

CHAPTER 11 | BAD SEX CAN BE GOOD—FOR OUR GENES

1.   Peck MS. Further along the road less travelled: the unending journey toward spiritual growth. London: Simon & Schuster UK; 1993. p. 226.

2.   O'Toole, Garson. The only unnatural sex act is that which one cannot perform. Quote investigator [Internet]. 2018 [cited 2018 Jan 6]. Available from: https://quoteinvestigator.com/2013/03/20/unnatural-act.

3.   Buss DM. Sex differences in human mate preferences: evolutionary hypotheses tested in 37 cultures. Behav Brain Sci. 1989;12(1):1–49.

4.   Li NP, Bailey JM, Kenrick DT, Linsenmeier JAW. The necessities and luxuries of mate preferences: testing the tradeoffs. J Pers Soc Psychol. 2002;82(6):947–55.

5.   Shakya HB, Christakis NA. Association of Facebook use with compromised well-being: a longitudinal study. Am J Epidemiol. 2017 Feb 1;185(3):203–11.

6.   Kenrick DT, Gutierres SE, Goldberg LL. Influence of popular erotica on ratings of strangers and mates. J Exp Soc Psychol. 1989;25(2): 159–67.

7. Hazen C, Diamond LM. The place of attachment in human mating. Rev Gen Psychol Spec Issue Adult Attach. 2000;4(2):186–204.

8. Zeifman D, Hazan C. Attachment: the bond in pair-bonds. In: Simpson JA, Kenrick DT, editors. Evolutionary social psychology. Hillsdale (NJ): Lawrence Erlbaum Associates; 1997. pp. 237–63.

9. Tennov D. Love and limerence: the experience of being in love [Internet]. 1999 [cited 2017 Dec 17]. Available from: http://site.ebrary.com/id/10895438.

10. Bierce A. The devil's dictionary. Ware, Hertfordshire (UK): Wordsworth Editions Limited; 1996 [1906]. p. 162.

11. de Botton A. Why you will marry the wrong person. The New York Times [Internet]. 2016 May 28 [cited 2017 Jun 16]. Available from: https://www.nytimes.com/2016/05/29/opinion/sunday/why-you-will-marry-the-wrong-person.html?_r=0.

12. Kirkpatrick RC. The evolution of human homosexual behavior. Curr Anthropol. 2000 Jun 1;41(3):385–413.

13. Wilson EO. Sociobiology.

14. Boomsma JJ. Lifetime monogamy and the evolution of eusociality. Philos Trans R Soc B Biol Sci. 2009 Nov 12;364(1533):3191–207.

15. Emlen ST. An evolutionary theory of the family. Proc Natl Acad Sci. 1995 Aug 29;92(18):8092–9.

16. Bobrow D, Bailey JM. Is male homosexuality maintained via kin selection? Evol Hum Behav. 2001 Sep 1;22(5):361–8.

17. Roughgarden J. Homosexuality and evolution: a critical appraisal. In: Tibayrenc M, Ayala FJ, editors. On human nature [Internet]. San Diego (CA): Academic Press; 2017 [cited 2018 May 26]. pp. 495–516. Available from: https://www.sciencedirect.com/science/article/pii/B9780124201903000302.

18. Ruse M. Homosexuality: a philosophical inquiry. New York: Blackwell; 1988.

19. Roughgarden J. Homosexuality and evolution.

20. Bailey NW, Zuk M. Same-sex sexual behavior and evolution. Trends Ecol Evol. 2009 Aug 1;24(8):439–46.

21. Balthazart J. Sex differences in partner preferences in humans and animals. Phil Trans R Soc B. 2016 Feb 19;371(1688):20150118.

22. Sommer V, Vasey PL. Homosexual behaviour in animals: an evolutionary perspective. Cambridge (UK): Cambridge University Press; 2006.

23. Blanchard R. Fraternal birth order, family size, and male homosexuality: meta-analysis of studies spanning 25 years. Arch Sex Behav. 2018 Jan;47(1):1–15.

24. Bogaert AF, Skorska MN, Wang C, Gabrie J, MacNeil AJ, Hoffarth MR, et al. Male homosexuality and maternal immune responsivity to the Y-linked protein NLGN4Y. Proc Natl Acad Sci. 2017 Dec 11;201705895.

25. Blanchard R. Fraternal birth order, family size, and male homosexuality.

26. Jannini EA, Burri A, Jern P, Novelli G. Genetics of human sexual behavior: where we are, where we are going. Sex Med Rev. 2015 Apr 1;3(2):65–77.

27. Stevens A, Price J. Evolutionary psychiatry: a new beginning. Hove (UK): Routledge; 2015.

28. Bailey NW, Zuk M. Same-sex sexual behavior and evolution.

29. Buss DM. The evolution of desire: strategies of human mating. Rev ed. New York: Basic Books; 2003.

30. Troisi A. Sexual disorders in the context of Darwinian psychiatry. J Endocrinol Invest. 2003;26(3 Suppl):54–7.

31. Betzig L, Mulder MB, Turke P. Human reproductive behaviour: a Darwinian perspective. New York: Cambridge University Press; 1988.

32. Daly M, Wilson M. Sex, evolution, and behavior. 2nd ed. Boston: Willard Grant Press; 1983.

33. Symons D. The evolution of human sexuality. New York: Oxford University Press; 1979.

34. Haselton MG. The sexual overperception bias: evidence of a systematic bias in men from a survey of naturally occurring events. J Res Personal. 2003;37(1):34–47.

35. Aronsson H. Sexual imprinting and fetishism: an evolutionary hypothesis. In: De Block A, Adriaens PR, editors. Maladapting minds: philosophy, psychiatry, and evolutionary theory. New York: Oxford University Press; 2011. pp. 65-90.

36.   Natterson-Horowitz B, Bowers K. Zoobiquity: the astonishing connection between human and animal health. New York: Vintage; 2013.

37.   Erectile dysfunction drugs analysis by product (Viagra, Levitra/Staxyn, Stendra/Spedra, Zydena, Vitaros), and segment forecasts to 2022 [Internet]. 2016 [cited 2017 Dec 17]. Available from: https://www.grand viewresearch.com/industry-analysis/erectile-dysfunction-drugs-market.

38.   Baker R, Bellis M. Human sperm competition: ejaculation manipulation by females and a function for the female orgasm. Animal Behavior. 1993;46(5):887–909.

39.   Lee H-J, Macbeth AH, Pagani JH, Young WS. Oxytocin: the great facilitator of life. Prog Neurobiol. 2009 Jun;88(2):127–51.

40.   Levin RJ. The human female orgasm: a critical evaluation of its proposed reproductive functions. Sexual and Relationship Therapy. 2011 Nov 1;26(4):301–14.

41.   Lloyd EA. The case of the female orgasm: bias in the science of evolution. Cambridge (MA): Harvard University Press; 2009.

42.   Pavličev M, Wagner G. The evolutionary origin of female orgasm. J Exp Zoolog B Mol Dev Evol. 2016 Sep 1;326(6):326–37.

43.   Wagner GP, Pavličev M. What the evolution of female orgasm teaches us. J Exp Zoolog B Mol Dev Evol. 2016;326(6):325.

44.   Wagner GP, Pavličev M. Origin, function, and effects of female orgasm: all three are different. J Exp Zoolog B Mol Dev Evol. 2017 Jun 1;328(4):299–303.

45.   Dunn KM, Cherkas LF, Spector TD. Genetic influences on variation in female orgasmic function: a twin study. Biol Lett. 2005 Sep 22; 1(3):260–3.

46.   Zietsch BP, Miller GF, Bailey JM, Martin NG. Female orgasm rates are largely independent of other traits: implications for "female orgasmic disorder" and evolutionary theories of orgasm. J Sex Med. 2011; 8(8):2305–16.

47.   Laumann EO, Paik A, Rosen RC. Sexual dysfunction in the United States: prevalence and predictors. JAMA. 1999 Feb 10;281(6):537–44.

48.   Waldinger MD, Quinn P, Dilleen M, Mundayat R, Schweitzer DH, Boolell M. Original research—ejaculation disorders: a multinational

population survey of intravaginal ejaculation latency time. J Sex Med. 2005 Jul 1;2(4):492–7.

49. Waldinger MD, Zwinderman AH, Olivier B, Schweitzer DH. Proposal for a definition of lifelong premature ejaculation based on epidemiological stopwatch data. J Sex Med. 2005 Jul 1;2(4):498–507.

50. Gallup GG, Burch RL, Zappieri ML, Parvez RA, Stockwell ML, Davis JA. The human penis as a semen displacement device. Evol Hum Behav. 2003 Jul 1;24(4):277–89.

51. Gallup GG, Burch RL. Semen displacement as a sperm competition strategy in humans. Evol Psychol. 2004 Jan 1;2(1):245–54.

52. Pham MN, DeLecce T, Shackelford TK. Sperm competition in marriage: semen displacement, male rivals, and spousal discrepancy in sexual interest. Personal Individ Differ. 2017 Jan 15;105(Suppl C):229–32.

53. Dewsbury DA, Pierce JD. Copulatory patterns of primates as viewed in broad mammalian perspective. Am J Primatol. 1989 Jan 1;17(1):51–72.

54. Hong LK. Survival of the fastest: on the origin of premature ejaculation. J Sex Res. 1984 May 1;20(2):109–22.

55. Gallup GG, Burch RL. Semen displacement as a sperm competition strategy in humans.

56. Parker GA, Pizzari T. Sperm competition and ejaculate economics. Biol Rev. 2010 Nov 1;85(4):897–934.

57. Wallen K, Lloyd EA. Female sexual arousal: genital anatomy and orgasm in intercourse. Horm Behav. 2011 May;59(5):780–92.

58. Laumann EO, Paik A, Rosen RC. Sexual dysfunction in the United States.

59. Wallen K, Lloyd EA. Female sexual arousal: genital anatomy and orgasm in intercourse. Horm Behav. 2011 May;59(5):780–92.

60. Armstrong EA, England P, Fogarty ACK. Accounting for women's orgasm and sexual enjoyment in college hookups and relationships. Am Sociol Rev. 2012 Jun 1;77(3):435–62.

61. Laumann EO, Paik A, Rosen RC. Sexual dysfunction in the United States.

62. Moynihan R. The making of a disease: female sexual dysfunction. BMJ. 2003 Jan 4;326(7379):45–7.

63. Narjani AE. Considérations sur les causes anatomiques de la frigidité chez la femme. Brux Méd. 1924;27:768–78.

64. Bertin C. Marie Bonaparte, a life. New York: Harcourt; 1982.

65. Storr A. An unlikely analyst. The New York Times [Internet]. 1983 Feb 6 [cited 2017 Jul 31]. Available from: http://www.nytimes.com/1983/02/06/books/an-unlikely-analyst.html.

66. Young-Bruehl E. Freud on women. New York: Random House; 2013.

67. Bonaparte M. Les deux frigidités de la femme. Bull Société Sexol. 1933;5:161–70.

68. Moore A. Relocating Marie Bonaparte's clitoris. Aust Fem Stud. 2009 Jun;24(60):149–65.

69. Wallen K, Lloyd EA. Female sexual arousal: genital anatomy and orgasm in intercourse. Horm Behav. 2011 May;59(5):780–92.

70. Woodroffe R, Vincent A. Mother's little helpers: patterns of male care in mammals. Trends Ecol Evol. 1994 Aug 1;9(8):294–7.

71. Alexander RD. How did humans evolve?: reflections on the uniquely unique species. Mus Zool Univ Mich. 1990;1:1–38.

72. Buchan JC, Alberts SC, Silk JB, Altmann J. True paternal care in a multi-male primate society. Nature. 2003 Sep;425(6954):179–81.

73. Kaplan HS, Lancaster JB. An evolutionary and ecological analysis of human fertility, mating patterns, and parental investment [Internet]. Washington (DC): National Academies Press; 2003 [cited 2018 Jan 7]. Available from: https://www.ncbi.nlm.nih.gov/books/NBK97292.

74. Buss DM. The evolution of desire.

75. Troisi A. Sexual disorders in the context of Darwinian psychiatry.

76. Betzig L, Mulder MB, Turke P. Human reproductive behaviour.

77. Daly M, Wilson M. Sex, evolution, and behavior.

78. Lancaster JB, Kaplan H. Human mating and family formation strategies: The effects of variability among males in quality and the allocation of mating effort and parental investment. Topics in primatology. 1992; 1:21–33.

79. Low BS. Ecological and social complexities in human monogamy. In: Reichard UH, Boesch C, editors. Monogamy: mating strategies and

partnerships in birds, humans, and other mammals. Cambridge (UK): Cambridge University Press; 2003. pp. 161–76.

80. Dunbar RI. Coevolution of neocortical size, group size and language in humans. Behav Brain Sci. 1993;16(4):681–94.

81. Mitteroecker P, Huttegger SM, Fischer B, Pavlicev M. Cliff-edge model of obstetric selection in humans. Proc Natl Acad Sci. 2016 Dec 20; 113(51):14680–5.

82. Boyd R, Richerson PJ. Culture and the evolutionary process. Chicago: University of Chicago Press; 1985.

83. Dunbar RIM, Knight C, Power C. The evolution of culture: an interdisciplinary view. New Brunswick (NJ): Rutgers University Press; 1999.

84. Low BS. Ecological and social complexities in human monogamy.

85. Geary DC, Flinn MV. Evolution of human parental behavior and the human family. Parent Sci Pract. 2001;1(1–2):5–61.

86. Burley N. The evolution of concealed ovulation. Am Nat. 1979 Dec 1;114(6):835–58.

87. Pawłowski B. Loss of oestrus and concealed ovulation in human evolution: the case against the sexual-selection hypothesis. Curr Anthropol. 1999 Jun 1;40(3):257–76.

88. Strassmann BI. Sexual selection, paternal care, and concealed ovulation in humans. Ethol Sociobiol. 1981 Jan 1;2(1):31–40.

89. Pawłowski B. Loss of oestrus and concealed ovulation in human evolution.

90. Reis HT, Patrick BC. Attachment and intimacy: component processes. In: Higgins ET, Kruglanski AW, editors. Social psychology: handbook of basic principles. New York: Guilford Press; 1996. pp. 523–63.

91. Carter CS. Oxytocin pathways and the evolution of human behavior. Annu Rev Psychol. 2014;65(1):17–39.

92. Young LJ, Wang Z. The neurobiology of pair bonding. Nat Neurosci. 2004 Oct;7(10):1048–54.

93. Donaldson ZR, Young LJ. Oxytocin, vasopressin, and the neurogenetics of sociality. Science. 2008 Nov 7;322(5903):900–4.

94. Fisher H. Anatomy of love: a natural history of mating, marriage, and why we stray. New York: W. W. Norton; 1992.

95.   Buss DM. The evolution of desire.

96.   Buss DM, Larsen RJ, Westen D, Semmelroth J. Sex differences in jealousy: evolution, physiology, and psychology. Psychol Sci. 1992;3:251–5.

97.   Flinn MV, Low BS. Resource distribution, social competition, and mating patterns in human societies. Ecol Asp Soc Evol. 1986;217–43.

98.   Klinger E. Consequences of commitment to and disengagement from incentives. Psychol Rev. 1975;82:1–25.

99.   Daly M, Wilson M. Sex, evolution, and behavior.

100. Gangestad SW, Thornhill R. Female multiple mating and genetic benefits in humans: investigations of design. In: Kappeler PM, van Schaik CP, editors. Sexual selection in primates: new and comparative perspectives. Cambridge (UK): Cambridge University Press; 2004. pp. 90–116.

101. Buss DM. The dangerous passion: why jealousy is as necessary as love or sex. New York: Free Press; 2000.

102. Betzig LL. Despotism and differential reproduction: a Darwinian view of history. New York: Aldine; 1986.

103. Betzig L. Means, variances, and ranges in reproductive success: comparative evidence. Evol Hum Behav. 2012 Jul;33(4):309–17.

104. Betzig L. Eusociality in history. Hum Nat. 2014 Mar;25(1):80–99.

105. Zerjal T, Xue Y, Bertorelle G, Wells RS, Bao W, Zhu S, et al. The genetic legacy of the Mongols. Am J Hum Genet. 2003 Mar 1;72(3):717–21.

106. Webster TH, Sayres MAW. Genomic signatures of sex-biased demography: progress and prospects. Curr Opin Genet Dev. 2016 Dec;41:62–71.

107. Betzig L. Eusociality in history.

108. Twenge JM, Sherman RA, Wells BE. Changes in American adults' sexual behavior and attitudes, 1972–2012. Arch Sex Behav. 2015 Nov 1;44(8):2273–85.

109. Jasienska G. The fragile wisdom: an evolutionary view on women's biology and health. Cambridge (MA): Harvard University Press; 2013.

110. Juul F, Chang VW, Brar P, Parekh N. Birth weight, early life weight gain and age at menarche: a systematic review of longitudinal studies. Obes Rev. 2017 Nov 1;18(11):1272–88.

111. Vitzthum VJ. The ecology and evolutionary endocrinology of reproduction in the human female. Am J Phys Anthropol. 2009 Jan 1;140(Suppl 49):95–136.

112. Stearns PN. Jealousy: the evolution of an emotion in American history. New York: New York University Press; 1989.

113. Buss DM. The dangerous passion.

114. Millward J. Deep inside: a study of 10,000 porn stars and their careers [Internet]. 2013 [cited 2017 Dec 17]. Available from: http://jon millward.com/blog/studies/deep-inside-a-study-of-10000-porn-stars.

115. Naked capitalism. The Economist [Internet]. 2015 Sep 26 [cited 2017 Dec 17]. Available from: https://www.economist.com/news /international/21666114-internet-blew-porn-industrys-business-model -apart-its-response-holds-lessons.

116. Marcus BS. Changes in a woman's sexual experience and expectations following the introduction of electric vibrator assistance. J Sex Med. 2011 Dec 1;8(12):3398–406.

117. Scheutz M, Arnold T. Are we ready for sex robots? In: The Eleventh ACM/ IEEE International Conference on Human Robot Interaction [Internet]. Piscataway (NJ): IEEE Press; 2016 [cited 2017 Dec 17]. pp. 351–8. Available from: http://dl.acm.org/citation.cfm?id=2906831.2906891.

CHAPTER 12 | PRIMAL APPETITES

1. Fortuna JL. Sweet preference, sugar addiction and the familial history of alcohol dependence: shared neural pathways and genes. J Psychoactive Drugs. 2010 Jun 1;42(2):147–51.

2. Alcock J, Maley CC, Aktipis CA. Is eating behavior manipulated by the gastrointestinal microbiota?: evolutionary pressures and potential mechanisms. BioEssays. 2014 Oct 1;36(10):940–9.

3. Ogden CL, Carroll MD. Prevalence of overweight, obesity, and extreme obesity among adults: United States, trends 1976–1980 through 2007–2008. National Center for Health Statistics [Internet]. 2010 June. Available from: https://www.cdc.gov/nchs/data/hestat/obesity_adult_ 07_08/obesity_adult_07_08.pdf.

4. Flegal KM, Carroll MD, Kit BK, Ogden CL. Prevalence of obesity and

trends in the distribution of body mass index among US adults, 1999–2010. JAMA. 2012 Feb 1;307(5):491–7.

5. Higginson AD, McNamara JM. An adaptive response to uncertainty can lead to weight gain during dieting attempts. Evol Med Public Health. 2016 Jan 1;2016(1):369–80.

6. Booth HP, Prevost AT, Gulliford MC. Impact of body mass index on prevalence of multimorbidity in primary care: cohort study. Fam Pract. 2014 Feb 1;31(1):38–43.

7. Sturm R, Wells KB. Does obesity contribute as much to morbidity as poverty or smoking? Public Health. 2001;115(3):229–35.

8. Allison DB, Fontaine KR, Manson JE, Stevens J, VanItallie TB. Annual deaths attributable to obesity in the United States. JAMA. 1999 Oct 27;282(16):1530–8.

9. Marketdata Enterprises. Weight loss market sheds some dollars in 2013 [Internet]. 2014 [cited 2017 Jun 25]. Available from: https://www .marketdataenterprises.com/wp-content/uploads/2014/01/Diet-Market -2014-Status-Report.pdf.

10. Wang YC, McPherson K, Marsh T, Gortmaker SL, Brown M. Health and economic burden of the projected obesity trends in the USA and the UK. The Lancet. 2011 Aug 27;378(9793):815–25.

11. Power ML, Schulkin J. The evolution of obesity. Baltimore: Johns Hopkins University Press; 2009.

12. Berrington de Gonzalez A, Hartge P, Cerhan JR, Flint AJ, Hannan L, MacInnis RJ, et al. Body-mass index and mortality among 1.46 million white adults. N Engl J Med. 2010 Dec 2;363(23):2211–9.

13. Higginson AD, McNamara JM. An adaptive response to uncertainty can lead to weight gain during dieting attempts.

14. Dulloo AG, Jacquet J, Montani J-P, Schutz Y. How dieting makes the lean fatter: from a perspective of body composition autoregulation through adipostats and proteinstats awaiting discovery. Obes Rev. 2015 Feb 1;16:25–35.

15. Hill AJ. Does dieting make you fat? Br J Nutr. 2004;92(Suppl 1):S15–8.

16. Fothergill E, Guo J, Howard L, Kerns JC, Knuth ND, Brychta R, et al. Persistent metabolic adaptation 6 years after "The Biggest Loser" competition. Obesity. 2016 Aug 1;24(8):1612–9.

17. Corwin RL, Avena NM, Boggiano MM. Feeding and reward: perspectives from three rat models of binge eating. Physiol Behav. 2011 Jul 25;104(1):87–97.

18. Frankl VE. Man's search for meaning. New York: Simon & Schuster; 1985.

19. Bruch H. The golden cage: the enigma of anorexia nervosa. Cambridge (MA): Harvard University Press; 2001.

20. Brandenburg BMP, Andersen AE. Unintentional onset of anorexia nervosa. Eat Weight Disord. 2007 Jun 1;12(2):97–100.

21. Habermas T. In defense of weight phobia as the central organizing motive in anorexia nervosa: historical and cultural arguments for a culture-sensitive psychological conception. Int J Eat Disord. 1996 May 1;19(4):317–34.

22. Keating C. Theoretical perspective on anorexia nervosa: the conflict of reward. Neurosci Biobehav Rev. 2010 Jan 1;34(1):73–9.

23. Tozzi F, Sullivan PF, Fear JL, McKenzie J, Bulik CM. Causes and recovery in anorexia nervosa: the patient's perspective. Int J Eat Disord. 2003 Mar;33(2):143–54.

24. Bulik CM, Sullivan PF, Tozzi F, Furberg H, Lichtenstein P, Pedersen NL. Prevalence, heritability, and prospective risk factors for anorexia nervosa. Arch Gen Psychiatry. 2006 Mar;63(3):305–12.

25. Kaye WH, Wierenga CE, Bailer UF, Simmons AN, Bischoff-Grethe A. Nothing tastes as good as skinny feels: the neurobiology of anorexia nervosa. Trends Neurosci. 2013 Feb;36(2):110–20.

26. Weiss KM. Tilting at quixotic trait loci (QTL): an evolutionary perspective on genetic causation. Genetics. 2008 Aug;179(4):1741–56.

27. Norn M. Myopia among the Inuit population of East Greenland. Longitudinal study 1950–1994. Acta Ophthalmol Scand. 1997;75(6):723–5.

28. Boraska V, Franklin CS, Floyd JA, Thornton LM, Huckins LM, Southam L, et al. A genome-wide association study of anorexia nervosa. Mol Psychiatry. 2014 Oct;19(10):1085–94.

29. Duncan L, Yilmaz Z, Gaspar H, Walters R, Goldstein J, Anttila V, et al. Significant locus and metabolic genetic correlations revealed in genome-wide association study of anorexia nervosa. Am J Psychiatry. 2017 May 12;174(9):850–8.

30.   Surbey M. Anorexia nervosa, amenorrhea, and adaptation. Ethol Sociobiol. 1987;8(Suppl 1):47–61.

31.   Vitzthum VJ. The ecology and evolutionary endocrinology of reproduction in the human female. Am J Phys Anthropol. 2009 Jan 1;140(Suppl 49):95–136.

32.   Ellison PT. Energetics and reproductive effort. Am J Hum Biol. 2003 May 1;15(3):342–51.

33.   Jasienska G. Energy metabolism and the evolution of reproductive suppression in the human female. Acta Biotheor. 2003;51(1):1–18.

34.   Myerson M, Gutin B, Warren MP, May MT, Contento I, Lee M, et al. Resting metabolic rate and energy balance in amenorrheic and eumenorrheic runners. Med Sci Sports Exerc. 1991 Jan;23(1):15–22.

35.   Abed RT. The sexual competition hypothesis for eating disorders. Br J Med Psychol. 1998 Dec 1;71(4):525–47.

36.   Faer LM, Hendriks A, Abed RT, Figueredo AJ. The evolutionary psychology of eating disorders: female competition for mates or for status? Psychol Psychother Theory Res Pract. 2005;78(3):397–417.

37.   Singh D. Body shape and women's attractiveness. Hum Nat. 1993 Sep 1;4(3):297–321.

38.   Faer LM, Hendriks A, Abed RT, Figueredo AJ. The evolutionary psychology of eating disorders: female competition for mates or for status?

39.   Guisinger S. Adapted to flee famine: adding an evolutionary perspective on anorexia nervosa. Psychol Rev. 2003;110(4):745–61.

40.   Rosenvinge JH, Pettersen G. Epidemiology of eating disorders, part I: introduction to the series and a historical panorama. Adv Eat Disord. 2015 Jan 2;3(1):76–90.

41.   Klein DA, Boudreau GS, Devlin MJ, Walsh BT. Artificial sweetener use among individuals with eating disorders. Int J Eat Disord. 2006 May 1;39(4):341–5.

42.   Just T, Pau HW, Engel U, Hummel T. Cephalic phase insulin release in healthy humans after taste stimulation? Appetite. 2008 Nov 1;51(3):622–7.

43.   Veedfald S, Plamboeck A, Deacon CF, Hartmann B, Knop FK, Vilsbøll T, et al. Cephalic phase secretion of insulin and other enteropancreatic

hormones in humans. American Journal of Physiology-Gastrointestinal and Liver Physiology. 2015 Oct 22;310(1):G43–51.

44. Rozengurt E, Sternini C. Taste receptor signaling in the mammalian gut. Curr Opin Pharmacol. 2007 Dec 1;7(6):557–62.

45. Pepino MY. Metabolic effects of non-nutritive sweeteners. Physiol Behav. 2015 Dec 1;152:450–5.

46. Fowler SP, Williams K, Resendez RG, Hunt KJ, Hazuda HP, Stern MP. Fueling the obesity epidemic?: artificially sweetened beverage use and long-term weight gain. Obesity. 2008;16(8):1894–900.

47. Mattes RD, Popkin BM. Nonnutritive sweetener consumption in humans: effects on appetite and food intake and their putative mechanisms. Am J Clin Nutr. 2009 Jan 1;89(1):1–14.

48. Renwick AG, Molinary SV. Sweet-taste receptors, low-energy sweeteners, glucose absorption and insulin release. Br J Nutr. 2010 Nov;104(10): 1415–20.

49. Azad MB, Abou-Setta AM, Chauhan BF, Rabbani R, Lys J, Copstein L, et al. Nonnutritive sweeteners and cardiometabolic health: a systematic review and meta-analysis of randomized controlled trials and prospective cohort studies. Can Med Assoc J. 2017 Jul 17;189(28):E929–39.

50. Barker DJ, Gluckman PD, Godfrey KM, Harding JE, Owens JA, Robinson JS. Fetal nutrition and cardiovascular disease in adult life. The Lancet. 1993 Apr 10;341(8850):938–41.

51. Gluckman PD, Hanson MA, Spencer HG. Predictive adaptive responses and human evolution. Trends Ecol Evol. 2005;20(10):527–33.

52. Gluckman PD, Hanson MA, Bateson P, Beedle AS, Law CM, Bhutta ZA, et al. Towards a new developmental synthesis: adaptive developmental plasticity and human disease. The Lancet. 2009 May 9;373(9675):1654–7.

53. Guerrero-Bosagna C. Transgenerational epigenetic inheritance: past exposures, future diseases. In: Rosenfeld CS, editor. The epigenome and developmental origins of health and disease [Internet]. Boston: Academic Press; 2016 [cited 2017 Dec 19]. pp. 425–37. Available from: https://www.sciencedirect.com/science/article/pii/B9780128013830000219.

54. Rosenfeld CS. Nutrition and epigenetics: evidence for multi- and transgenerational effects. In: Burdge G, Lillycrop K, editors. Nutrition, epigenetics and health. New Jersey: World Scientific; 2017. pp. 133–57.

55. Lea AJ, Altmann J, Alberts SC, Tung J. Developmental constraints in a wild primate. Am Nat. 2015 Jun 1;185(6):809–21.

56. Crespi BJ. Vicious circles: positive feedback in major evolutionary and ecological transitions. Trends Ecol Evol. 2004 Dec;19(12):627–33.

57. Nettle D, Bateson M. Adaptive developmental plasticity: what is it, how can we recognize it and when can it evolve? Proc Biol Sci. 2015 Aug 7;282(1812):20151005.

58. Nussbaum MC. The therapy of desire: theory and practice in Hellenistic ethics. Princeton (NJ): Princeton University Press; 1994.

CHAPTER 13 | GOOD FEELINGS FOR BAD REASONS

1. Centers for Disease Control and Prevention. Fact sheets—Alcohol use and your health [Internet]. [cited 2018 Aug 16]. Available from: https://www.cdc.gov/alcohol/fact-sheets/alcohol-use.htm.

2. Grant BF, Stinson FS, Dawson DA, Chou SP, Dufour MC, Compton W, et al. Prevalence and co-occurrence of substance use disorders and independent mood and anxiety disorders: results from the National Epidemiologic Survey on Alcohol and Related Conditions. Arch Gen Psychiatry. 2004;61(8):807–18.

3. Substance Abuse and Mental Health Services Administration (SAMHSA). 2015 National Survey on Drug Use and Health (NSDUH). Table 5.6B—Substance use disorder in past year among persons aged 18 or older, by demographic characteristics: percentages, 2014 and 2015. Available at: https://www.samhsa.gov/data/sites/default/files /NSDUH-DetTabs-2015/NSDUH-DetTabs-2015/NSDUH -DetTabs-2015.htm#tab5-6b.

4. Centers for Disease Control and Prevention. Tobacco-related mortality [Internet]. 2016 [cited 2017 Jul 17]. Available from: http://www.cdc .gov/tobacco/data_statistics/fact_sheets/health_effects/tobacco_related _mortality.

5. Hill EM, Newlin DB. Evolutionary approaches to addiction. Addiction. 2002 Apr;97(4):375–9.

6. Hyman SE. Addiction: a disease of learning and memory. FOCUS. 2007 Apr 1;5(2):220–8.

7. Nesse RM, Berridge KC. Psychoactive drug use in evolutionary perspective. Science. 1997;278(5335):63–6.

8. Dudley R. Evolutionary origins of human alcoholism in primate frugivory. Q Rev Biol. 2000;75(1):3–15.

9. Sullivan RJ, Hagen EH. Psychotropic substance-seeking: evolutionary pathology or adaptation? Addiction. 2002 Apr 1;97(4):389–400.

10. Chevallier J. The great medieval water myth. Les Leftovers [Internet]. 2013 [cited 2017 Dec 20]. Available from: https://leslefts.blogspot.com .au/2013/11/the-great-medieval-water-myth.html.

11. Dudley R. Ethanol, fruit ripening, and the historical origins of human alcoholism in primate frugivory. Integr Comp Biol. 2004 Aug;44(4): 315–23.

12. Nesse RM. Evolution and addiction. Addiction. 2002 Apr;97(4):470–1.

13. Hayden B, Canuel N, Shanse J. What was brewing in the Natufian?: an archaeological assessment of brewing technology in the Epipaleolithic. J Archaeol Method Theory. 2013 Mar 1;20(1):102–50.

14. Sullivan RJ, Hagen EH. Psychotropic substance-seeking: evolutionary pathology or adaptation? Addiction. 2002 Apr 1;97(4):389–400.

15. Roulette CJ, Mann H, Kemp BM, Remiker M, Roulette JW, Hewlett BS, et al. Tobacco use vs. helminths in Congo basin hunter-gatherers: self-medication in humans? Evol Hum Behav. 2014 Sep 1;35(5):397–407.

16. Ruiz-Lancheros E, Viau C, Walter TN, Francis A, Geary TG. Activity of novel nicotinic anthelmintics in cut preparations of *Caenorhabditis elegans*. Int J Parasitol. 2011;41(3–4):455–61.

17. Gardner EL. What we have learned about addiction from animal models of drug self-administration. Am J Addict. 2000 Oct 1;9(4):285–313.

18. Sullivan RJ, Hagen EH. Psychotropic substance-seeking.

19. Hagen EH, Sullivan RJ, Schmidt R, Morris G, Kempter R, Hammerstein P. Ecology and neurobiology of toxin avoidance and the paradox of drug reward. Neuroscience. 2009;160(1):69–84.

20. Hagen EH, Roulette CJ, Sullivan RJ. Explaining human recreational use of "pesticides": the neurotoxin regulation model of substance use vs. the hijack model and implications for age and sex differences in drug consumption. Front Psychiatry [Internet]. 2013 [cited 2017 Dec 20];4.

Available from: http://journal.frontiersin.org/article/10.3389/fpsyt
.2013.00142/abstract.

21. Turke PW, Betzig LL. Those who can do: wealth, status, and reproductive success on Ifaluk. Ethology and Sociobiology 1985;6(2):79–87. Available from: https://doi.org/10.1016/0162-3095(85)90001-9.

22. McLaughlin GT. Cocaine: the history and regulation of a dangerous drug. Cornell Rev. 1972;58(3):537–73.

23. Markel H. An anatomy of addiction: Sigmund Freud, William Halsted, and the miracle drug cocaine. New York: Vintage; 2011.

24. Davenport-Hines R. The pursuit of oblivion: a social history of drugs. London: Weidenfeld & Nicolson; 2012.

25. Brownstein MJ. A brief history of opiates, opioid peptides, and opioid receptors. Proc Natl Acad Sci. 1993;90(12):5391–3.

26. Brown RH. The opium trade and opium policies in India, China, Britain, and the United States: historical comparisons and theoretical interpretations. Asian J Soc Sci. 2002;30(3):623–56.

27. Braswell SR. American meth: a history of the methamphetamine epidemic in America. Lincoln (NE): iUniverse; 2006.

28. Pubchem. Carefentanil [Internet]. 2017 [cited 2017 Dec 20]. Available from: https://pubchem.ncbi.nlm.nih.gov/compound/62156.

29. McLaughlin K. Underground labs in China are devising potent new opiates faster than authorities can respond. Science [Internet]. 2017 Mar 29 [cited 2017 Dec 20]. Available from: http://www.sciencemag.org/news/2017/03/underground-labs-china-are-devising-potent-new-opiates-faster-authorities-can-respond.

30. Berridge KC, Robinson TE. The mind of an addicted brain: neural sensitization of wanting versus liking. Curr Dir Psychol Sci. 1995; 4(3):71–6.

31. Kendler KS, Maes HH, Sundquist K, Ohlsson H, Sundquist J. Genetic and family and community environmental efects on drug abuse in adolescence: a Swedish national twin and sibling study. Am J Psychiatry. 2014 Feb 1;171(2):209–17.

32. Young SE, Rhee SH, Stallings MC, Corley RP, Hewitt JK. Genetic and environmental vulnerabilities underlying adolescent substance use and problem use: general or specific? Behav Genet. 2006;36(4):603–15.

33. Alexander BK, Hadaway PF. Opiate addiction: the case for an adaptive orientation. Psychol Bull. 1982;92(2):367–81.

34. Zucker RA. Genes, brain, behavior, and context: the developmental matrix of addictive behavior. In: Stoltenberg S, editor. Genes and the motivation to use substances [Internet]. New York: Springer; 2014 [cited 2017 Dec 20]. pp. 51–69. Available from: https://link.springer.com/chapter/10.1007/978-1-4939-0653-6_4.

35. Volkow ND, Koob GF, McLellan AT. Neurobiologic advances from the brain disease model of addiction. N Engl J Med. 2016 Jan 28; 374(4):363–71.

CHAPTER 14 | MINDS UNBALANCED ON FITNESS CLIFFS

1. Wiener N. Cybernetics; or, control and communication in the animal and the machine. Cambridge (MA): Technology Press; 1948. p. 151.

2. Smoller JW, Finn CT. Family, twin, and adoption studies of bipolar disorder. Am J Med Genet C Semin Med Genet. 2003 Nov 15;123 C(1): 48–58.

3. Sullivan RJ, Allen JS. Natural selection and schizophrenia. Behav Brain Sci. 2004 Dec;27(6):865–6.

4. Sandin S, Lichtenstein P, Kuja-Halkola R, Larsson H, Hultman CM, Reichenberg A. The familial risk of autism. JAMA. 2014 May 7;311(17): 1770–7.

5. Smoller JW, Finn CT. Family, twin, and adoption studies of bipolar disorder.

6. Sandin S, et al. The familial risk of autism.

7. Lichtenstein P, Björk C, Hultman CM, Scolnick E, Sklar P, Sullivan PF. Recurrence risks for schizophrenia in a Swedish national cohort. Psychol Med. 2006 Oct;36(10):1417–25.

8. Kendler KS, Thornton LM, Gardner CO. Stressful life events and previous episodes in the etiology of major depression in women: an evaluation of the "kindling" hypothesis. Am J Psychiatry. 2000 Aug 1; 157(8):1243–51.

9. Ellison Z, van Os J, Murray R. Special feature: childhood personality

characteristics of schizophrenia: manifestations of, or risk factors for, the disorder? J Personal Disord. 1998 Sep 1;12(3):247–61.

10. Johnson EC, Border R, Melroy-Greif WE, de Leeuw CA, Ehringer MA, Keller MC. No evidence that schizophrenia candidate genes are more associated with schizophrenia than noncandidate genes. Biol Psychiatry [Internet]. 2017 Jul 13 [cited 2017 Sep 15]. Available from: http://www.sciencedirect.com/science/article/pii/S0006322317317729.

11. Sanders AR, Duan J, Levinson DF, Shi J, He D, Hou C, et al. No significant association of 14 candidate genes with schizophrenia in a large European ancestry sample: implications for psychiatric genetics. Am J Psychiatry. 2008 Apr 1;165(4):497–506.

12. Anttila V, Bulik-Sullivan B, Finucane HK, Bras J, Duncan L, Escott-Price V, et al. Analysis of shared heritability in common disorders of the brain. 2016 Apr 16 [cited 2017 Jun 19]. Available from: http://biorxiv.org/lookup/doi/10.1101/048991.

13. Kendler KS. What psychiatric genetics has taught us about the nature of psychiatric illness and what is left to learn. Mol Psychiatry. 2013 Oct;18(10):1058–66.

14. Corvin A, Sullivan PF. What next in schizophrenia genetics for the Psychiatric Genomics Consortium? Schizophr Bull. 2016 May 1;42(3): 538–41.

15. Forstner AJ, Hecker J, Hofmann A, Maaser A, Reinbold CS, Mühleisen TW, et al. Identification of shared risk loci and pathways for bipolar disorder and schizophrenia. PLOS ONE. 2017 Feb 6;12(2): e0171595.

16. Eichler EE, Flint J, Gibson G, Kong A, Leal SM, Moore JH, et al. Missing heritability and strategies for finding the underlying causes of complex disease. Nat Rev Genet. 2010 Jun;11(6):446–50.

17. Manolio TA, Collins FS, Cox NJ, Goldstein DB, Hindorff LA, Hunter DJ, et al. Finding the missing heritability of complex diseases. Nature. 2009 Oct 8;461(7265):747–53.

18. Nolte IM, van der Most PJ, Alizadeh BZ, de Bakker PI, Boezen HM, Bruinenberg M, et al. Missing heritability: is the gap closing? An analysis of 32 complex traits in the Lifelines Cohort Study. Eur J Hum Genet EJHG. 2017 Jun;25(7):877–85.

19. Gaugler T, Klei L, Sanders SJ, Bodea CA, Goldberg AP, Lee AB, et al. Most genetic risk for autism resides with common variation. Nat Genet. 2014 Aug;46(8):881–5.

20. Gratten J, Wray NR, Keller MC, Visscher PM. Large-scale genomics unveils the genetic architecture of psychiatric disorders. Nat Neurosci. 2014;17(6):782–90.

21. Kendler KS. What psychiatric genetics has taught us about the nature of psychiatric illness and what is left to learn. Mol Psychiatry. 2013 Oct;18(10):1058–66.

22. Woo HJ, Yu C, Kumar K, Reifman J. Large-scale interaction effects reveal missing heritability in schizophrenia, bipolar disorder and post-traumatic stress disorder. Transl Psychiatry. 2017 Apr 11;7(4):e1089.

23. Gaugler T et al. Most genetic risk for autism resides with common variation.

24. Cardno AG, Owen MJ. Genetic relationships between schizophrenia, bipolar disorder, and schizoaffective disorder. Schizophr Bull. 2014 May 1;40(3):504–15.

25. Malaspina D, Harlap S, Fennig S, Heiman D, Nahon D, Feldman D, et al. Advancing paternal age and the risk of schizophrenia. Arch Gen Psychiatry. 2001 Apr 1;58(4):361–7.

26. Reichenberg A, Gross R, Weiser M, Bresnahan M, Silverman J, Harlap S, et al. Advancing paternal age and autism. Arch Gen Psychiatry. 2006 Sep 1;63(9):1026–32.

27. Gratten J, Wray NR, Peyrot WJ, McGrath JJ, Visscher PM, Goddard ME. Risk of psychiatric illness from advanced paternal age is not predominantly from de novo mutations. Nat Genet. 2016 Jul;48(7):718–24.

28. Pedersen CB, McGrath J, Mortensen PB, Petersen L. The importance of father's age to schizophrenia risk. Mol Psychiatry. 2014 May;19 (5):530–1.

29. Bundy H, Stahl D, MacCabe JH. A systematic review and meta-analysis of the fertility of patients with schizophrenia and their unaffected relatives. Acta Psychiatr Scand. 2011;123(2):98–106.

30. Power RA, Kyaga S, Uher R, MacCabe JH, Långström N, Landen M, et al. Fecundity of patients with schizophrenia, autism, bipolar disorder, depression, anorexia nervosa, or substance abuse vs their unaffected siblings. JAMA Psychiatry. 2013 Jan 1;70(1):22–30.

31. Ibid.

32. Keller MC, Miller G. Resolving the paradox of common, harmful, heritable mental disorders: which evolutionary genetic models work best? Behav Brain Sci. 2006 Aug;29(4):385–404.

33. Crespi B, Badcock CR. Psychosis and autism as diametrical disorders of the social brain. Behav Brain Sci. 2008 Jun;31(3):241–61; discussion 261–320.

34. Crespi BJ. Revisiting Bleuler: relationship between autism and schizophrenia. Br J Psychiatry. 2010 Jun;196(6):495; author reply 495–6.

35. Wilkins JF, Haig D. What good is genomic imprinting: the function of parent-specific gene expression. Nat Rev Genet. 2003;4(5):359–68.

36. Haig D. Transfers and transitions: parent-offspring conflict, genomic imprinting, and the evolution of human life history. Proc Natl Acad Sci. 2010 Jan 26;107 (Suppl 1):1731–5.

37. Patten MM, Úbeda F, Haig D. Sexual and parental antagonism shape genomic architecture. Proc R Soc Lond B Biol Sci. 2013;280(1770): 20131795.

38. Crespi BJ. The evolutionary etiologies of autism spectrum and psychotic affective spectrum disorders. In: Evolutionary thinking in medicine [Internet]. Cham (Switzerland): Springer; 2016 [cited 2018 Jan 2]. p. 299–327. Available from: https://link.springer.com/chapter/10.1007/978-3-319-29716-3_20.

39. Crespi BJ. Autism, psychosis, and genomic imprinting: recent discoveries and conundrums. Curr Opin Behav Sci. 2018;25:1–7.

40. Crespi B, Summers K, Dorus S. Adaptive evolution of genes underlying schizophrenia. Proc R Soc Lond B Biol Sci. 2007 Nov 22;274(1627): 2801–10.

41. Dinsdale NL, Hurd PL, Wakabayashi A, Elliot M, Crespi BJ. How are autism and schizotypy related?: evidence from a non-clinical population. PLOS ONE. 2013;8(5):e63316.

42. Byars SG, Stearns SC, Boomsma JJ. Opposite risk patterns for autism and schizophrenia are associated with normal variation in birth size: phenotypic support for hypothesized diametric gene-dosage effects. Proc R Soc B. 2014 Nov 7;281(1794):20140604.

43. Lai M-C, Lombardo MV, Auyeung B, Chakrabarti B, Baron-Cohen S.

Sex/gender differences and autism: setting the scene for future research. J Am Acad Child Adolesc Psychiatry. 2015 Jan 1;54(1):11–24.

44. Baron-Cohen S, Knickmeyer RC, Belmonte MK. Sex differences in the brain: implications for explaining autism. Science. 2005 Nov 4; 310(5749):819–23.

45. van Dongen J, Boomsma DI. The evolutionary paradox and the missing heritability of schizophrenia. Am J Med Genet B Neuropsychiatr Genet. 2013 Mar 1;162(2):122–36.

46. Polimeni J, Reiss JP. Evolutionary perspectives on schizophrenia. Can J Psychiatry. 2003;48(1):34–9.

47. Stevens A. Prophets, cults and madness. London: Gerald Duckworth & Co.; 2000.

48. Nettle D, Clegg H. Schizotypy, creativity and mating success in humans. Proc R Soc Lond B Biol Sci. 2006;273(1586):611–5.

49. Greenwood TA. Positive traits in the bipolar spectrum: the space between madness and genius. Mol Neuropsychiatry. 2016;2(4):198–212.

50. Jamison KR. Touched with fire: manic-depressive illness and the artistic temperament. New York: Free Press; 1993.

51. Higier RG, Jimenez AM, Hultman CM, Borg J, Roman C, Kizling I, et al. Enhanced neurocognitive functioning and positive temperament in twins discordant for bipolar disorder. Am J Psychiatry. 2014;171(11): 1191–8.

52. Polimanti R, Gelernter J. Widespread signatures of positive selection in common risk alleles associated to autism spectrum disorder. PLOS Genet. 2017 Feb 10;13(2):e1006618.

53. Zheutlin AB, Viehman RW, Fortgang R, Borg J, Smith DJ, Suvisaari J, et al. Cognitive endophenotypes inform genome-wide expression profiling in schizophrenia. Neuropsychology. 2016;30(1):40–52.

54. Woo HJ, Yu C, Kumar K, Reifman J. Large-scale interaction effects reveal missing heritability in schizophrenia, bipolar disorder and post-traumatic stress disorder. Transl Psychiatry. 2017 Apr 11;7(4):e1089.

55. Srinivasan S, Bettella F, Hassani S, Wang Y, Witoelar A, Schork AJ, et al. Probing the association between early evolutionary markers and schizophrenia. PLOS ONE. 2017 Jan 12;12(1):e0169227.

56. Chen H, Li C, Zhou Z, Liang H. Fast-evolving human-specific neural enhancers are associated with aging-related diseases. Cell Syst. 2018 May;6(5):604–11.

57. Corbett S, Courtiol A, Lummaa V, Moorad J, Stearns S. The transition to modernity and chronic disease: mismatch and natural selection.

58. Judd LL, Akiskal HS. The prevalence and disability of bipolar spectrum disorders in the US population: re-analysis of the ECA database taking into account subthreshold cases. J Affect Disord. 2003 Jan 1;73(1):123–31.

59. Merikangas KR, Akiskal HS, Angst J, Greenberg PE, Hirschfeld RM, Petukhova M, et al. Lifetime and 12-month prevalence of bipolar spectrum disorder in the National Comorbidity Survey replication. Arch Gen Psychiatry. 2007;64(5):543–52.

60. Wilson DR. Evolutionary epidemiology and manic depression. Br J Med Psychol. 1998;71(4):375–95.

61. Abed RT, Abbas MJ. A reformulation of the social brain theory for schizophrenia: the case for out-group intolerance. Perspect Biol Med. 2011 Apr 28;54(2):132–51.

62. Stevens A, Price J. Evolutionary psychiatry: a new beginning. 2nd ed. Hove (UK): Psychology Press; 2000.

63. Jablensky A, Sartorius N, Ernberg G, Anker M, Korten A, Cooper JE, et al. Schizophrenia: manifestations, incidence and course in different cultures. A World Health Organization ten-country study. Psychol Med Monogr Suppl. 1992 Jan;20:1–97.

64. Jongsma HE, Gayer-Anderson C, Lasalvia A, Quattrone D, Mulè A, Szöke A, et al. Treated incidence of psychotic disorders in the multinational EU-GEI Study. JAMA Psychiatry [Internet]. 2017 Dec 6 [cited 2018 Jan 2]. Available from: https://jamanetwork.com/journals/jama psychiatry/fullarticle/2664479.

65. McGrath JJ. Variations in the incidence of schizophrenia: data versus dogma. Schizophr Bull. 2006 Jan 1;32(1):195–7.

66. Torrey EF, Bartko JJ, Yolken RH. *Toxoplasma gondii* and other risk factors for schizophrenia: an update. Schizophr Bull. 2012 May 1; 38(3):642–7.

67. Brown AS, Begg MD, Gravenstein S, Schaefer CA, Wyatt RJ, Bresnahan M, et al. Serologic evidence of prenatal influenza in the etiology of schizophrenia. Arch Gen Psychiatry. 2004 Aug 1;61(8):774–80.

68. Kendell RE, Kemp IW. Maternal influenza in the etiology of schizophrenia. Arch Gen Psychiatry. 1989;46(10):878–82.

69. Kunugi H, Nanko S, Takei N, Saito K, Hayashi N, Kazamatsuri H. Schizophrenia following in utero exposure to the 1957 influenza epidemics in Japan. Am J Psychiatry. 1995;152(3):450–2.

70. Brüne M. Social cognition and behaviour in schizophrenia. Soc Brain Evol Pathol. 2003;277–313.

71. Crespi B, Summers K, Dorus S. Adaptive evolution of genes underlying schizophrenia. Proc R Soc Lond B Biol Sci. 2007 Nov 22;274(1627): 2801–10.

72. Crow TJ. Is schizophrenia the price that *Homo sapiens* pays for language? Schizophr Res. 1997;28(2):127–41.

73. Brüne M. "Theory of mind" in schizophrenia: a review of the literature. Schizophr Bull. 2005;31(1):21–42.

74. Corvin A, Sullivan PF. What next in schizophrenia genetics for the Psychiatric Genomics Consortium? Schizophr Bull. 2016 May;42(3):538–41.

75. Crespi BJ. The Evolutionary etiologies of autism spectrum and psychotic affective spectrum disorders. In: Evolutionary thinking in medicine [Internet]. Cham (Switzerland): Springer; 2016 [cited 2018 Jan 2]. pp. 299–327. (Advances in the Evolutionary Analysis of Human Behaviour). Available from: https://link.springer.com/chapter/10.1007/978-3-319-29716-3_20

76. Feinberg I. Schizophrenia: caused by a fault in programmed synaptic elimination during adolescence? Journal of Psychiatric Research. 1982 Jan 1;17(4):319–34.

77. Kavanagh DH, Tansey KE, O'Donovan MC, Owen MJ. Schizophrenia genetics: emerging themes for a complex disorder. Mol Psychiatry. 2015 Feb;20(1):72–6.

78. Keller MC. Evolutionary perspectives on genetic and environmental risk factors for psychiatric disorders. Annual Review of Clinical Psychology. 2018;14:471–93.

79. Lee SH, Byrne EM, Hultman CM, Kähler A, Vinkhuyzen AA, Ripke

S, et al. New data and an old puzzle: the negative association between schizophrenia and rheumatoid arthritis. Int J Epidemiol. 2015 Oct 1;44(5):1706–21.

80. Pearlson GD, Folley BS. Schizophrenia, psychiatric genetics, and Darwinian psychiatry: an evolutionary framework. Schizophr Bull. 2007;34(4):722–33.

81. Polimeni J, Reiss J. Evolutionary perspectives on schizophrenia. Can J Psychiatry. 2003;48(1):34–9.

82. Power RA, Steinberg S, Bjornsdottir G, Rietveld CA, Abdellaoui A, Nivard MM, et al. Polygenic risk scores for schizophrenia and bipolar disorder predict creativity. Nature Neuroscience. 2015 Jul;18(7):953–5.

83. van Dongen J, Boomsma DI. The evolutionary paradox and the missing heritability of schizophrenia. Am J Med Genet. 2013 Mar 1;162(2):122–36.

84. Burns JK. An evolutionary theory of schizophrenia: cortical connectivity, metarepresentation, and the social brain. Behav Brain Sci. 2005; 27(6):831–55.

85. Nesse RM. Cliff-edged fitness functions and the persistence of schizophrenia (commentary). Behav Brain Sci. 2004;27(6):862–3.

86. Lack D. The evolution of reproductive rates. In: Huxley J, Hardy AC, Ford EB, editors. Evolution as a process. London: George Allen and Unwin; 1954. Vol. 1, pp. 143–56.

87. Lack D, Gibb J, Owen DF. Survival in relation to brood-size in tits. Proc Zool Soc Lond. 1957 Jun 1;128(3):313–26.

88. Nesse RM. Cliff-edged fitness functions and the persistence of schizophrenia (commentary).

89. Bumpus HC. The elimination of the unfit as illustrated by the introduced sparrow, *Passer domesticus*. Biol Lect Mar Biol Lab Woods Hole. 1899;6:209–26.

90. Crespi BJ. Autism, psychosis, and genomic imprinting.

91. Crespi BJ, Go MC. Diametrical diseases reflect evolutionary-genetic tradeoffs: evidence from psychiatry, neurology, rheumatology, oncology, and immunology. Evol Med Public Health. 2015 Sep 9;2015(1):216–53.

92. Wilson AJ, Rambaut A. Breeding racehorses: what price good genes? Biol Lett. 2008 Apr 23;4(2):173–5.

93. Crow TJ. Is schizophrenia the price that *Homo sapiens* pays for language?

94. Brüne M. Social cognition and behaviour in schizophrenia.

95. Brüne M. "Theory of mind" in schizophrenia.

96. Nesse R. Cliff-edged fitness landscapes make complex genetic disease inevitable. In preparation.

97. Mitteroecker P, Huttegger SM, Fischer B, Pavlicev M. Cliff-edge model of obstetric selection in humans. Proc Natl Acad Sci. 2016 Dec 20;113(51):14680–5.

98. lvarez-Lario B, Macarrn-Vicente J. Uric acid and evolution. Rheumatology. 2010;49:2010–5.

99. Tomasetti C, Vogelstein B. Variation in cancer risk among tissues can be explained by the number of stem cell divisions. Science. 2015 Jan 2; 347(6217):78–81.

100. Friedman N, Ito S, Brinkman BAW, Shimono M, DeVille REL, Dahmen KA, et al. Universal critical dynamics in high resolution neuronal avalanche data. Phys Rev Lett. 2012 May 16;108(20):208102.

101. Vercken E, Wellenreuther M, Svensson EI, Mauroy B. Don't fall off the adaptation cliff: when asymmetrical fitness selects for suboptimal traits. PLOS ONE. 2012 Apr 11;7(4):e34889.

102. Metcalf CJE, Tate AT, Graham AL. Demographically framing trade-offs between sensitivity and specificity illuminates selection on immunity. Nat Ecol Evol. 2017 Nov;1(11):1766–72.

103. Schizophrenia Working Group of the Psychiatric Genomics Association. Biological insights from 108 schizophrenia-associated genetic loci. Nature. 2014 Jul;511(7510):421.

104. Awasthi M, Singh S, Pandey VP, Dwivedi UN. Alzheimer's disease: an overview of amyloid beta dependent pathogenesis and its therapeutic implications along with in silico approaches emphasizing the role of natural products. J Neurol Sci. 2016 Feb 15;361:256–71.

105. Kumar DKV, Choi SH, Washicosky KJ, Eimer WA, Tucker S, Ghofrani J, et al. Amyloid-β peptide protects against microbial infection in mouse and worm models of Alzheimer's disease. Sci Transl Med. 2016;8(340): 340ra72.

106. Stephan AH, Barres BA, Stevens B. The complement system: an unex-

pected role in synaptic pruning during development and disease. Annu Rev Neurosci. 2012;35(1):369–89.

107. Readhead B, Haure-Mirande J-V, Funk CC, Richards MA, Shannon P, Haroutunian V, et al. Multiscale analysis of independent Alzheimer's cohorts finds disruption of molecular, genetic, and clinical networks by human herpesvirus. Neuron [Internet]. 2018 Jun [cited 2018 Jun 23]. Available from: https://linkinghub.elsevier.com/retrieve/pii /S0896627318304215.

108. Nesse RM, Finch CE, Nunn CL. Does selection for short sleep duration explain human vulnerability to Alzheimer's disease? Evol Med Public Health. 2017 Jan 1;2017(1):39–46.

109. Wiener N. Cybernetics.

110. Solomon RL. The opponent-process theory of acquired motivation: the costs of pleasure and the benefits of pain. Am Psychol. 1980;35(8): 691–712.

111. Meredith KE. Heirloom of agony: a new theory about why happiness hurts and what you can do about it. Privately published; 2017.

EPILOGUE

1. Robinson, M. The Niagara Gorge kite contest. Kite history [Internet]. 2005 [cited 2018 Jan 15]. Available from: http://kitehistory.com/Miscel laneous/Homan_Walsh.htm.

2. Alcock J. The triumph of sociobiology. New York: Oxford University Press; 2001.

3. Alcock J. Ardent adaptationism. Nat Hist. 1987 Apr;96(4):4.

4. Gould SJ, Lewontin RC. The spandrels of San Marco and the Panglossian paradigm: a critique of the adaptationist programme. Proc R Soc Lond. 1979;205:581–98.

5. Segerstråle UCO. Defenders of the truth: the battle for science in the sociobiology debate and beyond. New York: Oxford University Press; 2000.

6. Pigliucci M, Kaplan J. The fall and rise of Dr. Pangloss: adaptationism and the Spandrels paper 20 years later. Trends Ecol Evol. 2000;15(2):66–70.

7. Queller DC. The spaniels of St. Marx and the Panglossian paradox: a critique of a rhetorical programme. Q Rev Biol. 1995;70:485–9.

8. Nesse RM. Ten questions for evolutionary studies of disease vulnerability. Evol Appl. 2011;4(2):264–77.

9. Troisi A. Mental health and well-being: clinical applications of Darwinian psychiatry. Appl Evol Psychol. 2012;276.

10. Troisi A, McGuire MT. Darwinian psychiatry: it's time to focus on clinical questions. Clin Neuropsychiatry. 2006;3:85–6.

11. Brüne M. Textbook of evolutionary psychiatry and psychosomatic medicine: the origins of psychopathology. New York: Oxford University Press; 2015.

12. Hjemdal O, Hagen R, Solem S, Nordahl H, Kennair LEO, Ryum T, et al. Metacognitive therapy in major depression: an open trial of comorbid cases. Cogn Behav Pract. 2017 Aug 1;24(3):312–8.

13. Gilbert P. The origins and nature of compassion focused therapy. Br J Clin Psychol. 2014;53(1):6–41.

14. Gilbert P. Human nature and suffering. Hove (UK): Lawrence Erlbaum; 1989.

15. Gilbert P, Bailey KG. Genes on the couch: explorations in evolutionary psychotherapy. Philadelphia: Taylor & Francis; 2000.

ACKNOWLEDGMENTS

This book is a product of selection. I have lobbed ideas to colleagues and friends in conversations and drafts for decades, and they have tossed them back or away. Those conversations and comments have carved away much nonsense and confusion and helped me to capture ideas that otherwise would have gotten away. Barbara Smuts, Linda A. W. Brakel, and Richard Nisbett deserve special thanks. Barb is a psychologist and primatologist whose work and friendship have inspired me. Linda is psychoanalyst/ psychiatrist/philosopher who for years joined Barb and me in weekly discussions that shaped my ideas and who provided wonderful critical comments on drafts of these chapters. Dick is a social psychologist whose work and friendship have inspired me and whose comments on a draft of this book were invaluable.

My students and colleagues at the University of Michigan have provided wonderful encouragement and criticism. Generations of psychiatry residents took my course on evolution and mental disorders. One group read a whole draft of a previous version and provided cogent suggestions; it included Ryan Edwards, Lauren Edwards, Srijan Sen, Margit Burmeister, Paul Wright, and Shweta Ramdas. This version of the book is so different that they will not recognize it. Professors of psychiatry who inspired my research career at the University of Michigan include John Greden, Bernard Carroll, George Curtis, Kevin Kerber, James Abelson, and Oliver Cameron.

The University of Michigan provided a fabulous intellectual environment in the last twenty years of the twentieth century. The evolutionary biologist Richard Alexander brought together a nucleus of scientists to debate the crucial issues about evolution and behavior. That group developed into the Evolution and Human Behavior Program, including Barbara Smuts, Richard Wrangham, Bobbi Low, Warren Holmes, David Buss, and me. Younger affiliated scientists, including Beverly Strassmann, Paul Turke, Laura Betzig, and Paul Ewald, have gone on to stellar careers. After that group disbanded, the university provided funds, thanks to Nancy Cantor, that allowed me to continue as the director of the Evolution and Human Adaptation Program. Many others at the university were also sophisticated evolutionary thinkers, including the psychologist Phoebe Ellsworth and the philosophers Allen Gibbard and Peter Railton, whose evolution and ethics lunches set me straight on many matters. The university also made possible leaves that allowed creation of this book, including one at the Wissenschaftskolleg zu Berlin, where the environment was extraordinarily conducive to creative thinking. UK philosophers and evolution experts Helena Cronin and Janet Radcliffe Richards provided friendship and conversations that were even more inspiring than their wonderful books.

Conversations with John Holland, Bob Axelrod, Bobbi Low, and Carl Simon proved seminal about complexity theory, and regular lunch conversations with the geneticist Jim Neel over many years provided an advanced education in genetics and a model of generosity from a world-leading scientist to a curious doctor. Visitors, including Bill Hamilton, George Williams, Bill Irons, Napoleon Chagnon, Martin Daly, and Margo Wilson, expanded our vision. The person at Michigan who did the most to make my work possible was Nancy Cantor; in her administrative position she arranged for half of my appointments to move from the medical center to the main campus, where I was able to do the work needed to develop evolutionary medicine.

Many friends and colleagues provided detailed commentary on chapters, some on the entire book, line by line. Your reading experience has been greatly improved as a result of the generous and detailed critiques provided by Sylvia Bonner, Annette Hollander, Richard Nisbett, Carl Carlson, Holly Carlson, Linda Brakel, Holly Smith, and Paul St. John-Smith. Tyler Quigley spent an entire summer editing and helping me find missing references. Maria Klingler and Chelsea Landolin are careful readers whose comments were as encouraging as they were critical. Julia Heiman, Marlene Zuk, Laura Betzig, and Hanna Kokko provided crucial critiques of the sex chapter.

Conversations and friendships with evolutionary psychiatry leaders have inspired many ideas and made this work possible. A few of them are Daniel Stein, Martin Brüne, John Price, Russell Gardner, Riadh Abed, Paul St. John-Smith, Daniel Wilson, Daniel Nettle, Paul Gilbert, Leon Sloman, Douglas Kramer, Jay Feierman, Pieter Adriaens, John Beahrs, Jerry Wakefield, Allan Horowitz, Jay Belsky, Kalman Glantz, Eiko Fried, Matthew Keller, Andy Thompson, and most of all Brant Wenegrat, Melvin Konner, Alfonso Troisi, and Michael McGuire, whose seminal books about evolutionary psychiatry set this field in motion decades ago.

I hope this book will be recognized as a fine example of the "third culture" developed so well by my agents John Brockman and Katinka Matson, who is also a talented artist. Their work and their Edge.org blog have created a new publishing space for popular books that advance serious new science. I am especially grateful to Katinka for her patience and sage advice at many phases of the process.

Finally, the two editors who provided the most help and support to get this manuscript in shape are my wonderful wife, the novelist Margaret Nesse, and my wonderful editor at Dutton, Stephen Morrow. Warmest thanks to them and everyone else I can never repay. I hope they and all others who have helped will take satisfaction in seeing this book do what it can to advance our understanding of mental disorders and to find better ways to treat them.

INDEX

ABOUT THE AUTHOR

Randolph Nesse, MD, is a cofounder of the field of evolutionary medicine, a new field launched twenty-five years ago with his coauthored book *Why We Get Sick*, which has sold more than 100,000 copies and been translated into eight languages. He has served on the faculty of the University of Michigan as professor of psychiatry, professor of psychology, and research professor. In 2014 he moved to the University of Arizona, where he currently serves as the founding director of the Center for Evolution and Medicine. He is the current president of the International Society for Evolution, Medicine, and Public Health, and is the editor of *The Evolution and Medicine Review*. More information is available at RandophNesse.com and @RandyNesse on Twitter.